UPDATE ON MULTIPLE MYELOMA

Edited by **Khalid Ahmed Al-Anazi**

Update on Multiple Myeloma
http://dx.doi.org/10.5772/intechopen.72220
Edited by Khalid Ahmed Al-Anazi

Contributors

Craig Wallington-Beddoe, Douglas Coghlan, Rafael Ríos-Tamayo, María José Sánchez Pérez, Dolores Sánchez Rodríguez, Yoe-Ling Chang-Chan, Milda Rudzianskiene, Viktoras Rudzianskas, Ruta Dambrauskiene, Rolandas Gerbutavicius, Ogbonna Collins Nwabuko, Roberto Ria, Antonio Giovanni Solimando, Azzurra Sportelli, Angelo Vacca, Assunta Melaccio, Zeeshan Ahmed, Afshan Rasheed, Muhammad Shariq Shaikh, Asghar Nasir, Tariq Moatter, Khalid Ahmed Al-Anazi

First published in London, United Kingdom, 2019 by IntechOpen
IntechOpen is the global imprint of INTECHOPEN LIMITED, registered in England and Wales, registration number: 11086078, The Shard, 25th floor, 32 London Bridge Street
London, SE19SG – United Kingdom
Printed in Croatia

British Library Cataloguing-in-Publication Data
A catalogue record for this book is available from the British Library

Additional hard copies can be obtained from orders@intechopen.com

Update on Multiple Myeloma, Edited by Khalid Ahmed Al-Anazi
p. cm.
Print ISBN 978-1-78985-217-2
Online ISBN 978-1-78985-218-9

For EU product safety concerns :
IN TECH d.o.o., Prolaz Marije Krucifikse Kozulić 3, 51000 Rijeka, Croatia,
info@intechopen.com or visit our website at intechopen.com.

Meet the editor

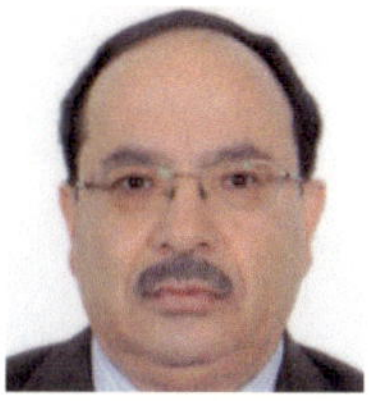

Dr. Khalid Ahmed Al-Anazi is a consultant hemato-oncologist and the Chairman of the Department of Adult Hematology and Hematopoietic Stem Cell Transplantation (HSCT) at King Fahad Specialist Hospital (KFSH) in Dammam, Saudi Arabia.
He graduated from the College of Medicine, King Saud University (KSU) in Riyadh, in 1986. After passing his Boards in Internal Medicine, he trained in clinical hematology and HSCT at King's College Hospital, University of London, UK. He has 4 years of experience in internal medicine and 26 years of experience in adult clinical hematology and HSCT at Riyadh Armed Forces Hospital, then King Faisal Specialist Hospital and Research Centre (KFSH&RC) in Riyadh, King Khalid University Hospital and College of Medicine, KSU in Riyadh, and KFSH in Dammam, Saudi Arabia.
He received the award of best teacher in the Department of Medicine at the College of Medicine and KKUH in Riyadh in 2014. During his work at KFSH&RC in Riyadh and KFSH in Dammam, he was heavily involved in hemato-oncology and HSCT and he contributed to the success and achievements at both institutions in addition to the establishment of the adult HSCT program at KFSH in Dammam in 2010. He has 85 publications, including retrospective studies, review articles, book chapters, and electronic books, and he is a reviewer for 23 international medical journals. He is the Editor-in-Chief of the *Journal of Stem Cell Biology and Transplantation* and the *Journal of Molecular Genetics and Medicine* in addition to being an associate editor of 26 other medical journals in HSCT, hematology, cancer, and infectious diseases.

Contents

Preface

Over the past two decades, the outcome of patients with multiple myeloma has improved substantially due to the increased understanding of disease biology, introduction of advanced diagnostics and several novel therapies, evolution of new therapeutic strategies, and recent improvement in supportive care.

This book represents an update on multiple myeloma. It is divided into three sections that cover a wide range of topics, which include: epidemiology and pathogenesis of the disease, genetic targets and pathways, resistance to novel therapies, angiogenesis and anti-angiogenesis, hematopoietic stem cell transplantation, role of radiology and radiotherapy in myeloma, infectious complications, and management of myeloma in resource-poor countries. Each chapter is written by scientists and clinicians with expertise in the field.

I would like to thank the authors for their valuable contributions, as well as the publishing manager Lada Bozic and IntechOpen staff for their remarkable efforts that ultimately made this book project a reality.

Khalid Ahmed Al-Anazi
Oncology Center
King Fahad Specialist Hospital
Dammam, Saudi Arabia

Section 1

Introduction and Epidemiology of Multiple Myeloma

Chapter 1

Introductory Chapter: Multiple Myeloma in the Era of Novel Therapeutics

Khalid Ahmed Al-Anazi

Additional information is available at the end of the chapter

http://dx.doi.org/10.5772/intechopen.82174

1. Introduction

Multiple myeloma (MM), the second most common hematologic malignancy (HM), is a malignant B-cell neoplasm that is characterized by clonal expansion of plasma cells in the bone marrow (BM) with subsequent production of monoclonal immunoglobulins [1–8]. The disease has several complications including anemia; renal dysfunction or failure; bone involvement including osteopenia, lytic lesions, and pathological fractures; hypercalcemia; immunodeficiency; and various infectious complications [1, 4, 5, 7–12]. The incidence of MM has increased since the year 1990 with the largest increase in resource-poor countries [13]. MM is a heterogeneous disease even in its etiology, and there are several risk factors for the disease that include old age; obesity; ionizing radiation; exposure to solvents and pesticides; agricultural occupations; autoimmune disorders such as pernicious anemia and ankylosing spondylitis; monoclonal gammopathy of undetermined significance; and familial predisposition [14–18]. One hallmark of MM is the presence of heterogeneous chromosomal aberrations and numerous genetic mutations that not only can help in risk stratifying the disease but also can affect management and prognosis to a large extent [7, 8, 19]. Recently, MM is stratified according to stage of the disease, plasma cell labeling index, cytogenetics, and gene expression profiling [20–22].

Over the past two decades, the outcomes of patients with MM have improved substantially even in patients with relapsed or refractory (RR) disease [1–4, 23–28]. The remarkable improvement in the outcome of MM is due to the following reasons: (1) the evolution of advanced technology that facilitated understanding biology of the disease and helped in the diagnosis, risk stratification, and follow-up of patients; (2) the introduction of several novel therapies, monoclonal antibodies, and immunotherapies; (3) the widespread utilization of high-dose (HD) chemotherapy followed by autologous stem cell transplantation (HSCT); (4) the recent improvements in supportive care and antimicrobial therapies; and (5) the evolution of new therapeutic strategies such as consolidation and maintenance treatments as well as total or continuous therapy [1–5, 24–29]. Currently, the following novel therapies are available for patients with MM: (1) immunomodulatory agents such as thalidomide, lenalidomide, and pomalidomide; (2) proteasome inhibitors such as bortezomib, carfilzomib, and ixazomib; (3) monoclonal antibodies such as daratumumab and elotuzumab; and (4) histone deacetylase inhibitors such as panobinostat and vorinostat [1–5, 26–29]. Other novel therapeutic options that are available for patients with RR-MM include chimeric antigen receptor T cells as well as other cellular and immunotherapies such as the use of specific antigen-presenting cells to overcome immune incompetence and engineered T cells as well as natural killer cell products [30–32].

Several studies and meta-analyses have shown that the most beneficial induction therapies in terms of overall response rate, overall survival (OS), and progression-free survival (PFS) in transplant-eligible patients with newly diagnosed MM are (1) bortezomib, lenalidomide, and dexamethasone (VRD), (2) bortezomib, cyclophosphamide, and dexamethasone, and (3) bortezomib, thalidomide, and dexamethasone [1, 33–35]. However, the standard induction therapy in patients with newly diagnosed MM is the VRD triplet regimen [4, 8]. Also, autologous HSCT is the standard of care for transplant eligible patients either upfront or at relapse [4, 8, 27]. Therefore, HD chemotherapy followed by autologous HSCT, which is an integral part in the treatment of the disease, is considered the standard of care for patients with MM who are eligible for HSCT [36–39]. With the recent advances in supportive care, autologous HSCT has been extended to include older patients with MM and those with comorbid medical conditions such as renal failure (RF) [37, 38]. Nevertheless, autologous HSCT and novel therapies are complementary to each other in the management of patients with MM [37, 40].

Studies have shown that post-HSCT consolidation and maintenance treatments can further improve the outcome of patients with MM [8, 27, 41]. In particular, the use of either proteasome inhibitors such as bortezomib or immunomodulatory drugs such as lenalidomide in the maintenance therapy is associated with increased OS and PFS [42–46]. However, for transplant-eligible patients, stratified maintenance therapy based on risk features and depth of response is recommended [47]. Monitoring disease response at various stages of treatment is essential, and studies have shown that monitoring of minimal residual disease (MRD) is associated with longer PFS and OS [48, 49]. Patients with high-risk (HR) cytogenetics require not only specific induction therapies but also autologous HSCT as well as consolidation and maintenance therapies [50, 51]. For such patients, deeper responses should be obtained as several studies and meta-analyses have shown that MRD negativity is a strong predictor of clinical outcome and is associated with long-term survival [49, 52, 53].

The numerous treatment modalities that are available for patients with MM have shown their efficacy, but they have their own adverse effects that include BM suppression and infectious complications that may be life-threatening [9, 10, 54].

Also, there is very limited access to effective care in many countries particularly in sub-Saharan Africa. Additionally, the available novel therapies are rather expensive, and the economic burden of the disease is huge [13, 14, 55–57].

Progression of MM is related to the underlying BM microenvironment and to the genetic heterogeneity of the disease [7, 19]. Studies have shown that the main causes of death in patients with MM are infections, comorbid medical conditions such as RF, having RR disease, and the presence of HR features such as adverse cytogenetics or advanced stage of the disease at presentation [54, 58, 59]. The second-line treatment for patients with RR-MM is rather heterogeneous [60]. Different novel therapeutic agents that are usually given in various combinations are currently available for the treatment of patients with RR disease [61, 62]. However, in the setting of RR disease, treatment options become more complex, but the aim should be to provide the patient with specific drug combination so as to gain clinical benefit while minimizing drug toxicity [63]. Additionally, studies have shown clinical benefit for continued therapy. However, improved outcome is paralleled by certain barriers such as drug toxicity and evolution of drug resistance [64, 65].

Current treatment standards for patients with RR-MM include (1) salvage therapy using a combination of novel agents, (2) salvage autologous HSCT, (3) allogeneic HSCT in highly selected patients with RR-MM, and (4) post-HSCT consolidation and maintenance therapies [39, 66–68]. The available novel drug combinations that have been shown to be effective in RR disease include (1) daratumumab, lenalidomide, and dexamethasone, (2) daratumumab, bortezomib, and dexamethasone, (3) carfilzomib-based combinations with panobinostat or elotuzumab, and (4) pomalidomide-based combinations with carfilzomib or dexamethasone [24, 66, 69–72]. However, the choice of therapeutic regimen should take disease-related factors and patient-related factors into consideration [62, 63, 73].

Life expectancy in patients with MM has recently increased due to the availability of large numbers of novel agent with different mechanisms of action against the disease [3, 24, 27, 74]. For example, in the year 2015, five new novel agents were approved for the treatment of RR-MM [24]. Unfortunately, despite the progress achieved in the diagnostics and therapeutics including the plethora of new novel agents and despite the remarkable improvements in supportive care and stem cell therapies, the disease remains mostly incurable as patients usually experience disease relapse after enjoying a certain period of disease control [1, 3–5, 24, 28, 74, 75].

Hopefully, the following will optimize antimyeloma management in the near future: (1) better understanding of the biology of the disease, (2) characterization of genetic and molecular basis of the disease, (3) incorporation of risk stratification in the management of newly diagnosed MM patients, (4) availability of several novel agents as well as monoclonal antibodies and effective management of their adverse effects, (5) availability of safer autologous HSCT, (6) improvement of supportive care and management of comorbid medical conditions, and (7) designing new novel therapies to restore autologous antimyeloma immunity and to target protein degradation as well as aberrant biology [4, 65, 76–78]. Finally, it is essential to reduce the costs of the novel therapies so that patients with low income can afford them and make benefit from utilizing them particularly in the setting of RR-MM [13, 79–81].

Author details

Khalid Ahmed Al-Anazi

Address all correspondence to: kaa_alanazi@yahoo.com

Department of Hematology and Hematopoietic Stem Cell Transplantation, Oncology Center, King Fahad Specialist Hospital, Dammam, Saudi Arabia

References

[1] Naymagon L, Abdul-Hay M. Novel agents in the treatment of multiple myeloma: A review about the future. Journal of Hematology & Oncology. 2016;**9**(1):52. DOI: 10.1186/s13045-016-0282-1

[2] Holstein SA, McCarthy PL. Immunomodulatory drugs in multiple myeloma: Mechanisms of action and clinical experience. Drugs. 2017;**77**(5):505-520. DOI: 10.1007/s40265-017-0689-1

[3] Larocca A, Mina R, Gay F, Bringhen S, Boccadoro M. Emerging drugs and combinations to treat multiple myeloma. Oncotarget. 2017;**8**(36):60656-60672. DOI: 10.18632/oncotarget.19269. eCollection 2017 Sep 1

[4] Raza S, Safyan RA, Rosenbaum E, Bowman AS, Lentzsch S. Optimizing current and emerging therapies in multiple myeloma: A guide for the hematologist. Therapeutic Advances in Hematology. 2017;**8**(2):55-70. DOI: 10.1177/2040620716680548. Epub 2016 Dec 9

[5] Mimura N, Hideshima T, Anderson KC. Novel therapeutic strategies for multiple myeloma. Experimental Hematology. 2015;**43**(8):732-741. DOI: 10.1016/j.exphem.2015.04.010. Epub 2015 Jun 26

[6] Rajkumar SV, Kumar S. Multiple myeloma: Diagnosis and treatment. Mayo Clinic Proceedings. 2016;**91**(1):101-119. DOI: 10.1016/j.mayocp.2015.11.007

[7] Fairfield H, Falank C, Avery L, Reagan MR. Multiple myeloma in the marrow: Pathogenesis and treatments. Annals of the New York Academy of Sciences. 2016;**1364**:32-51. DOI: 10.1111/nyas.13038

[8] Rajkumar SV. Multiple myeloma: 2016 update on diagnosis, risk-stratification, and management. American Journal of Hematology. 2016;**91**(7):719-734. DOI: 10.1002/ajh.24402

[9] Nucci M, Anaissie E. Infections in patients with multiple myeloma in the era of high-dose therapy and novel agents. Clinical Infectious Diseases. 2009;**49**(8):1211-1225. DOI: 10.1086/605664

[10] Teh BW, Harrison SJ, Worth LJ, Spelman T, Thursky KA, Slavin MA. Risks, severity and timing of infections in patients with multiple myeloma: A longitudinal cohort study in the era of immunomodulatory drug therapy. British Journal of Haematology. 2015;**171**(1):100-108. DOI: 10.1111/bjh.13532. Epub 2015 Jun 24

[11] Heher EC, Rennke HG, Laubach JP, Richardson PG. Kidney disease and multiple myeloma. Clinical Journal of the American Society of Nephrology. 2013;**8**(11):2007-2017. DOI: 10.2215/CJN.12231212. Epub 2013 Jul 18

[12] Katagiri D, Noiri E, Hinoshita F. Multiple myeloma and kidney disease. Scientific World Journal. 2013;**2013**:487285. DOI: 10.1155/2013/487285. eCollection 2013

[13] Cowan AJ, Allen C, Barac A, Basaleem H, Bensenor I, Curado MP, et al. Global burden of multiple myeloma: A systematic analysis for the global burden of disease study 2016. JAMA Oncology. 2018;**4**(9):1221-1227. DOI: 10.1001/jamaoncol.2018.2128. Epub 2018 May 16

[14] Curado MP, Oliveira MM, Silva DRM, Souza DLB. Epidemiology of multiple myeloma in 17 Latin American countries: An update. Cancer Medicine. 2018;**7**(5):2101-2108. DOI: 10.1002/cam4.1347. Epub 2018 Mar 24

[15] Becker N. Epidemiology of multiple myeloma. Recent Results in Cancer Research. 2011;**183**:25-35. DOI: 10.1007/978-3-540-85772-3_2

[16] Sergentanis TN, Zagouri F, Tsilimidos G, Tsagianni A, Tseliou M, Dimopoulos MA, et al. Risk factors for multiple myeloma: A systematic review of meta-analyses. Clinical Lymphoma, Myeloma & Leukemia. 2015;**15**(10):563-577.e1-563-577.e3. DOI: 10.1016/j.clml.2015.06.003. Epub 2015 Jun 19

[17] Kazandjian D. Multiple myeloma epidemiology and survival: A unique malignancy. Seminars in Oncology. 2016;**43**(6):676-681. DOI: 10.1053/j.seminoncol.2016.11.004. Epub 2016 Nov 10

[18] Raluy M, Ramagopalan S, Panjabi S, Lambrelli D. Epidemiology and clinical characteristics of patients with multiple myeloma in the United Kingdom. Blood. 2014;**124**:2048

[19] Shay G, Hazlehurst L, Lynch CC. Dissecting the multiple myeloma-bone microenvironment reveals new therapeutic opportunities. Journal of Molecular Medicine. 2016;**94**(1): 21-35. DOI: 10.1007/s00109-015-1345-4. Epub 2015 Oct 1

[20] Hanbali A, Hassanein M, Rasheed W, Aljurf M, Alsharif F. The evolution of prognostic factors in multiple myeloma. Advances in Hematology. 2017;**2017**:4812637. DOI: 10.1155/2017/4812637. Epub 2017 Feb 21

[21] Johnson SK, Heuck CJ, Albino AP, Qu P, Zhang Q, Barlogie B, et al. The use of molecular-based risk stratification and pharmacogenomics for outcome prediction and personalized therapeutic management of multiple myeloma. International Journal of Hematology. 2011;**94**(4):321-333. DOI: 10.1007/s12185-011-0948-y. Epub 2011 Oct 15

[22] Chng WJ, Dispenzieri A, Chim CS, Fonseca R, Goldschmidt H, Lentzsch S, et al. IMWG consensus on risk stratification in multiple myeloma. Leukemia. 2014;**28**(2):269-277. DOI: 10.1038/leu.2013.247. Epub 2013 Aug 26

[23] Thorsteinsdottir S, Dickman PW, Landgren O, Blimark C, Hultcrantz M, Turesson I, et al. Dramatically improved survival in multiple myeloma patients in the recent decade: Results from a Swedish population-based study. Haematologica. 2018;**103**(9):e412-e415. DOI: 10.3324/haematol.2017.183475. Epub ahead of print

[24] Dingli D, Ailawadhi S, Bergsagel PL, Buadi FK, Dispenzieri A, Fonseca R, et al. Therapy for relapsed multiple myeloma: Guidelines from the Mayo stratification for myeloma and risk-adapted therapy. Mayo Clinic Proceedings. 2017;**92**(4):578-598. DOI: 10.1016/j.mayocp.2017.01.003. Epub 2017 Mar 11

[25] Kharfan-Dabaja MA, Hamadani M, Reljic T, Nishihori T, Bensinger W, Djulbegovic B, et al. Comparative efficacy of tandem autologous versus autologous followed by allo geneic hematopoietic cell transplantation in patients with newly diagnosed multiple myeloma: A systematic review and meta-analysis of randomized controlled trials. Journal of Hematology & Oncology. 2013;**6**:2. DOI: 10.1186/1756-8722-6-2

[26] Anderson KC. Progress and paradigms in multiple myeloma. Clinical Cancer Research. 2016;**22**(22):5419-5427. DOI: 10.1158/1078-0432.CCR-16-0625

[27] Gay F, Engelhardt M, Terpos E, Wäsch R, Giaccone L, Auner HW, et al. From transplant to novel cellular therapies in multiple myeloma: European myeloma network guidelines and future perspectives. Haematologica. 2018;**103**(2):197-211. DOI: 10.3324/haematol.2017.174573. Epub 2017 Dec 7

[28] Sonneveld P, De Wit E, Moreau P. How have evolutions in strategies for the treatment of relapsed/refractory multiple myeloma translated into improved outcomes for patients? Critical Reviews in Oncology/Hematology. 2017;**112**:153-170. DOI: 10.1016/j.critrevonc.2017.02.007. Epub 2017 Feb 14

[29] Orlowski RZ, Lonial S. Integration of novel agents into the care of patients with multiple myeloma. Clinical Cancer Research. 2016;**22**(22):5443-5452. DOI: 10.1158/1078-0432.CCR-16-0861. Epub 2016 Nov 14

[30] Garfall AL, Stadtmauer EA, Hwang WT, Lacey SF, Melenhorst JJ, Krevvata M, et al. Anti-CD19 CAR T cells with high-dose melphalan and autologous stem cell transplantation for refractory multiple myeloma. JCI Insight. 2018;**3**(8):pii: 120505. DOI: 10.1172/jci.insight.120505. Epub ahead of print

[31] Danylesko I, Beider K, Shimoni A, Nagler A. Novel strategies for immunotherapy in multiple myeloma: Previous experience and future directions. Clinical & Developmental Immunology. 2012;**2012**:753407. DOI: 10.1155/2012/753407. Epub 2012 May 10

[32] Rasche L, Weinhold N, Morgan GJ, van Rhee F, Davies FE. Immunologic approaches for the treatment of multiple myeloma. Cancer Treatment Reviews. 2017;**55**:190-199. DOI: 10.1016/ctrv.2017.03.010. Epub 2017 Apr 6

[33] Wang X, Li Y, Yan X. Efficacy and safety of novel agent-based therapies for multiple myeloma: A meta-analysis. BioMed Research International. 2016;**2016**:6848902. DOI: 10.1155/2016/6848902. Epub 2016 Feb 1

[34] Zeng ZH, Chen JF, Li YX, Zhang R, Xiao LF, Meng XY. Induction regimens for transplant-eligible patients with newly diagnosed multiple myeloma: A network meta-analysis of randomized controlled trials. Cancer Management and Research. 2017;**9**:287-298. DOI: 10.2147/CMAR.S138932. eCollection 2017

[35] Kouroukis TC, Baldassarre FG, Haynes AE, Imrie K, Reece DE, Cheung MC. Bortezomib in multiple myeloma: Systematic review and clinical considerations. Current Oncology. 2014;**21**(4):e573-e603. DOI: 10.3747/co.21.1798

[36] Al-Anazi KA. Autologous hematopoietic stem cell transplantation for multiple myeloma without cryopreservation. Bone Marrow Research. 2012;**2012**:917361. DOI: 10.1155/2012/917361. Epub 2012 May 28

[37] Costa LJ, Zhang MJ, Zhong X, Dispenzieri A, Lonial S, Krishnan A, et al. Trends in utilization and outcomes of autologous transplantation as early therapy for multiple myeloma. Biology of Blood and Marrow Transplantation. 2013;**19**(11):1615-1624. DOI: 10.1016/j.bbmt.2013.08.002. Epub 2013 Aug 11

[38] Mahajan S, Tandon N, Kumar S. The evolution of stem-cell transplantation in multiple myeloma. Therapeutic Advances in Hematology. 2018;**9**(5):123-133. DOI: 10.1177/2040620718761776. Epub 2018 Mar 5

[39] Mactier CE, Islam MS. Haematopoietic stem cell transplantation as first-line treatment in myeloma: A global perspective of current concepts and future possibilities. Oncology Reviews. 2012;**6**(2):e14. DOI: 10.4081/oncol.2012.e14. eCollection 2012 Oct 2

[40] Cavo M. A third-generation IMiD for MM. Blood. 2011;**118**(11):2931-2932. DOI: 10.1182/blood-2011-07-364315

[41] Facon T. Maintenance therapy for multiple myeloma in the era of novel agents. Hematology. American Society of Hematology. Education Program. 2015;**2015**:279-285. DOI: 10.1182/asheducation-2015.1.279

[42] Ye X, Huang J, Pan Q, Li W. Maintenance therapy with immunomodulatory drugs after autologous stem cell transplantation in patients with multiple myeloma: A meta-analysis of randomized controlled trials. PLoS One. 2013;**8**(8):e72635. DOI: 10.1371/journal.pone.0072635. eCollection 2013

[43] Lee HS, Min CK. Optimal maintenance and consolidation therapy for multiple myeloma in actual clinical practice. The Korean Journal of Internal Medicine. 2016;**31**(5):809-819. DOI: 10.3904/kjim.2016. 110. Epub 2016 Sep 1

[44] Li J-L, Fan G-Y, Liu Y-J, Zeng Z-H, Huang J-J, Yang Z-M, et al. Long-term efficacy of maintenance therapy for multiple myeloma: A quantitative synthesis of 22 randomized controlled trials. Frontiers in Pharmacology. 2018;**9**:430. DOI: 10.3389/fphar.2018.00430. Epub 2018 Apr 30

[45] Mian I, Milton DR, Shah N, Nieto Y, Popat UR, Kebriaei P, et al. Prolonged survival with a longer duration of maintenance lenalidomide after autologous hematopoietic stem cell transplantation for multiple myeloma. Cancer. 2016;**122**(24):3831-3837. DOI: 10.1002/cncr.30366. Epub 2016 Sep 28

[46] Liu J, Yang H, Liang X, Wang Y, Hou J, Liu Y, et al. Meta-analysis of the efficacy of treatments for newly diagnosed and relapsed/refractory multiple myeloma with del(17p). Oncotarget. 2017;**8**(37):62435-62444. DOI: 10.18632/oncotarget.18722. eCollection 2017 Sep 22

[47] Lipe B, Vukas R, Mikhael J. The role of maintenance therapy in multiple myeloma. Blood Cancer Journal. 2016;**6**(10):e485. DOI: 10.1038/bcj.2016.89

[48] Landgren O, Rajkumar SV. New developments in diagnosis, prognosis, and assessment of response in multiple myeloma. Clinical Cancer Research. 2016;**22**(22):5428-5433. DOI: 10.1158/1078-0432.CCR-16-0866

[49] Fulciniti M, Munshi NC, Martinez-Lopez J. Deep response in multiple myeloma: A critical review. BioMed Research International. 2015;**2015**:832049. DOI: 10.1155/2015/832049. Epub 2015 Dec 10

[50] Sonneveld P, Avet-Loiseau H, Lonial S, Usmani S, Siegel D, Anderson KC, et al. Treatment of multiple myeloma with high-risk cytogenetics: A consensus of the International Myeloma

Working Group. Blood. 2016;**127**(24):2955-2962. DOI: 10.1182/blood-2016-01-631200. Epub 2016 Mar 21

[51] Kazmi SM, Nusrat M, Gunaydin H, Cornelison AM, Shah N, Kebriaei P, et al. Outcomes among high-risk and standard-risk multiple myeloma patients treated with high-dose chemotherapy and autologous hematopoietic stem-cell transplantation. Clinical Lymphoma, Myeloma & Leukemia. 2015;**15**(11):687-693. DOI: 10.1016/j.clml. 2015.07.641. Epub 2015 Aug 5

[52] Landgren O, Devlin S, Boulad M, Mailankody S. Role of MRD status in relation to clinical outcomes in newly diagnosed multiple myeloma patients: A meta-analysis. Bone Marrow Transplantation. 2016;**51**(12):1565-1568. DOI: 10.1038/bmt.2016. 222. Epub 2016 Sep 5

[53] Munshi NC, Avet-Loiseau H, Rawstron AC, Owen RG, Child JA, Thakurta A, et al. Association of minimal residual disease with superior survival outcomes in patients with multiple myeloma: A meta-analysis. JAMA Oncology. 2017;**3**(1):28-35. DOI: 10.1001/jamaoncol.2016.3160

[54] Mai EK, Haas EM, Lücke S, Löpprich M, Kunz C, Pritsch M, et al. A systematic classification of death causes in multiple myeloma. Blood Cancer Journal. 2018;**8**(3):30. DOI: 10.1038/s41408-018-0068-5

[55] MacEwan JP, Batt K, Yin W, Peneva D, Sison S, Vine S, et al. Economic burden of multiple myeloma among patients in successive lines of therapy in the United States. Leukemia & Lymphoma. 2018;**59**(4):941-949. DOI: 10.1080/10428194. 2017.1361035. Epub 2017 Aug 13

[56] Robinson D Jr, Orlowski RZ, Stokes M, He J, Huse S, Chitnis A, et al. Economic burden of relapsed or refractory multiple myeloma: Results from an international trial. European Journal of Haematology. 2017;**99**(2):119-132. DOI: 10.1111/ejh.12876. Epub 2017 May 11

[57] Pandya S, Clancy Z, Shrestha S, Wang L, Ni Q, Baser O. Economic burden of early progression in newly-diagnosed multiple myeloma patients. Journal of Clinical Oncology. 2018;**36**(15 suppl):e20040. DOI: 10.1200/JCO.2018.36.15_suppl.e20040. Epub 2018 June 01

[58] Gregersen H, Vangsted AJ, Abildgaard N, Andersen NF, Pedersen RS, Frølund UC, et al. The impact of comorbidity on mortality in multiple myeloma: A Danish nationwide population-based study. Cancer Medicine. 2017;**6**(7):1807-1816. DOI: 10.1002/cam4.1128. Epub 2017 Jun 22

[59] Blimark C, Holmberg E, Mellqvist UH, Landgren O, Björkholm M, Hultcrantz M, et al. Multiple myeloma and infections: A population-based study on 9253 multiple myeloma patients. Haematologica. 2015;**100**(1):107-113. DOI: 10.3324/haematol.2014.107714. Epub 2014 Oct 24

[60] Jagannath S, Abonour R, Durie BGM, Gasparetto C, Hardin JW, Narang M, et al. Heterogeneity of second-line treatment for patients with multiple myeloma in the connect MM registry (2010-2016). Clinical Lymphoma, Myeloma & Leukemia. 2018;**18**(7):480-485.e3. DOI: 10.1016/j.clml.2018.04.007. Epub 2018 May 4

[61] Botta C, Ciliberto D, Rossi M, Staropoli N, Cucè M, Galeano T, et al. Network meta-analysis of randomized trials in multiple myeloma: Efficacy and safety in relapsed/refractory patients. Blood Advances. 2017;**1**(7):455-466. DOI: 10.1182/bloodadvances.2016003905. eCollection 2017 Feb 28

[62] Nijhof IS, van de Donk NWCJ, Zweegman S, Lokhorst HM. Current and new therapeutic strategies for relapsed and refractory multiple myeloma: An update. Drugs. 2018;**78**(1):19-37. DOI: 10.1007/s40265-017-0841-y

[63] Cook G, Zweegman S, Mateos MV, Suzan F, Moreau P. A question of class: Treatment options for patients with relapsed and/or refractory multiple myeloma. Critical Reviews in Oncology/Hematology. 2018;**121**:74-89. DOI: 10.1016/j.critrevonc.2017.11.016. Epub 2017 Dec 5

[64] Hari P, Romanus D, Palumbo A, Luptakova K, Rifkin RM, Tran LM, et al. Prolonged duration of therapy is associated with improved survival in patients treated for relapsed/refractory multiple myeloma in routine clinical care in the United States. Clinical Lymphoma, Myeloma & Leukemia. 2018;**18**(2):152-160. DOI: 10.1016/j.clml.2017.12.012. Epub 2018 Jan 5

[65] Ludwig H, Delforge M, Facon T, Einsele H, Gay F, Moreau P, et al. Prevention and management of adverse events of novel agents in multiple myeloma: A consensus of the European myeloma network. Leukemia. 2018;**32**(7):1542-1560. DOI: 10.1038/s41375-018-0040-1. Epub 2018 May 2

[66] Chen R, Wang Y, Luan C, Gao C, Zhang X, Chen B. Effect of pomalidomide on relapsed/refractory multiple myeloma: A systematic review and meta-analysis. Journal of Cancer. 2017;**8**(10):1801-1808. DOI: 10.7150/jca.17999. eCollection 2017

[67] Giralt S, Garderet L, Durie B, Cook G, Gahrton G, Bruno B, et al. American Society of Blood and Marrow Transplantation, European Society of Blood and Marrow Transplantation, Blood and Marrow Transplant Clinical Trials Network, and International Myeloma Working Group consensus conference on salvage hematopoietic cell transplantation in patients with relapsed multiple myeloma. Biology of Blood and Marrow Transplantation. 2015;**21**(12):2039-2051. DOI: 10.1016/j.bbmt.2015.09.016. Epub 2015 Sep 30

[68] Yin X, Tang L, Fan F, Jiang Q, Sun C, Hu Y. Allogeneic stem-cell transplantation for multiple myeloma: A systematic review and meta-analysis from 2007 to 2017. Cancer Cell International. 2018;**18**:62. DOI: 10.1186/s12935-018-0553-8. eCollection 2018

[69] Dimopoulos MA, Kaufman JL, White D, Cook G, Rizzo M, Xu Y, et al. A comparison of the efficacy of immunomodulatory-containing regimens in relapsed/refractory multiple myeloma: A network meta-analysis. Clinical Lymphoma, Myeloma & Leukemia. 2018; **18**(3):163-173.e6. DOI: 10.1016/j.clml. 2017.12.011. Epub 2018 Jan 5

[70] Liu L, Zhao N, Xu W, Sheng Z, Wang L. Pooled analysis of the reports of carfilzomib, panobinostat, and elotuzumab combinations in patients with refractory/relapsed multiple myeloma. Journal of Hematology & Oncology. 2016;**9**(1):54. DOI: 10.1186/s13045-016-0286-x

[71] Zou Y, Ma X, Yu H, Hu C, Fan L, Ran X. Carfilzomib/pomalidomide single-agent or in combination with other agents for the management of relapsed/refractory multiple myeloma: A meta-analysis of 37 trials. Oncotarget. 2017;**8**(24):39805-39817. DOI: 10.18632/oncotarget.10768

[72] Zhang T, Wang S, Lin T, Xie J, Zhao L, Liang Z, et al. Systematic review and meta-analysis of the efficacy and safety of novel monoclonal antibodies for treatment of relapsed/refractory multiple myeloma. Oncotarget. 2017;**8**(20):34001-34017. DOI: 10.18632/oncotarget.16987

[73] Cornell RF, Kassim AA. Evolving paradigms in the treatment of relapsed/refractory multiple myeloma: Increased options and increased complexity. Bone Marrow Transplantation. 2016;**51**(4):479-491. DOI: 10.1038/bmt.2015.307. Epub 2016 Jan 4

[74] Gonsalves WI, Milani P, Derudas D, Buadi FK. The next generation of novel therapies for the management of relapsed multiple myeloma. Future Oncology. 2017;**13**(1):63-75. DOI: 10.2217/fon-2016-0200. Epub 2016 Aug 11

[75] Latif A, Kapoor V, Sipra QUAR, Malik SU, Bilal J, Bin Riaz I, et al. Disease milestones through bibliometric analysis of the top 100 cited articles in multiple myeloma. Cureus. 2018;**10**(4):e2438. DOI: 10.7759/cureus.2438

[76] Saika TK. Developments in the field of myeloma in the last decade. Indian Journal of Hematology and Blood Transfusion. 2017;**33**(1):3-7. DOI: 10.1007/s12288-017-0777-0. Epub 2017 Jan 17

[77] Munshi NC, Anderson KC. New strategies in the treatment of multiple myeloma. Clinical Cancer Research. 2013;**19**(13):3337-3344. DOI: 10.1158/1078-0432.CCR-12-1881. Epub 2013 Mar 20

[78] Anderson KC. Vision statement for multiple myeloma: Future directions. Cancer Treatment and Research. 2016;**169**:15-22. DOI: 10.1007/978-3-319-40320-5_2

[79] Fonseca R, Abouzaid S, Bonafede M, Cai Q, Parikh K, Cosler L, et al. Trends in overall survival and costs of multiple myeloma, 2000-2014. Leukemia. 2017;**31**(9):1915-1921. DOI: 10.1038/leu.2016.380. Epub 2016 Dec 23

[80] de Souza JA, Muffly L. The overlooked cost of multiple myeloma. The Lancet Haematology. 2015;**2**(10):e394-e395. DOI: 10.1016/S2352-3026(15)00192-1. Epub 2015 Sep 17

[81] Yamabe K, Inoue S, Hiroshima C. Epidemiology and burden of multiple myeloma in Japan: A systematic review. Value in Health. 2015;**18**(7):A449. DOI: 10.1016/j.jval.2015. 09.1129. Epub 2015 Oct 20

Chapter 2

Epidemiology of Multiple Myeloma

Rafael Ríos-Tamayo, Dolores Sánchez Rodríguez,
Yoe-Ling Chang-Chan and
María-José Sánchez Pérez

Additional information is available at the end of the chapter

http://dx.doi.org/10.5772/intechopen.75396

Abstract

Multiple myeloma is a heterogeneous hematological malignancy in which epidemiology plays an increasingly important role. In recent years, an unprecedented intensive research, including both clinical and molecular epidemiology, has deepened the knowledge about its pathogenesis, risk factors, and prognostic factors, leading also to the approval of new drugs. Although the etiology remains largely unknown, among the confirmed risk factors, only obesity and the exposure to certain carcinogens are potentially preventable. Familial myeloma and occupational myeloma are topics of great interest. Most population-based cancer registries show a stable incidence or only a slight trend to increase. The diagnostic delay should be avoided as much as possible. Mortality rates, including early mortality, are progressively decreasing, although infection remains the leading cause of mortality. The outcome in terms of overall survival and health-related quality of life has remarkably improved, joining the group of potentially curable malignancies. Nowadays the clinical scenario is challenging. Clinical and epidemiological variables of interest should be standardized in clinical records. Patients should be included in a population-based registry network. The clinical coordination of a multidisciplinary team in a specialized unit is needed in order to maximize the outcome of every patient.

Keywords: multiple myeloma, epidemiology, population-based registry, incidence, risk factors, survival

1. Introduction

Multiple myeloma (MM) is a complex and heterogeneous disease [1–3], with variable survival. MM is a malignancy of terminally differentiated clonal plasma cells (PC) which are primarily localized in the bone marrow. In most cases, these PC are able to secrete a monoclonal immunoglobulin (Ig) protein (M protein) in the serum and/or urine. About 15–20% of MM patients secrete monoclonal light chains (LC) only, without expression of the normal Ig heavy chain, which constitutes LCMM [4], a subtype of MM-associated to poor outcome [5, 6]. True non-secretory MM represents only about 3% [7, 8].

The current definition of MM is based on the demonstration of 10% or more clonal bone marrow PC (or a biopsy-proven plasmacytoma) and one or more of the so-called myeloma defining events (MDE), including those events that evidence end-organ damage such as hypercalcemia, renal insufficiency, anemia, or osteolytic bone lesions (CRAB), or the presence of a biomarker of malignancy such as 60% or more clonal PC, 100 or more involved/uninvolved serum free light chain ratio (i/u FLCr), or more than one focal lesion on MRI.

Most patients with newly-diagnosed MM (NDMM) are preceded by a precursor disease (PD) [9, 10]. The most frequent PD is the monoclonal gammopathy of undetermined significance (MGUS), which is defined by a low M protein level (<30 g/L in serum or <500 mg/24-hour in urine), <10% of clonal bone marrow PC, and absence of CRAB or amyloidosis. Smoldering MM (SMM) is an asymptomatic plasma cell disorder. It is an intermediate entity between MGUS and MM, characterized by both the absence of MDE or amyloidosis, and a certain level of M protein (Ig G or A ≥ 30 g/L in serum or ≥500 mg in 24-hour urine) and/or 10–60% clonal bone marrow PC. The risk of progression to MM of MGUS and SMM is about 1 and 10% per year, respectively [11, 12].

The outcome of patients with NDMM in terms of overall survival (OS) is highly variable according to the type of study, selection criteria and calendar period. The real improvement in OS over time can be shown using population-based registries in which all incident cases are included with standardized rules and thorough follow-up [13–15]. Several well-established or emergent prognostic factors in relation to the disease, the host, the stage and the response to therapy are involved. However, the current risk stratification systems [16–20] cannot accurately predict the outcome in a particular patient.

Multilevel heterogeneity is a common denominator of MM. The epidemiological background [21, 22], the clinical presentation [23, 24], the genetic instability [25, 26] as well as clonal evolution [27, 28], and finally, the response to therapy [29, 30], are the most relevant levels of heterogeneity. All of them have a well-known impact on the outcome. Epidemiology is probably the first level of heterogeneity and its knowledge is key to understand MM outcome. Herein, an updated perspective on the epidemiology of MM will be highlighted.

2. Epidemiology of multiple myeloma

2.1. Incidence of multiple myeloma

MM incidence within a geographically determined population can be established by means of population-based cancer registries. The main goal of these registries is the identification of all incident cases of NDMM diagnosed among the residents of a defined geographical area [31]. The International Agency for Research on Cancer and the International Association of Cancer Registries provides high-quality statistics on the incidence of cancer from population-based registries around the world [32].

The incidence of MM is generally higher in more-developed countries. The estimated NDMM incident cases in the United States throughout 2017 is 30,280 (17,490 men and 12,790 women), representing 1.8% of all new cancer, with an incidence rate (per 100,000 inhabitants and age-standardized to the 2000 United States standard population) of 8 and 5.2 respectively, and a male/female ratio of 1.5 [33]. Similar or slightly lower age-standardized incidence rates can be found in European countries [31, 34–38]. Conversely, in Asian countries, the incidence is particularly low [39, 40]. There is a marked racial disparity in the incidence of MGUS and MM, with a two to threefold increased risk in blacks compared with whites, after adjusting for socioeconomic and other risk factors, suggesting a genetic predisposition [41].

Most population-based cancer registries show a stable or slightly increasing MM incidence over the last decades. In some registries, an improvement in case ascertainment may be the reason for the slight increase trend in the incidence. Based on data from the Surveillance, Epidemiology, and End Results Program [42] approximately 0.8% of the population will be diagnosed with MM at some point during their lifetime. On the other hand, as expected, the prevalence of MM has increased due to progressive improvement in OS.

2.2. Risk factors

MM is a multifactorial disease with a wide variety of risk factors including both environmental and genetic. Despite the growing interest in the field, the etiology of MM is poorly understood. However, many risk factors have been implicated, with variable levels of evidence [43, 44]. Herein, the main risk factors will be reviewed. Interestingly, some of these variables such as age, sex, race, and others, have a double behavior, as risk and prognostic factors. Remarkably, only two risk factors are potentially preventable. On the one hand, obesity is an increasingly common comorbidity. On the other hand, the exposition to certain chemical products, such as some herbicides, has been also demonstrated to be associated with the risk of developing MM.

2.2.1. Precursor disease

MM has a multistep pathogenesis [2, 45]. All MM patients are virtually preceded by a PD. Several PD can progress to MM, such as MGUS [46], SMM [12] or solitary plasmacytoma [47]. Despite the fact that MGUS is considered the main risk factor for MM, only few MM patients have a prior knowledge of MGUS at the time of the diagnosis of MM. Remarkably, in a Swedish nationwide study of 14,798 patients with MM, only 2.7% had previously diagnosed as having MGUS, but this subgroup showed significantly better OS [48]. Moreover, in the Granada (south of Spain) population-based cancer registry, all MM with any type of previously documented PD had a better outcome and this trend was maintained over the past three decades and it was not associated to diagnostic delay [49].

2.2.2. Age

The incidence of cancer in general and hematologic malignancies increases with age. The median age of MM at diagnosis is about 70 years [14, 38]. 72% of patients included in the Swedish Multiple Myeloma Registry were 65 years or older [38]. The median relative survival was 7.7 years for patients 65 years or younger, in comparison with 3.4 years for those with 66 years or older.

Several studies [50–54] have demonstrated that the advanced age is predictive of shorter OS. Aging is associated with a decrease in the tolerability to treatment, a higher rate of drug discontinuation due to adverse events and lower cumulative delivered-dose. All these circumstances may have an impact on the outcome. Survival in older adults with MM is also improving, but to a lesser extent than in young patients [14, 55].

Age, along with renal failure and certain comorbidities, is associated with early mortality [56, 57]. The number of comorbidities increases with aging, and this may be one of the reasons why elderly people with MM have a poor outcome.

2.2.3. Sex

Most but not all registries show a higher incidence of MM in men. Moreover, in several studies, men have a trend to poorer survival in relation to women [14, 54, 58, 59] although in most cases this is not statistically significant.

2.2.4. Race

The prognostic impact of race in OS is controversial. Racial disparities in outcomes may be related with biologic factors, individual factors, health behaviors, and structural barriers [60]. In a large study from the Surveillance, Epidemiology, and End Results (SEER), with more than 40,000 patients, the differences in OS between patients in the white and black race did not reach statistically significant differences [61]. A recent study from the Mayo Clinic did not found any survival difference by race but it showed considerable variability in MM therapeutics utilization with seeming inequity for racial-ethnic minorities [62]. A comprehensive study analyzing ethnically defined NDMM has shown molecular differences between African and European descent cases [63]. If this fact could have a clinical impact remains to be determined. Overall, the current evidence seems to confirm the conclusion of old studies pointing out that race is not a significant prognostic factor in MM, whereas the socioeconomic status may influence survival [64].

2.2.5. Socioeconomic status

In recent years, the socioeconomic status has been suggested to be a confusing variable in order to analyze more deeply the association between race and survival. However, there was not strong evidence until recently. Fiala et al. [65] showed that low socioeconomic status was independently associated with poorer OS in 562 patients at the Washington University School of Medicine, and this was confirmed in a large cohort of 45,505 patients from the SEER. The most likely hypothesis for this is that this subgroup of patients delay seeking medical attention and thus are farther advanced at presentation. Costa et al. [66] also studied a cohort of 10,161 patients from SEER highlighting the strong impact of social determinants of health, such as marital status (other than married), insurance status, and income. In this study, income and education were reported at the county level, not at the individual level. An important limitation of both studies is that comorbidities are not registered in the SEER database and therefore, its influence could not be explored.

Accordingly, all variables affecting outcomes, including sociodemographic factors, should be taken into account in order to make rigorous comparisons between different therapeutic approaches. A widening gap among socioeconomic status groups have been shown in the last two decades [67]. In this increasingly complex therapeutic scenario, it is imperative to focus on subgroups that may remain disadvantaged [68].

2.2.6. *Familial MM*

Family history is a well-defined risk factor for cancer. The demonstration of MM in two or more members of the same family is a rare occurrence. However, several reports during the past three decades [69–73] have analyzed the pattern of aggregation and pointed out a putative autosomal dominant mode of genetic transmission, reporting an excess familial risk for MM of about 2- to 4-fold and supporting a role for germline susceptibility genes, shared environmental influences, or an interaction of both. A variation in the presence of defining clinical features in MM patients according to family history of hematologic malignancy has been described [74, 75]. MM showed an association with breast and prostate cancer, and colorectal cancer families, suggesting that MM shares genetic susceptibility with many cancers [76].

2.2.7. *Occupational MM*

To facilitate international comparisons of occupational statistics, the definitions of all groups of occupations should be standardized [77]. The risk of MM has been associated with several manufacturing occupations and industries [78], such as machine operators and tenders, textile, food and beverage preparation, bakers and pastry cooks [79], printing and cleaning [80], hairdressers [81], and others. A meta-analysis including 5 cohort studies and 13 case–control studies on occupational exposure to dichloromethane, a widespread used solvent, showed an excess risk of MM [82].

Agriculture plays an important economic role in both developed and developing countries. There is a growing body of evidence about the association between farming and the risk of MM [83–85]. Despite methodological issues in some studies, the exposure to potential or confirmed carcinogens such as herbicides and pesticides commonly used by agricultural workers have been pointed out as key determinants of the cancer risk observed in agricultural populations. Some studies found a different pattern of risk according to sex [86] or even in female spouses of pesticide applicators [87]. Glyphosate is the most commonly used herbicide in the world and recent meta-analysis points out a marginally significant positive association with MM [88].

2.2.8. *Obesity*

Obesity is one of the biggest problems in public health throughout the world. According to the WHO definition, obese individuals have a body mass index of 30 Kg/m^2 or higher [89]. A causal link between obesity and cancer has been shown. About 20% of cancers are obesity-related, even 40% including overweight [90].

About 32% of NDMM patients are obese [14] Four meta-analysis have shown a positive association between obesity and MM risk [91–94]. The impact of obesity on the number of obesity-attributable NDMM cases was estimated to be 1.3 as relative risk and about 10% as population attributable risk [95]. On the other hand, the association of obesity with higher all-cause mortality is consistent [96], although the role of obesity as prognostic factor in MM is controversial. However, evidence suggests that obesity could have a negative impact on MM outcome [97].

2.2.9. *Type 2 diabetes*

Obesity and type 2 diabetes share close ties [98]. Approximately one fifth of NDMM have type 2 diabetes. The association between type 2 diabetes and MM has been evaluated in one meta-analysis [99] showing a trend toward significantly increased odds of MM in patients with type 2 diabetes. Moreover, some genetic variants may influence the risk of developing MM [100]. There is increasing evidence regarding the role of type 2 diabetes as an independent prognostic factor in MM at both clinical and genomic level [101, 102].

2.2.10. *Alcohol*

Alcohol consumption is a major cause of disease and death worldwide. More than 5% of the total number of cancer cases are alcohol-attributable [103]. However, the role of alcohol intake in the MM risk is unclear. Interestingly several studies, including two meta-analyses, have shown a protective effect in terms of MM risk [104–107].

2.2.11. *Smoking*

Smoking is not considered a risk factor for MM [108, 109]. Surprisingly, a recent study shows a potential interaction between certain single nucleotide polymorphisms and smoking associated with increase MM risk [110].

2.2.12. *Diet*

The current evidence about this topic is not strong due to the inherent difficulties and characteristics of the studies. Notwithstanding, some issues can be highlighted. A high consumption of fish is inversely associated with MM risk [111]. The consumption of green tea seems to have a protective effect in some [43] but not all studies [112]. Combined fruit and vegetable consumption has been associated with decreased non-Hodgkin lymphoma risk but it did not reach statistical significance for MM [113]. Remarkably, a diet-induced obesity promotes an MM-like condition [114]. Despite the potentially important role of diet and nutrition in cancer prevention, the current evidence is inconsistent [115].

2.2.13. *Physical activity*

The literature surrounding MM and physical activity are very limited [116]. Leisure-time physical activity was associated with lower risks of many cancer types, including MM [117, 118]. The effectiveness of participation in exercise programs remains unclear for patients with MM [119].

2.2.14. Other risk factors

Little evidence supports the infection with hepatitis B and C viruses [120, 121], environmental factors [122], or the use of drugs [123], as risk factors for MM.

Besides obesity and type 2 diabetes, other conditions such as autoimmune diseases [124], thyroid disease [125], or inflammatory disorders [126], may increase the MM risk.

Autoimmune diseases constitute a heterogeneous group of disorders, which jointly affect 5–10% of the population. In relation to the potential association of autoimmune diseases and MM, an individualized approach must be implemented. A significant increase in MM incidence after ankylosing spondylitis and systemic sclerosis was showed [124]. A few cases of immune thrombocytopenia purpura associated with MM at the time of MM diagnosis have been reported [127]. In a Swedish cohort study, a significant increase of MM was demonstrated in women previously diagnosed with pernicious anemia [128]. A history of the autoimmune disease has been recently associated with impaired OS in MM and MGUS [129].

Host-related immunodeficiency is known to play a role in the development of MM [130]. More than 8% of NDMM have a prior or synchronous malignancy [14]. MM is associated with many other malignancies, including colorectal, breast and prostate cancers, non-thyroid endocrine tumors, leukemia and cancer of unknown primary [76]. The prognosis of patients with a second or third cancer is inferior [131]. Sometimes, NDMM and other hematological neoplasm such as myelodysplastic syndrome are diagnosed at the same time in the same patient [132]. Increased life expectancy has led to renewed concerns about the long-term risk of second primary malignancies [133].

2.3. Survival

OS remains the key end-point in both clinical trials and real-life patients. Survival in MM is highly variable and depends on prognostic factors, which can be categorized into four groups: host-related, disease-related, staging and therapy. Among host-related factors, comorbidity plays an important role. However, the analysis of prognostic factors is beyond the aim of this chapter. Notwithstanding, it must be emphasized that many of the above-mentioned risk factors can also behave as prognostic factors, as is the case of age. In this regard, less than 3% of patients with MM are younger than 40 years, showing similar clinical features to the whole MM population, except for a higher proportion of LCMM [134]. On the other hand, renal impairment is a common presenting complication of MM with a negative impact on the outcome; despite this, there has been a major improvement in OS in these patients, although the risk of early death remains high [135]. Moreover, the size and type of institution where the patients are treated may have an impact on the outcome in some studies [38, 136, 137]. OS has continuously improved over the past decades due to better supportive care and advances in therapy. Population-based studies are needed to accurately estimate OS in real-life patients [14, 35, 38]. An important gap exists between the outcome of these patients and those included in clinical trials, which have to fulfill specific selection criteria. Although some patients can achieve deep responses and become long-term survivors, being some of them cured, the goal of curing MM in a significant proportion of patients is still far away. In the current scenario, getting and maintaining a minimal residual disease has become the primary objective of therapy before cure [29]. In the meantime, the importance of improving quality of life should be pointed out [138].

2.4. Mortality

Based on data from the SEER Program [42], MM is the fourteenth leading cause of cancer death in the United States. The number of deaths was 3.3 per 100,000 men and women per year (age-adjusted rates), based on 2010–2014 deaths.

Comorbidity has also an impact on mortality, in particular, early mortality [57]. Infection remains as the first cause of death in most studies, frequently associated with aging, renal failure, and relapse. Therefore, every effort to avoid serious infection should be taken into account. In this regard, prophylactic antibiotics [139] and vaccines are key measures.

2.5. Prevention

Little is known about effective measures to avoid the development of MM. Early treatment of asymptomatic patients with high-risk SMM or even high-risk MGUS, now only in the context of clinical trials, may prevent the appearance of MM, increasing the probability of cure [140].

Currently, the potentially preventable risk factors for MM are obesity and the exposure to MM-related carcinogens, particularly in the context of farming. Efforts should be made to fight globally and effectively against these risk factors.

On the other hand, the prevention of treatment-related adverse events is a matter of concern [141].

3. Conclusions

- MM is a very complex and heterogeneous disease. Heterogeneity is largely responsible for the great variability in the outcome of patients and can be stratified in several levels. Epidemiology should be considered the first level of heterogeneity. Therefore, the knowledge of the epidemiological background should be taken into account in both real-life and clinical trials settings to accurately assess the outcome, allowing a precise comparison between studies.
- MM epidemiology is an exciting research topic. In the era of precision and personalized medicine, both clinical and molecular epidemiology should be integrated as a mandatory step in the optimized workup of every patient.
- MM is a multistep malignancy. Virtually all patients with NDMM had a previous precursor disease. However, the proportion of NDMM patients with a previously known precursor disease is remarkably small. Both MGUS and SMM have also a heterogeneous pattern of risk progression. Early treatment in high-risk SMM is expected to increase the rate of cure.

- MM is a multifactorial condition. Many risk factors are involved with variable levels of evidence. The meta-analysis is located at the top of the pyramid of evidence, having largely contributed to highlight the role of potential or plausible risk factors.
- MM is a rapidly changing field. In the last decade, the pathogenesis, diagnosis, prognosis, and treatment of MM have dramatically changed. The knowledge of the epidemiological perspective can help to better understand current and future challenges, leading to an optimized MM care.

Author details

Rafael Ríos-Tamayo[1,2,3,4,5]*, Dolores Sánchez Rodríguez[1,7], Yoe-Ling Chang-Chan[4,6] and María-José Sánchez Pérez[4,5,6]

*Address all correspondence to: rriost33@gmail.com

1 Monoclonal Gammopathies Unit, University Hospital Virgen de las Nieves, Granada, Spain

2 Department of Hematology, University Hospital Virgen de las Nieves, Granada, Spain

3 Genomic Oncology Area, GENYO, Centre for Genomics and Oncological Research, Pfizer/University of Granada/Andalusian Regional Government, PTS, Granada, Spain

4 Biosanitary Research Institute of Granada (Ibs.GRANADA), University Hospitals of Granada/University of Granada, Granada, Spain

5 CIBER of Epidemiology of Public Health (CIBERESP), Madrid, Spain

6 Granada Cancer Registry, Andalusian School of Public Health, Granada, Spain

7 FIBAO, Granada, Spain

References

[1] Rajkumar SV, Dimopoulos MA, Palumbo A, Bladé J, Merlini G, Mateos MV, et al. International myeloma working group updated criteria for the diagnosis of multiple myeloma. The Lancet Oncology. 2014;**15**:e538-e548. DOI: 10.1016/S1470-2045(14)70442-5

[2] Bianchi G, Munshi NC. Pathogenesis beyond the cancer clone(s) in multiple myeloma. Blood. 2015;**125**:3049-3058. DOI: 10.1182/blood-2014-11-568881

[3] Kumar SK, Rajkumar V, Kyle RA, van Duin M, Sonneveld P, Mateos MV, et al. Multiple myeloma. Nature Reviews Disease Primers. 2017;**3**:17046. DOI: 10.1038/nrdp.2017.46

[4] Kyle RA, Rajkumar SV. Criteria for diagnosis, staging, risk stratification and response assessment of multiple myeloma. Leukemia. 2009;**23**:3-9. DOI: 10.1038/leu.2008.291

[5] Ríos-Tamayo R, Sánchez MJ, García de Veas JL, Rodríguez T, Puerta JM, Chang-Chan YL, et al. Light chain multiple myeloma: A single institution series. Journal of Leukemia. 2015;**3**:184. DOI: 10.4172/2329-6917.1000184

[6] Zhang JJ, Sun WJ, Huang ZX, Chen SL, Zhong YP, Hu Y, et al. Light chain multiple myeloma, clinic features, responses to therapy and survival in a long-term study. World Journal of Surgical Oncology. 2014;**12**:234. DOI: 10.1186/1477-7819-12-234

[7] Bladé J, Kyle RA. Nonsecretory myeloma, immunoglobulin D myeloma, and plasma cell leukemia. Hematology/Oncology Clinics of North America. 1999;**13**:1259-1272

[8] Chawla SS, Kumar SK, Dispenzieri A, Greenberg AJ, Larson DR, Kyle RA, et al. Clinical course and prognosis of non-secretory multiple myeloma. European Journal of Hematology. 2015;**95**:57-64. DOI: 10.1111/ejh.12478

[9] Landgren O, Kyle RA, Pfeiffer RM, Katzmann JA, Caporaso NE, Hayes RB, et al. Monoclonal gammopathy of undetermined significance (MGUS) consistently precedes multiple myeloma: a prospective study. Blood. 2009;**113**:5412-5417. DOI: 1182/blood-2008-12-194241

[10] Weiss BM, Abadie J, Verma P, Howard RS, Kuehl M. A monoclonal gammopathy precedes multiple myeloma in most patients. Blood. 2009;**113**:5418-5422. DOI: 10.1182/blood-2008-12-195008

[11] Kyle RA, Therneau TM, Rajkumar SV, Offord JR, Larson DR, Plevak MF, et al. A long-term study of prognosis in monoclonal gammopathy of undetermined significance. The New England Journal of Medicine. 2002;**346**:564-569

[12] Rajkumar SV, Landgren O, Mateos MV. Smoldering multiple myeloma. Blood. 2015;**125**: 3069-3075. DOI: 10.1182/blood-2014-09-568899

[13] Kristinsson SY, Landgren O, Dickman PW, Derolf AR, Björkholm M. Patterns of survival in multiple myeloma: A population-based study of patients diagnosed in Sweden from 1973 to 2003. Journal of Clinical Oncology. 2007;**25**:1993-1999. DOI: 10.1200/JCO.2006.09.0100

[14] Ríos-Tamayo R, Sánchez MJ, Puerta JM, Sainz J, Chang-Chan DY, Rodríguez T, et al. Trends in survival of multiple myeloma: A thirty-year population-based study in a single institution. Cancer Epidemiology. 2015;**39**:693-699. DOI: 10.1016/j.canep.2015.08.002

[15] Turesson I, Velez R, Kristinsson SY, Landgren O. Patterns of improved survival in patients with multiple myeloma in the twenty-first century: A population-based study. Journal of Clinical Oncology. 2010;**28**:830-834. DOI: 10.1200/JCO.2009.25.4177

[16] Greipp PR, San Miguel J, Durie BGM, Crowley JJ, Barlogie B, Bladé J, et al. International staging system for multiple myeloma. Journal of Clinical Oncology. 2005;**23**:3412-3420. DOI: 10.1200/JCO.2005.04.242

[17] Palumbo A, Avet-Loiseau H, Oliva S, Lokhorst HM, Goldschmidt H, Rosiñol L, et al. Revised international staging system forMultiple myeloma: A report from international myeloma working group. Journal of Clinical Oncology. 2015;**33**:2863-2869. DOI: 10.1200/JCO.2015.61.2267

[18] Ríos-Tamayo R, Romero A, Puerta JM, González PA, López-Fernández E, Moratalla L, et al. ISS versus R-ISS for risk stratification of multiple myeloma patients undergoing autologous stem cell transplant. Journal of Leukemia. 2015;**3**:189. DOI: 10.4172/2329-6917.1000189

[19] Chng WJ, Dispenzieri A, Chim C-S, Fonseca R, Goldschmidt H, Lentzsch S, et al. IMWG consensus on risk stratification in multiple myeloma. Leukemia. 2014;**28**:269-277. DOI: 10.1038/leu.2013.247

[20] Usmani SZ, Rodriguez-Otero P, Bhutani M, Mateos MV, San Miguel J. Defining and treating high-risk multiple myeloma. Leukemia. 2015;**29**:2119-2125. DOI: 10.1038/leu.2015.209

[21] Alexander DD, Mink PJ, Adami HO, Cole P, Mandel JS, Oken MM, et al. Multiple myeloma: A review of the epidemiologic literature. International Journal of Cancer. 2007;**120**: 40-61. DOI: 10.1002/ijc.22718

[22] Kyle RA, Rajkumar SV. Epidemiology of the plasma-cell disorders. Best Practice and Research Clinical Haematology. 2007;**20**:637-664. DOI: 10.1016/j.beha.2007.08.001

[23] Greenberg AJ, Rajkumar SV, Therneau TM, Singh PP, Dispenzieri A, Kumar SK. Relationship between initial clinical presentation and the molecular cytogenetic classification of myeloma. Leukemia. 2014;**28**:398-403. DOI: 10.1038/leu.2013.258

[24] Ríos-Tamayo R, Sainz J, Alba AM, Cruz AJ, Pérez JA, Morente E, et al. The impact of the type of myeloma-defining event on early mortality and survival. In: EHA 21th;9-12 June 2016; Copenhagen. Denmark: Haematologica. 2016;**100**(s.1):pp. 544-545

[25] Egan JB, Shi C-X, Tembe W, Christoforides A, Kurdoglu A, Sinari S, et al. Whole-genome sequencing of multiple myeloma from diagnosis to plasma cell leukemia reveals genomic initiating events, evolution, and clonal tides. Blood. 2012;**120**:1060-1066. DOI: 10.1182/blood-2012-01-405977

[26] Corre J, Munshi N, Avet-Loiseau H. Genetics of multiple myeloma: Another heterogeneity level? Blood. 2015;**125**:1870-1876. DOI: 10.1182/blood-2014-10-567370

[27] Keats JJ, Chesi M, Egan JB, Garbitt VM, Palmer SE, Braggio E, et al. Clonal competition with alternating dominant in multiple myeloma. Blood. 2012;**120**:1067-1076. DOI: 10.1182/blood-2012-01-405985

[28] Melchor L, Brioli A, Wardell CP, Murison A, Potter NE, Kaiser MF, et al. Single-cell genetic analysis reveals the composition of initiating clones and phylogenetic patterns of branching and parallel evolution in myeloma. Leukemia. 2014;**28**:1705-1715. DOI: 10.1038/leu.2014.13

[29] Lahuerta JJ, Paiva B, Vidriales MB, Cordón L, Cedena MT, Puig N, et al. Depth of response in multiple myeloma: A pooled analysis of three PETHEMA/GEM clinical trials. Journal of Clinical Oncology. 2017;**35**:2900-2910. DOI: 10.1200/JCO.2016.69.2517

[30] Kumar S, Paiva B, Anderson KC, Durie B, Landgren O, Moreau P, et al. International myeloma working group consensus criteria for response and minimal residual disease assessment in multiple myeloma. The Lancet Oncology. 2016;**17**:e328-e346. DOI: 10.1016/S1470-2045(16)30206-6

[31] Galceran J, Ameijide A, Carulla M, Mateos A, Quirós JR, Rojas D, et al. Cancer incidence in Spain, 2015. Clinical & Translational Oncology. 2017;**19**:799-825. DOI: 10.1007/s12094-016-1607-9

[32] Bray F, Colombet M, Mery L, Piñeros M, Znaor A, Zanetti R, Ferlay J, editors. Cancer Incidence in Five Continents, Vol. XI (electronic version). Lyon: International Agency for Research on Cancer; 2017. Available from: http://ci5.iarc.fr. [Accessed December 9, 2017]

[33] Siegel RL, Miller KD, Jemal A. Cancer statistics, 2017. CA: a Cancer Journal for Clinicians. 2017;**67**:7-30. DOI: 10.3322/caac.21387

[34] Vélez R, Turesson I, Landgren O, Kristinsson SY, Cuzick J. Incidence of multiple myeloma in Great Britain, Sweden, and Malmö, Sweden: The impact of differences in case ascertainment on observed incidence trends. BMJ Open. 2016;**6**:e009584. DOI: 10.1136/bmjopen-2015-009584

[35] Turesson I, Vélez R, Kristinsson SY, Landgren O. Patterns of multiple myeloma during the past 5 decades: Stable incidence rates for all age groups in the population but rapidly changing age distribution in the clinic. Mayo Clinic Proceedings. 2010;**85**:225-230. DOI: 10.4065/mcp.2009.0426

[36] Renshaw C, Ketley N, Møller H, Davies EA. Trends in the incidence and survival of multiple myeloma in South East England 1985-2004. BMC Cancer. 2010;**10**:74. DOI: 0.1186/1471-2407-10-74

[37] Maluskova D, Svobodova I, Kucerova M, Brozova L, Muzik J, Jarkopvsky J, et al. Epidemiology of multiple myeloma in the Czech Republic. Klin Oncol. 2017;**30**(Suppl 2):2S35-2S42. DOI: 10.14735/amko20172S35

[38] Blimark CH, Turesson I, Genell A, Ahlberg L, Björkstrand B, Carlson K, et al. Outcome and survival of myeloma patients diagnosed 2008-2015. Real world data on 4904 patients from the Swedish myeloma registry (SMR). Haematologica. 2018;**103**:506-513. DOI: 10.3324/haematol.2017.178103

[39] Huang SY, Yao M, Tang JL, Lee WC, Tsay W, Cheng AL, et al. Epidemiology of multiple myeloma in Taiwan. Increasing incidence for the past 25 years and higher prevalence of extramedullary myeloma in patients younger than 55 years. Cancer. 2007;**110**:896-905. DOI: 10.1002/cncr.22850

[40] Lee JH, Lee DS, Lee JJ, Chang YH, Jin JY, Jo DY, et al. Multiple myeloma in Korea: Past, present, and future perspectives. Experience of the Korean multiple myeloma working party. International Journal of Haematology. 2010;**92**:52-57. DOI: 10.1007/s12185-010-0617-6

[41] Greenberg AJ, Vachon CM, Rajkumar SV. Disparities in the prevalence, pathogenesis and progression of monoclonal gammopathy of undetermined significance and multiple myeloma between blacks and whites. Leukemia. 2012;**26**:609-614. DOI: 10.1038/leu.2011.368

[42] National Cancer Institute. Surveillance, Epidemiology, and End Results Program [Internet]. 2017. Available from: http://www.seer.cancer.gov [Accessed: December 10, 2017]

[43] Wang Q, Wang Y, Ji Z, Chen X, Pan Y, Gao G, et al. Risk factors for multiple myeloma: A hospital-based case–control study in Northwest China. Cancer Epidemiology. 2012; **36**:439-444. DOI: 10.1016/j.canep.2012.05.002

[44] Sergentanis TN, Zagouri F, Tsilimidos G, Tsagianni A, Tseliou M, Dimopoulos MA, et al. Risk factors for multiple myeloma: A systematic review of meta-analyses. Clinical Lymphoma Myeloma and Leukemia. 2015;**15**:563-577. DOI: 10.1016/j.clml.2015.06.003

[45] Palumbo A, Anderson K. Multiple myeloma. The New England Journal of Medicine. 2011;**364**:1046-1060. DOI: 10.1056/NEJMra1011442

[46] Kyle RA, Therneau TM, Rajkumar SV, Larson DR, Plevak MF, Offord JR, et al. Prevalence of monoclonal gammopathy of undetermined significance. The New England Journal of Medicine. 2006;**354**:1362-1369. DOI: 10.1056/NEJMoa054494

[47] Katodritou E, Terpos E, Symeonidis AS, Pouli A, Kelaidi C, Kyrtsonis MC, et al. Clinical features, outcome, and prognostic factors for survival and evolution to multiple myeloma of solitary plasmacytomas: A report of the Greek myeloma study group in 97 patients. American Journal of Hematology. 2014;**89**:803-808. DOI: 10.1002/ajh.23745

[48] Sigurdardottir EE, Turesson I, Lund SH, Lindqvist EK, Mailankody S, Korde N, et al. The role of diagnosis and clinical follow-up of monoclonal gammopathy of undetermined significance on survival in multiple myeloma. JAMA Oncology. 2015;**1**:168-174. DOI: 10.1001/jamaoncol.2015.23

[49] Ríos-Tamayo R, Sainz J, Jurado M, Puerta JM, González PA, Romero A, et al. Multiple myeloma with prior precursor disease shows better outcome. In: 57th Meeting of The American Hematology Association; 5-8 December 2015; Orlando. EEUU : Blood. 2015;**126**. Abstract 1756

[50] Bringhen S, Mateos MV, Zweegman S, Larocca A, Falcone AP, Oriol A, et al. Age and organ damage correlate with poor survival in myeloma patients: Meta-analysis of 1435 individual patient data from 4 randomized trials. Haematologica. 2013;**98**:980-987. DOI: 10.3324/haematol.2012.075051

[51] Chretien ML, Hebraud B, Cances-Lauwers V, Hulin C, Marit G, Leleu X, et al. Age is a prognostic factor even among patients with multiple myeloma younger than 66 years treated with high-dose melphalan: The IFM experience on 2316 patients. Haematologica. 2014;**99**:1236-1238. DOI: 10.3324/haematol.2013.098608

[52] Wildes TM, Rosko A, Tuchman SA. Multiple myeloma in older adults: Better prospects, more challenges. Journal of Clinical Oncology. 2014;**32**:2531-2540. DOI: 10.1200/JCO.2014.55.1028

[53] Kumar SK, Dispenzieri A, Lacy MQ, Gertz MA, Buadi FK, Pandey S, et al. Continued improvement in survival in multiple myeloma: Changes in early mortality and outcomes in older patients. Leukemia. 2014;**28**:1122-1128. DOI: 10.1038/leu.2013.313

[54] Liwing J, Uttervall K, Lund J, Aldrin A, Blimark C, Carlson K, et al. Improved survival in myeloma patients: Starting to close in on the gap between elderly patients and a matched normal population. British Journal of Haematology. 2014;**164**:684-693. DOI: 10.1111/bjh.12685

[55] Kristinsson SY, Anderson WF, Landgren O. Improved long-term survival in multiple myeloma up to the age of 80 years. Leukemia. 2014;**28**:1346-1348. DOI: 10.1038/leu.2014.23

[56] Augustson BM, Begum G, Dunn JA, Barth NJ, Davies F, Morgan G, et al. Early mortality after diagnosis of multiple myeloma: Analysis of patients entered onto the United Kingdom Medical Research Council trials between 1980 and 2002-Medical Research Council adult leukaemia working party. Journal of Clinical Oncology. 2005;**23**:9219-9226. DOI: 10.1200/JCO.2005.03.2086

[57] Ríos-Tamayo R, Sainz J, Martínez-López J, Puerta JM, Chang-Chan DY, Rodríguez T, et al. Early mortality in multiple myeloma: The time-dependent impact of comorbidity. A population-based study in 621 real-life patients. American Journal of Hematology. 2016;**91**:700-705. DOI: 10.1002/ajh.24389

[58] Kumar SK, Rajkumar SV, Dispenzieri A, Lacy MQ, Hayman SR, Buadi FK, et al. Improved survival in multiple myeloma and the impact of novel therapies. Blood. 2008;**111**:2516-2520. DOI: 10.1182/blood-2007-10-116129

[59] Yusuf AA, Natwick T, Werther W, Felici D, Mahue M, Bridges KR, et al. A retrospective analysis to examine factors associated with mortality in Medicare beneficiaries newly diagnosed with multiple myeloma. Current Medical Research and Opinion. 2016;**12**:1989-1996. DOI: 10.1080/03007995.2016.1226166

[60] Kirtane K, Lee SJ. Racial and ethnic disparities in hematologic malignancies. Blood. 2017; **130**:1699-1705. DOI: 10.1182/blood-2017-04-778225

[61] Kaya H, Peressini B, Jawed I, Martincic D, Elaimy AL, Lamoreaux WT, et al. Impact of age, race and decade of treatment on overall survival in a critical population analysis of 40,000 multiple myeloma patients. International Journal of Hematology. 2012;**95**:64-70. DOI: 10.1007/s12185-011-0971-z

[62] Ailawadhi S, Frank RD, Advani P, Swaika A, Temkit M, Menghani R, et al. Racial disparity in utilization of therapeutic modalities among multiple myeloma patients: A SEER-medicare analysis. Cancer Med-US. 2017;**6**:2876-2885. DOI: 10.1002/cam4.1246

[63] Manojlovic Z, Christofferson A, Liang WS, Aldrich J, Washington M, Wong S, et al. Comprehensive molecular profiling of 718 multiple myelomas reveals significant differences in mutation frequencies between African and European descent cases. PLoS Genetics. 2017;**13**:e1007087. DOI: 10.1371/journal.pgen.1007087

[64] Savage D, Lindenbaum J, Van Ryzin J, Struening E, Garret J. Race, poverty, and survival in multiple myeloma. Cancer. 1984;**54**:3085-3094

[65] Fiala MA, Finney JD, Liu J, Stockerl-Goldstein KE, Tomasson MH, Vij R, et al. Socioeconomic status is independently associated with overall survival in patient with multiple myeloma. Leukemia & Lymphoma. 2015;**56**:2643-2649. DOI: 10.3109/10428194.2015.1011156

[66] Costa LJ, Brill IK, Brown EE. Impact of marital status, insurance status, income, and race/ethnicity on the survival of younger patients diagnosed with multiple myeloma in the United States. Cancer. 2016;**122**:3183-3190. DOI: 10.1002/cncr.30183

[67] Sun T, Wang S, Sun H, Wen J, An G, Li J. Improved survival in multiple myeloma, with a diminishing racial gap and a widening socioeconomic status gap over three decades. Leukemia & Lymphoma. 2018;**59**:49-58. DOI: 10.1080/10428194.2017.1335398

[68] Ailawadhi S, Bhatia K, Aulakh S, Meghji Z, Chanan-Khan A. Equal treatment and outcomes for everyone with multiple myeloma: Are we there yet? Current Hematologic Malignancy Reports. 2017;**12**:309-316. DOI: 10.1007/s11899-017-0393-y

[69] Lynch HT, Ferrarar K, Barlogie B, Coleman EA, Lynch JF, Weisenburger D, et al. Familial myeloma. The New England Journal of Medicine. 2008;**359**:152-157. DOI: 10.1056/NEJMoa0708704

[70] Landgren O, Kristinsson SY, Goldin LR, Caporaso NE, Blimark C, Mellqvist UH, et al. Risk of plasma cell and lymphoproliferative disorders among 14 621 first-degree relatives of 4458 patients with monoclonal gammopathy of undetermined significance in Sweden. Blood. 2009;**114**:791-795. DOI: 10.1182/blood-2008-12-191676

[71] Altieri A, Chen B, Bermejo LR, Castro F, Hemminki K. Familial risks and temporal incidence trends of multiple myeloma. European Journal of Cancer. 2006;**42**:1661-1670. DOI: 10.1016/j.ejca.2005.11.033

[72] Coleman EA, Lynch H, Enderlin C, Stewart B, Thomé SD, Kennedy R, et al. Initial report of family registry of multiple myeloma. Cancer Nursing. 2009;**32**:456-464. DOI: 10.1097/NCC.0b013e3181a90168

[73] Vachon CM, Kyle RA, Therneau TM, Foreman BJ, Larson DR, Colby CL, et al. Increased risk of monoclonal gammopathy in first-degree relatives of patients with multiple myeloma or monoclonal gammopathy of undetermined significance. Blood. 2009;**114**:785-790. DOI: 10.1182/blood-2008-12-192575

[74] Van Valkenburg MAE, Pruitt GI, Brill IK, Costa L, Ehtsham M, Justement IT, et al. Family history of hematologic malignancies and risk of multiple myeloma: Differences by race and clinical features. Cancer Cause Control. 2016;**27**:81-91. DOI: 10.1007/s10552-015-0685-2

[75] Schinasi LH, Brown EE, Camp NJ, Wang SS, Hofmann JN, Chiu BC, et al. Multiple myeloma and family history of lymphohaematopoietic cancers: Results from the international multiple myeloma consortium. British Journal of Haematology. 2016;**175**:87-101. DOI: 10.1111/bjh.14199

[76] Frank C, Fallah M, Chen T, Mai EK, Sundquist J, Försti A, et al. Search for familial clustering of multiple myeloma with any cancer. Leukemia. 2016;**30**:627-632. DOI: 10.1038/leu.2015.279

[77] International Labour Organization. International Standard Classification of Occupations: ISCO-08. Geneva: ILO; 2012. V1. 420pp

[78] Gold LS, Milliken K, Stewart P, Purdue M, Severson R, Seixas N, et al. Occupation and multiple myeloma: An occupation and industry analysis. American Journal of Industrial Medicine. 2010;**53**:768-779. DOI: 10.1002/ajim.20857

[79] Lope V, Pérez-Gómez B, Aragonés N, López-Abente G, Gustavsson P, Plato N, et al. Occupation, exposure to chemicals, sensitizing agents, and risk of multiple myeloma in Sweden. Cancer Epidemiology, Biomarkers & Prevention. 2008;**17**:3123-3127. DOI: 10.1158/1055-9965.EPI-08-0343

[80] Perrotta C, Staines A, Codd M, Kleefeld S, Crowley D, Mannetje AT, et al. Multiple myeloma and lifetime occupation: Results from the EPILYMPH study. Journal of Occupational Medical Toxicology. 2012;**7**:25. DOI: 10.1186/1745-6673-7-25

[81] Takkouche B, Regueira-Méndez C, Montes-Martínez A. Risk of cancer among hairdressers and related workers: A meta-analysis. International Journal of Epidemiology. 2009;**38**:1512-1531. DOI: 10.1093/ije/dyp283

[82] Liu T, Xu Q, Zhang CH, Zhang P. Occupational exposure to methylene chloride and risk of cancer: A meta-analysis. Cancer Cause Control. 2006;**24**:2037-2049. DOI: 10.1007/s10552-013-0283-0

[83] Khuder SA, Mutgi AB. Meta-analyses of multiple myeloma and farming. American Journal of Industrial Medicine. 1997;**32**:510-516

[84] Perrotta C, Staines A, Cocco P. Multiple myeloma and farming. A systematic review of 30 years of research. Where next? Journal of Occupational Medicine and Toxicology. 2008;**3**:27. DOI: 10.1186/1745-6673-3-27

[85] Ghafari M, Cheraghi Z, Doosti-Irani A. Occupational risk factors among Iranian farmworkers: A review of the available evidence. Epidemiology and Health. 2017;**39**:e2017027. DOI: 10.4178/epih.e2017027

[86] Kachuri L, Harris MA, MacLeod JS, Tjepkema M, Peters PA, Demers PA. Cancer risks in a population-based study of 70,570 agricultural workers: Results from the Canadian census health and environment cohort (CanCHEC). BMC Cancer. 2017;**17**:343. DOI: 10.1186/s12885-017-3346-x

[87] Louis LM, Lerro CC, Friesen MC, Andreotti G, Koutros S, Sandler DP, et al. A prospective study of cancer risk among agricultural health study farm spouses associated with personal use of organochlorine insecticides. Environmental Health. 2017;**16**:95. DOI: 10.1186/s12940-017-0298-1

[88] Chang ET, Delzell E. Systematic review and meta-analysis of glyphosate exposure and risk of lymphohematopoietic cancers. Journal of Environmental Science and Health. Part. B. 2016;**51**:402-428. DOI: 10.1080/03601234.2016.1142748

[89] Ríos-Tamayo R, Sainz J, Jiménez-Moleón JJ, Jurado M. Obesity and multiple myeloma: What do the data tell us? Journal of Leukemia. 2014;**2**:e109. DOI: 10.4172/2329-6917.1000e109

[90] Brook C, Thomas CC, Henley SJ, Massetti GM, Galuska DA, Agurs-Collins T, et al. Vital signs: Trends in incidence of cancers associated with overweight and obesity — United States, 2005-2014. MMWR 2017;**66**:39. Available from: https://www.cdc.gov/mmwr. [Accessed: October 3, 2017]

[91] Larsson SC, Wolk A. Body mass index and risk of multiple myeloma: A meta-analysis. International Journal of Cancer. 2007;**121**:2512-2516. DOI: 10.1002/ijc.22968

[92] Renehan AG, Tyson M, Egger M, Heller RF, Zwahlen M. Body-mass index and incidence of cancer: A systematic review and meta-analysis of prospective observational studies. Lancet. 2008;**371**:569-578. DOI: 10.1016/S0140-6736(08)60269-X

[93] Wallin A, Larsson SC. Body mass index and risk of multiple myeloma: A meta-analysis of prospective studies. European Journal of Cancer. 2011;**47**:1606-1615. DOI: 10.1016/j.ejca.2011.01.020

[94] Ríos-Tamayo R, Jiménez-Moleón JJ, Sainz J, López F, Rivera AB, Sánchez MJ, et al. Multiple myeloma and obesity: A meta-analysis. In: EHA 16th;9-12 June 2011; London. UK: Haematologica -The Hematology Journal. 2011;**96**,s2:pp. s585-586

[95] Polednak AP. Estimating the number of U.S. incident cancers attributable to obesity and the impact on temporal trends in incidence rates for obesity-related cancers. Cancer Detection and Prevention. 2008;**32**:190-199. DOI: 10.1016/j.cdp.2008.08.004

[96] The Global BMI Mortality Collaboration. Body-mass index and all-cause mortality: Individual participant-data meta-analysis of 239 prospective studies in four continents. Lancet. 2016;**388**:776-786. DOI: 10.1016/S0140-6736(16)30175-1

[97] Yang L, Drake BF, Colditz GA. Obesity and other cancers. Journal of Clinical Oncology. 2016;**34**:4231-4237. DOI: 10.1200/JCO.2016.68.4837

[98] Ríos-Tamayo R, Sainz J, Jiménez-Moleón JJ, Jurado M. Type 2 diabetes and multiple myeloma: The latest insights. Journal of Leukemia. 2014;**2**:e110. DOI: 10.4172/2329-6917.1000e110

[99] Castillo JJ, Mull N, Reagan JL, Nemr S, Mitri J. Increased incidence of non-Hodgkin lymphoma, leukemia, and myeloma in patients with diabetes mellitus type 2: A meta-analysis of observational studies. Blood. 2012;**119**:4845-4850. DOI: 10.1182/blood-2011-06-362830

[100] Ríos-Tamayo R, Lupiañez CB, Campa D, Martino A, Martínez-López J, Martínez-Bueno M, et al. Type 2 diabetes-related variants influence the risk of developing multiple myeloma: Results from the IMMEnSE consortium. Endocrine-Related Cancer. 2015;**22**:545-559. DOI: 10.1530/ERC-15-0029

[101] Wu W, Merriman K, Nabaah A, Seval N, Seval D, Lin H, et al. The association of diabetes and anti-diabetic medications with clinical outcomes in multiple myeloma. British Journal of Cancer. 2014;**111**:628-636. DOI: 10.1038/bjc.2014.307

[102] Ríos-Tamayo R, Lupiañez CB, Campa D, Hielscher T, Weinhold N, Martínez-López J, et al. A common variant within the HNF1B gene is associated with overall survival of multiple myeloma patients: Results from the IMMEnSE consortium and meta-analysis. Oncotarget. 2016;**7**:59029-59048. DOI: 10.18632/oncotarget.10665

[103] Praud D, Rota M, Rehm J, Shield K, Zatonski W, Hashibe M, et al. Cancer incidence and mortality attributable to alcohol consumption. International Journal of Cancer. 2016;**138**:1380-1387. DOI: 10.1002/ijc.29890

[104] Psaltopoulou T, Sergentanis TN, Sergentanis IN, Karadimitris A, Terpos E, Dimopoulos MA. Alcohol intake, alcoholic beverage type and multiple myeloma risk: A meta-analysis of 26 observational studies. Leukemia & Lymphoma. 2015;**56**:1484-1501. DOI: 10.3109/10428194.2014.956312

[105] Rota M, Porta L, Pelucchi C, Negri E, Bagnardi V, Bellocco R, et al. Alcohol drinking and multiple myeloma risk – A systematic review and meta-analysis of the dose–risk relationship. European Journal of Cancer Prevention. 2014;**23**:113-121. DOI: 10.1097/CEJ.0000000000000001

[106] Andreotti G, Birmann B, De Roos AJ, Spinelli J, Cozen W, Camp NJ, et al. A pooled analysis of alcohol consumption and risk of multiple myeloma in the international multiple myeloma consortium. Cancer Epidemiology, Biomarkers & Prevention. 2013;**22**:1620-1627. DOI: 10.1158/1055-9965.EPI-13-0334

[107] Ji J, Sundquist J, Sundquist K. Alcohol consumption has a protective effect against hematological malignancies: A population-based study in Sweden including 420,489 individuals with alcohol use disorders. Neoplasia. 2014;**16**:229-234. DOI: 10.1016/j.neo.2014.03.003

[108] Andreotti G, Birmann B, Cozen W, De Roos AJ, Chiu BCH, Costas L, et al. A pooled analysis of cigarette smoking and risk of multiple myeloma from the international multiple myeloma consortium. Cancer Epidemiology, Biomarkers & Prevention. 2014;**24**:631-634. DOI: 10.1158/1055-9965.EPI-14-1145

[109] Psaltopoulou T, Sergentanis TN, Kanellias N, Kanavidis P, Terpos E, Dimopoulos MA. Tobacco smoking and risk of multiple myeloma: A meta-analysis of 40 observational studies. International Journal of Cancer. 2013;**132**:2413-2431. DOI: 10.1002/ijc.27898

[110] Chen P, Du ZL, Zhang Y, Liu B, Gui Z, Lou JX, et al. Association of VEGF and VDR gene- gene and gene- smoking interaction on risk of multiple myeloma in Chinese Han population. Oncotarget. 2017;**8**:36509-36516. DOI: 10.18632/oncotarget.16510

[111] Wang YZ, Wu QJ, Zhu J, Wu L. Fish consumption and risk of myeloma: A meta-analysis of epidemiological studies. Cancer Cause Control. 2015;**26**:1307-1314. DOI: 10.1007/s10552-015-0625-1

[112] Ugai T, Matsuo K, Sawada N, Iwasaki M, Yamaji T, Shimazu T, et al. Coffee and green tea consumption and subsequent risk of malignant lymphoma and multiple myeloma in Japan: The Japan public health Center-based prospective study. Cancer Epidemiology, Biomarkers & Prevention. 2017;**26**:1352-1356. DOI: 10.1158/1055-9965.EPI-17-0231

[113] Sergentanis TN, Psaltopoulou T, Ntanasis-Stathopoulos I, Liaskas A, Tzanninis IG, Dimopoulos MA. Consumption of fruits, vegetables, and risk of hematological malignancies: A systematic review and meta-analysis of prospective studies. Leukemia Lymphoma. 2018;**59**:434-447. DOI: 10.1080/10428194.2017.1339873

[114] Lwin ST, Olechnowicz SWZ, Fowler JA, Edwards CM. Diet-induced obesity promotes a myeloma-like condition. Leukemia. 2015;**29**:507-510. DOI: 10.1038/leu.2014.295

[115] Mayne ST, Playdon MC, Rock CL. Diet, nutrition, and cancer: Past, present and future. Nature Reviews. Clinical Oncology. 2016;**13**:504-515. DOI: 10.1038/nrclinonc.2016.24

[116] Smith L, McCourt O, Henrich M, Paton B, Yong K, Wardle J, et al. Multiple myeloma and physical activity: A scoping review. BMJ Open. 2015;**5**:e009576. DOI: 10.1136/bmjopen-2015-009576

[117] Moore SC, Lee IM, Weiderpass E, Campbell PT, Sampson JN, Kitahara CM, et al. Association of leisure-time physical activity with risk of 26 types of cancer in 1.44 million adults. JAMA Internal Medicine. 2016;**176**:816-825. DOI: 10.1001/jamainternmed.2016.1548

[118] Patel AV, Hildebrand JS, Campbell PT, Teras LR, Craft LL, McCullough ML, et al. Leisure-time spent sitting and site-specific cancer incidence in a large U.S. cohort. Cancer Epidemiology, Biomarkers & Prevention. 2015;**24**:1350-1359. DOI: 10.1158/1055-9965.EPI-15-0237

[119] Gan JH, Sim CYL, Santorelli LA. The effectiveness of exercise programmes in patients with multiple myeloma: A literature review. Critical Reviews in Oncology/Hematology. 2016;**98**:275-289. DOI: 10.1016/j.critrevonc.2015.11.005

[120] Franceschi S, Lise M, Trépo C, Berthillon P, Chuang SC, Nieters A, et al. Infection with hepatitis B and C viruses and risk of lymphoid malignancies in the European prospective investigation into cancer and nutrition (EPIC). Cancer Epidemiology, Biomarkers & Prevention. 2011;**20**:208-214. DOI: 10.1158/1055-9965.EPI- 10-0889

[121] Abe SK, Inoue M, Sawada N, Iwasaki M, Shimazu T, Yamaji T, et al. Hepatitis B and C virus infection and risk of lymphoid malignancies: A population-based cohort study (JPHC study). Cancer Epidemiology. 2015;**39**:562-566. DOI: 10.1016/j.canep.2015.06.002

[122] Wen J, Tao W, Kuiatse I, Lin P, Feng Y, Jones RJ, et al. Dynamic balance of multiple myeloma clonogenic side population cell percentages controlled by environmental conditions. International Journal of Cancer. 2015;**136**:991-1002. DOI: 10.1002/ijc.29078

[123] Nuyujukian DS, Voutsinas J, Bernstein L, Wang SS. Medication use and multiple myeloma risk in Los Angeles County. Cancer Cause Control. 2014;**25**:1233-1237. DOI: 10.1007/s10552-014-0424-0

[124] Hemminki K, Liu X, Försti A, Ji J, Sundquist J, Sundquist K. Effect of autoimmune diseases on incidence and survival in subsequent multiple myeloma. Journal of Hematology & Oncology. 2012;**5**:59. DOI: 10.1186/1756-8722-5-59

[125] Dalamaga M, Karmaniolas K, Papadavid E, Pelecanos N, Migdalis I. Association of thyroid disease and thyroid autoimmunity with multiple myeloma risk: A case-control study. Leukemia Lymphoma. 2008;**49**:1545-1552. DOI: 10.1080/10428190802165946

[126] Brown LM, Gridley G, Check D, Landgren O. Risk of multiple myeloma and monoclonal gammopathy of undetermined significance among white and black male United States veterans with prior autoimmune, infectious, inflammatory, and allergic disorders. Blood. 2008;**111**:3388-3394. DOI: 10.1182/blood-2007-10-121285

[127] Faller E, Chapman L, Enright H, Browne P, McHugh J, Desmond R. Immune thrombocytopenia purpura associated with multiple myeloma. Annals of Hematology. 2016;**95**:1371-1372. DOI: 10.1007/s00277-016-2694-y

[128] Hsing AW, Hansson LE, McLaughlin JK, Nyren O, Blot WJ, Ekbom A, et al. Pernicious anemia and subsequent cancer. Cancer. 1993;**71**:745-750. DOI: 10.1002/10970142(19930201)71:3<745::AID-CNCR2820710316>3.0.CO;2-1

[129] Lindqvist EK, Landgren O, Lund SH, Turesson I, Hultcrantz M, Goldin L, et al. History of autoimmune disease is associated with impaired survival in multiple myeloma and monoclonal gammopathy of undetermined significance: A population-based study. Annals of Hematology. 2017;**96**:261-269. DOI: 10.1007/s00277-016-2859-8

[130] Dosani T, Mailankody S, Korde N, Manasanch E, Bhutani M, Tageja N, et al. Host-related immunodeficiency in the development of multiple myeloma. Leukemia Lymphoma. DOI: 10.1080/10428194.2017.1361026

[131] Munker R, Shi R, Lin D, Guo S, Hayes TG. Multiple myeloma and other malignancies: A pilot study from the Houston VA. Clinical Lymphoma Myeloma and Leukemia. 2014;**14**:102-106. DOI: 10.1016/j.clml.2013.10.006

[132] Ríos-Tamayo R, Solé F, Gascón F. Simultaneous occurrence of the 5q- syndrome and multiple myeloma. Clinical and Laboratory Haematology. 2000;**22**:49-51. DOI: 10.1046/j.1365-2257.2000.00274.x

[133] Musto P, Anderson KC, Attal M, Richardson PG, Badros A, Hou J, et al. Second primary malignancies in multiple myeloma: An overview and IMWG consensus. Annals of Oncology. 2017;**28**:228-245. DOI: 10.1093/annonc/mdw606

[134] Bladé J, Kyle RA, Greipp PR. Presenting features and prognosis in 72 patients with multiple myeloma who were younger than 40 years. British Journal of Haematology. 1996;**93**:345-351. DOI: 10.1046/j.1365-2141.1996.5191061.x

[135] Dimopoulos MA, Delimpasi S, Katodritou E, Vassou A, Kyrtsonis MC, Repossis P, et al. Significant improvement in the survival of patients with multiple myeloma presenting with severe renalnimpairment after the introduction of novel agents. Annals of Oncology. 2014;**25**:195-200. DOI: 10.1093/annonc/mdt483

[136] Ríos-Tamayo R, González-Silva M, Molina E, García-Fernández JR, Clavero ME, Durán JM, et al. The impact of the type of hospital on survival of multiple myeloma patients: The MICORE study. Revista Clínica Española. 2013;**213**:330-335. DOI: 10.1016/j.rce.2013.02.014

[137] Go RS, Bartley AC, Crowson CS, Shah ND, Habermann EB, Holton SJ, et al. Association between treatment facility volume and mortality of patients with multiple myeloma. Journal of Clinical Oncology. 2017;**35**:598-604. DOI: 10.1200/JCO.2016.68.3805

[138] Ríos-Tamayo R, Sainz J, Jurado M. Comparative baseline health-related quality of life in real-life patients with monoclonal gammopathies. Journal of Leukemia. 2015;**3**:196. DOI: 10.4172/2329-6917.1000196

[139] Drayson MT, Bowcock S, Planche T, Iqbal G, Wood J, Raynes K, et al. Tackling early morbidity and mortality in myeloma (TEAMM): Assessing the benefit of antibiotic prophylaxis and its effect on healthcare associated infections in 977 patients. In: 59th Meeting of The American Hematology Association; 3-6 December 2017;Atlanta. EEUU. Blood. 2017;**130**(Suppl 1). Abstract 903

[140] Mateos MV, Martínez-López J, Rodríguez-Otero P, Ocio EM, González MS, Oriol A, et al. Curative Strategy for High-Risk Smoldering Myeloma (GEM-CESAR): Carfilzomib, Lenalidomide and Dexamethasone (KRd) As Induction Followed By HDT-ASCT, Consolidation with Krd and Maintenance with Rd. In: 59th Meeting of The American Hematology Association; 3-6 December 2017;Atlanta. EEUU : Blood. 2017;**130**(Suppl 1). Abstract 402

[141] Ludwig H, Delforge M, Facon T, Einsele H, Gay F, Moreau P, et al. Prevention and management of adverse events of novel agents in multiple myeloma: A consensus of the European Myeloma Network. Leukemia. 2017. DOI: 10.1038/leu.2017.353

Section 2

Pathogenesis, Genetics and Resistance Mechanisms

Chapter 3

Therapeutic Targets and Signaling Pathways for Diagnosis of Myeloma

Zeeshan Ansar Ahmed, Ashgar Nasir,
Muhammad Shariq Shaikh, Tariq Moatter and
Afshan Asghar Rasheed

Additional information is available at the end of the chapter

http://dx.doi.org/10.5772/intechopen.81751

Abstract

Multiple myeloma (MM) is a malignancy of plasma cells that not only shows different clinical behavior but also depicts heterogeneous groups at molecular level. The prognosis of the disease has been dramatically changed with the arrival of new drugs in the past few years. In this context of better therapeutic agents, there are important challenges for accurate evaluation of patients by better prognostic and predictive tools. Transcriptomic studies have largely added to decipher MM heterogeneity, dividing MM patients into different subgroups according to prognosis. Micro-arrays and more recently RNA sequencing have helped in evaluating coding and non-coding genes, mutations, unique transcriptome convertors and different splicing events giving new information concerning biology, outcome and treatment options. Initial data from gene expression profiling studies have also pointed out genes that predict prognosis, i.e., CSK1-B, and can deliver pharmacogenomics and biologic vision into the pathophysiology, targeted treatment, and future direction. Importantly, we suggest that all prospective studies and clinical trials now accept genetic testing and risk stratification of MM patients. In this review, we discuss the part and effect of gene expression profiling in myeloma.

Keywords: multiple myeloma, monoclonal gammopathy of undetermined significance, smoldering multiple myeloma, gene expression profile

1. Background

In literature, multiple myeloma accounts 1% of all malignancies and almost 10% of all hematologic malignancies [1, 2]. Every year more than 20,000 new patients are diagnosed in the

United States [3]. The age-adjusted annual incidence in the United States has lingered similar for years at almost 4 per 100,000 [4]. Multiple myeloma is marginally more commonly reported in men than in women, and is twofold as common in African-Americans as compared with Caucasians [5]. At time of diagnosis of this disease, the median age is about 65 years [6].

2. Approach for diagnosis

The diagnosis of multiple myeloma requires the presence of one or more myeloma defining events (MDE) in addition to evidence of either 10% or more clonal plasma cells on bone marrow examination or a biopsy-proven plasmacytoma [7–12]. MDE consists of established CRAB (hypercalcemia, renal failure, anemia, or lytic bone lesions) features as well as three specific biomarkers: clonal bone marrow plasma cells ≥60%, serum free light chain (FLC) ratio ≥100 (provided involved FLC level is ≥100 mg/L), and more than one focal lesion on magnetic resonance imaging (MRI). Each of the new biomarkers is associated with an approximately 80% risk of progression to symptomatic end-organ damage in two or more independent studies. The updated criteria represent a paradigm shift since they allow early diagnosis and initiation of therapy before end-organ damage [13–16]. The rate of progression is influenced by the underlying cytogenetic type of disease; patients with t(4;14) translocation, del(17p), and gain(1q) are at a higher risk of progression from SMM to multiple myeloma [17–19].

When multiple myeloma is suspected clinically, patients should be tested for the presence of M proteins using a combination of tests that should include a serum protein electrophoresis (SPEP), serum immunofixation (SIFE), and the serum free light chain (FLC) assay [20]. Approximately 2% of patients with multiple myeloma have true non-secretory disease and have no evidence of an M protein on any of the above studies [6]. Bone marrow studies at the time of initial diagnosis should include fluorescent in situ hybridization (FISH) probes designed to detect t(11;14), t(4;14), t(14;16), t(6;14), t(14;20), trisomies, and del(17p) [21]. Conventional karyotyping to detect hypodiploidy and deletion 13 has value, but if FISH studies are done, additional value in initial risk-stratification is limited. Gene expression profiling (GEP) if available can provide additional prognostic value [22].

3. Molecular classification

Although multiple myeloma is still thought to be a single disease, it is in reality comprises of collection of variable cytogenetically distinct plasma cell malignancies [23–30]. On fluorescent in situ hybridization (FISH) studies of the bone marrow, approximately 40% of multiple myeloma cells have trisomies (trisomic multiple myeloma), while remaining have translocation involving the immunoglobulin heavy chain (IgH) locus present on chromosome 14q32 (IgH translocated multiple myeloma) [31–34]. In small subset of patients both trisomies and IgH translocations are found simultaneously. Trisomies and IgH translocations are primary cytogenetic abnormalities and observed at the time of establishment of MGUS. In addition, secondary cytogenetic abnormalities developed during the disease course of multiple myeloma, including gain(1q), del(1p), del(17p), del [13], RAS mutations, and secondary translocations of MYC. Both primary and secondary cytogenetic abnormalities can influence disease progression, response to treatment, and overall prognosis [30].

4. Prognostication

The median survival of this disease is approximately 6–7 years; especially ASCT (Autologous stem cell transplant) eligible patients 4 year survival rates exceed 80%. However, behavior ofmalignancies is unpredictable, prognosis depends on patient characteristics such as age, co-morbids as well as disease characteristics such as disease stage, biology (cytogenetic abnormalities), and response to therapy [35, 36] Stage, i.e., tumor burden in multiple myeloma, is being evaluated by using the Durie-Salmon Staging (DSS) and the International Staging System (ISS) [37–39]. Disease biology best assessed by molecular abnormalities of multiple myeloma and the presence or absence of secondary cytogenetic abnormalities such as del(17p), gain(1q), or del(1p) [21, 29]. In literature, it is emphasized that the interpretation and impact of cytogenetic abnormalities are different according to the disease phase [30]. The recent staging system, Revised International Staging System (RISS) combines stage and disease biology (presence of high risk cytogenetic abnormalities or elevated lactate dehydrogenase level) to better define not only prognosis but guide treatment options [40].

It is important to note that in order to ensure constant availability, only three widely available cytogenetic markers are used in the RISS. Patients with standard risk multiple myeloma have a median overall survival (OS) of >7 years while those with high risk disease have a median OS of approximately 3 years despite tandem autologous stem cell transplantation (ASCT) [41, 42]. In addition to cytogenetic risk factors, two other markers that are related with rapid disease progression are elevated serum lactate dehydrogenase and plasma leukemic cells in circulation [43].

5. Pathways involved in multiple myeloma

5.1. PI3K/MEK/ERK pathways in myeloma

The phosphatidylinositol 3-kinases (PI3Ks) are a group of intracellular enzymes that phosphorylate the 3-OH group at the inositol ring of phosphatidylinositol leads to activation of PI3K/AKT signaling pathway that is responsible for chemoresistance [44]. PI3K signaling is inhibited by Phosphatase and tensin homolog (PTEN) and activated by insulin like growth factor 1 (IGF-1) and interleukin-6 (IL-6) But there is no FDA approved PI3K inhibitors for MM [44]. Inhibition of this pathway alone is not showing meaningful clinical responses in studies. MEK/ERK pathway is co-functioning with the PI3K/AKT [45]. Both pathways decrease apoptosis [45]. Resistance to treatment develops secondary to cross talk between pathways [45]. Therefore, targeting both pathways together may be an effective therapeutic strategy and has been proved in certain cancers, i.e., in melanoma and renal cell carcinoma [45].

5.2. Ras/MAPK pathway in myeloma

Ras protein family (H, K and N-Ras) send downstream signals that attracts growth-factor-receptor bound protein 2 (Grp2) and sons of Seven less (SOS) [46]. The grp2/SOS combination then converts Ras to active form by changing GTP to GdP [46]. Activated Ras recruits Raf to the cell membrane by phosphorylation [46]. This process is antagonized by GTPase-activating proteins, which promote GTP hydrolysis and the formation of inactive Ras-GDP complexes [46].

Mitogen-activated protein kinases (MAPKs) are a family of expressed kinases that convey cell surface signals into the cell. MAPK pathways are activated via a phosphorylation cascade [47]. The most proximal kinase in these pathways, the MAPK kinase kinase (MAPKKK or MAP3k), engaged by extracellular signals, phosphorylates a dual specificity MAPK kinase (MAPKK or MAP2K), which in turn phosphorylates and actives the distil effector MAPK [47].

The Ras/MAPK pathway consists of the Ras proteins, a family of small G-coupled molecules, the Raf kinases (MAP3K), the MAP2K kinases (MEK1 and MEK2) and ERK1 and ERK2 [47]. The Ras/MAPK network is frequently deregulated in malignancy and causes uncontrolled cellular proliferation and resistance to drug [47]. MEK is present at a junction of the Ras/MAPK pathway [47]. Amplification of Ras/MAPK pathway leads to the aggressive tumor characteristics [45]. In MM, certain translocation points the overall prognosis. The t(4;14) translocation overexpresses fibroblast growth factor receptor 3 overexpression that activates the Ras/MAPK pathway that subsequently leads to decreased apoptosis [45]. Incidence of activating Ras mutations is between 32 and 50% in MM (K-Ras and N-Ras), are also deregulate this pathway [46]. Novel agent RO5126766 showed activity in *RAS*- and *RAF*-mutated malignancies (lung and gynecological cancers) [48]. It also showed partial response in myeloma patient in Maxime Chenard-Poirier study [48].

5.3. Bruton's tyrosine kinase (BTK)

Bruton's tyrosine kinase (BTK) belongs to Tec family of tyrosine kinases [49]. The Tec family comprises of BTK, BMX, ITK, TEC, and RLK. BTK is the most commonly studied member of the Tec family and is present in different stages of B cells [49]. But this protein is absent in T lymphocytes and normal plasma cells [50]. On B cells and myeloma cells BTK controls signal pathways including PI3K, PLCγ, and PKC in multiple myeloma [49]. These pathways play important functions in cell propagation, expansion, delineation and survival [49]. BTK attract MM cells toward stromal cell-derived factor-1 (SDF-1) which is present at high levels in the BM [49]. BTK expression is correlated with SDF-1 receptor CXCR4 in myeloma cells [51]. BTK inhibition leads to the inhibition of anti-apoptotic proteins Bcl-xL, survivin and FLIPL and stimulates caspase-controlled apoptotic death within the myeloma cells [52]. One of the BTK inhibitor, ibrutinib, inhibits MM cell growth, osteoclasts or mesenchymal stem cells growth in vitro [53]. As a single agent, BTK inhibitor CC-292 did not show anti-myeloma activity in vitro but reveals negative impact on osteoclasts function. Interestingly, high levels of BTK have been reported as a poor prognostic marker in MM patients [52]. Therefore, we need targeting agents against this protein (BTK) to not only control microenvironment but also malignant plasma cells [54].

5.4. HSP70

Pathways, like HSP70, ubiquitin-proteasome and unfolded protein response (UPR) and autophagy pathways help neoplastic cells to adjust according to stress that is produced by immunoglobulin overload in the endoplasmic reticulum (ER) [55]. Heat shock protein 70 is one of the pathways that increase survival of myeloma cells by inhibiting gh APAF-1 and caspase 9 [55]. HSP expression is activated by heat and other stressors, i.e., radiation and chemotherapy exposure [56]. HSP70 family comprises of 13 proteins. Proteins of this family are: HSPA1A and HSPA1B (called together as HSP70 or HSP72), HSPA5 (BIP), HSPA8 (HSC70), and HSPA9 [55]. Hsp proteins consist of an N-terminal ATPase domain, a C-terminal domain, and a middle portion. After binding of ATP, Hsp undergoes a conformational change [57]. The middle segment is binding site for protein kinase PKB/Akt and is implicated as the main site for client protein interactions [58].

Recent studies reveal that tumor cells with high levels of HSP70 have beneficial effect of proteasome inhibitors [55]. This protein represents a possible target to establish a new approach for multiple myeloma treatment [55]. HSF1 knockdown sensitizes myeloma cells to bortezomib treatment [55]. Bustany et al. study strongly suggests that HSF1(HSP) inhibitors might be promising agents in combination with bortezomib-based therapeutic protocols to treat MM patients with adverse prognosis or in relapse [59]. Bustany et al. study, strongly suggest that HSF1(HSP) inhibitors might be promising agents in combination with bortezomib-based therapeutic protocols to treat MM patients with adverse prognosis or in relapse [60].

5.5. MicroRNAs (miRNAs)

MicroRNAs (miRNAs) are a group of 18–24 nucleotides, non-coding RNA molecules. Mature one attaches to 3′′UTR non translated site and control gene expression by translation modification or mRNA degradation [61]. They have substantial impact on post-transcriptional negative regulation of oncogenes (e.g. MYC, MDM2) and tumor suppressor genes (e.g. TP53, PTEN) [62]. miR-145 is tumor suppressor miRNA in MM, miR-145 mimics inhibited p-AKT and p-PI3K, impairing proliferation and survival of MM cells [63]. Until now, around 700 miRNAs have been revealed in humans. Each miRNA can target at least 200 genes [64]. Anderson et al. identified a MM-specific miRNAs print that is evident by degradation of miRNAs -15a/-16 and over expression of miRNAs -222/-221/-382/-181a/-181b [64]. They also reported that these miRNAs control proliferation and growth of MM cells by inhibiting AKT serine/threonine protein-kinase (AKT3), ribosomal-protein-S6, MAP-kinases, and NF-_B-activator MAP3KIP3. Furthermore these miRNAs exerted their activity even on bone marrow microenvironment [64]. One of the poor prognostic cytogenetics in myeloma is deletion of chromosome 13 that has been associated with overexpression, of miRNA-17_92 cluster (located on chromosome 13) in these patients [80]. In another study, miRNA-15 and -16, were down-regulated in MM patients having ch13 deletion [63].

The miRNA analysis showed contrary relationship between five assumed target genes (RAD54L, CCNA2, CYSLTR2, RASGRF2 and HKDC1) [61]. Anti-MM effects are also linked with miR-137 and miR-197. Studies showed that miR-34 and miR-125a inhibitors upregulates p53 related miR-192 and -194 and inhibits oncogenesis and migration while enhance apoptosis [63]. miR-202 is down-regulated in bone marrow microenvironment and treatment with miR-202 mimics to inhibit growth by decreasing BCL-2 and BAFF levels [63].

5.6. Histone

Histone acetyl transferase (HAT) and histone deacetylase (HDAC) are enzymes that regulate expression of genes by moving acetyl from acetyl-CoA to the lysine residue of histones [65]. Subsequently, hyper acetylated histones aggravate transcription [65]. HDACs are enzymes that catalyze the removal of acetyl groups from amino lysines in histones, resulting in relaxation of the DNA around the histones and suppression of transcription [66]. HDACs are divided into five groups: class I (HDAC1, HDAC2, HDAC3, and HDAC8), class IIa (HDAC4, HDAC5, HDAC7, and HDAC9), class IIb (HDAC6 and HDAC10), class III (SIRT family), and class IV (HDAC11) [66]. Inhibiting HDAC converts histones in hyperacetylation form and leads to alter gene expression [67]. In malignant cells, many HDAC inhibitors (HDACi) have shown good anti-tumor activities with anti-proliferative, pro-apoptotic and anti-angiogenic properties [67]. SAHA (suberoylanilide hydroxamic acid) is one of the HDACi, showed antimyeloma activity by inhibiting proteasome and expression of its subunits, and increases myeloma cell sensitivity to Bortezomib [68]. Extrinsic and intrinsic apoptotic pathways, non-apoptotic cell death, i.e., autophagy pathways and cytokines and proteins implicated in multiple myeloma survival, progression and immune escape have been documented in myeloma cells treated with an HDACi [67]. The cellular pathways controlled by SAHA include IGFIGF-1RAkt, IL-6gp130 and proliferative/antiapoptotic factors (e.g., NF-B, XBP-1, and E2F-1) [68].

Myeloma cells have overexpression of antiapoptotic proteins Bcl2 and Mcl1 and down regulation of pro-apoptotic protein Bax [67]. These findings depict resistance to chemotherapeutic agents [67]. Treatment with depsipeptide in myeloma cell line resulted in a decrease of the anti-apoptotic proteins Mcl1, Bcl2, BclxL and an increase in Bax [67]. 5-azacitidine is a DNA methyltransferase inhibitor shows activity against myeloma [67]. Azacitidine and analogs such decitabine are interesting agents to investigate hypermethylation in tumorigenesis and the clinical efficacy is under investigation in phase II trials [67]. In S. B. Khan s study, depsipeptide (HDACi) induces apoptosis in MM cells and shows an additive effect with melphalan [65].

5.7. Microenvironment

Microenvironment is defined as surrounding cells and tissues can impact the growth of specific cells by changing the pH, oxygen levels, nutrients, and antiapoptotic factors [69]. when this microenvironment is dysfunctional leads to disease progression, particularly in cancer. Like in other parts of body, the bone marrow has own microenvironment [69]. That is classically defined as to have two niches: the endosteal (osteoblastic) niche and the vascular (sinusoidal) architecture [69]. The osteoblastic niche comprises of reticular cells, fibroblasts, and adipocytes [70]. They provide supportive matrix for stem cells [70]. The vascular niche has important functions in bone marrow: transfer oxygen, nutrients and growth factors to hematopoietic cells for proliferation and differentiation of cells; support of homing and recruitment through chemokines [70].

The BM milieu of MM consists of extracellular matrix, hematopoietic and nonhematopoietic cells along with cytokines, growth factors, and adhesion molecules [70]. The increased osteoclastic activity is secondary to increase cytokines, i.e., IL-6, IL-1b, tumor necrosis factor (TNF)-α, and parathyroid hormone-related protein [70]. Other causes of osteoclast activation are: Myeloma cells express RANKL, TNF-α, and inactivation of RANKL decoy receptor and OPG. The destroyed bone environment stimulates platelets to release TGF-β and IGF-I that will cause myeloma genesis [70]. Not only osteoclast is activated, osteoblasts are also inhibited in myeloma. Factors responsible for inhibiting osteoblast are TGF-β and IL-3 [70]. Extracellular matrix of the myeloma show increased expression of angiogenic factors and their receptors, i.e., vascular endothelial growth factor (VEGF) and VEGF receptor-2, fibroblast growth factor-2 (FGF-2) and FGF-2 receptor-2, platelet-derived growth factor receptor beta (PDGFR-β) and ECs-released VEGF and IL-8 [70]. In the bone microenvironment, myeloma cell are surrounded by immune competent cells [68]. Because of certain growth factors rapid expansion of immature myeloid cells which fail to differentiate and, impede immune system and leads to oncogenesis [68]. Specific CD8+ T cells has been recognized in microenvironment, inhibiting CD4 + −cell growth by releasing interferon gamma causing immunosuppression [68]. The T-cell activity is also suppressed by the activation of PD-1 receptor with its ligand [69].

The PI3K-Akt signaling has been demonstrated to phosphorylate HKII Hexokinase II to activate Glycolytic pathway in MM cells [69].

A number of intracellular signaling pathways, i.e., NF-κB, Akt, p38MAPK, protein p62, Pim-2 are over-in both MM cells and their BM microenvironment [69]. Pim kinases are also involved in drug resistance by activating drug efflux transporters [69]. Pim-1 phosphorylates the ATP-binding cassette (ABC) transporter ABCG2 that subsequently causes drug resistance [69]. The side population (SP) phenotype is a feature of stem cells in tissues. The SP cells are associated with the expression of genes involved in the glycolytic pathway including GLUT1, GLUT3, and PDK1 and the glycolysis appears to be highly accelerated in SP cells [69]. The inhibition of glycolysis via targeting these SP cells can disrupt the drug resistance [69].

Immune microenvironment consists of T Cells, NK and NKT Cells, dendritic cells, myeloid derived suppressor cells and adipocytes [70]. Reciprocal increase in IL-17, IL-17 induces myeloma tumor cell growth and inhibits immune function in myeloma patients [70]. Impaired differentiation and function of NK and NKT cells have been recognized in MM. A major contributing factor to this immune dysfunction is believed to be IL-6 mediated [70]. Myeloid-derived suppressor cells (MDSCs) expands during cancer, inflammation and infection and have ability to suppress T-cell responses (**Table 1**) [71]. Recently, it has been proposed that a 5-fold increase in MDSCs in newly diagnosed MM [70] **Tables 1–3**.

5.8. Marrow-infiltrating lymphocytes

Lymphocytes residing in the bone marrow are called marrow infiltrating lymphocytes [72]. These MILs need to be activated and expanded in vitro to destroy malignant cells. Difference between peripherally derived T lymphocytes and marrow derived lymphocytes is: MILs have a ability to recognize a wide variety of proteins on the surface of the tumor cells than do cells

Growth factors/cytokines	Possible mechanism of actions
PTH, VIT D3, IL-1, IL-11	Activates osteoblast and stromal cells
PD-1 on T cells	PD-L1 on myeloma cells
VEGF, IL-6 on stromal cells	Raf/MEK/ERK activation on myeloma cells
VEGF, TGF-β, FGF from stromal cells	Angiogenesis
G-CSF and IL-6 induced a higher level of phospho-STAT3 in neutrophils	Angiogenesis
IL-10	Plasma cell proliferation and angiogenesis
Wnt, Dickkopf Wnt signaling pathway 1 (DKK1), fibroblast growth factor (FGF)	Decreased increased osteoblast number Decreased bone mineral density
Downregulating expression of the RANK-L decoy receptor (OPG) Elevated levels of IL-6 induce RANK-L expression and decrease INFγ production	Osteoclastogenesis Bone resorption

Abbreviations: PTH, parathyroid hormone; VIT D3, Vitamin D3; IL-1, IL-11:Interleukin1/11; VEGF, vascular endothelial growth factor receptor; TGF-β, transforming growth factor beta; FGF, fibroblast growth factor; G-CSF, granulocyte colony stimulating factor; RANK-L, receptor activator of nuclear factor kappa beta.Source: Mondello et al. [71].

Table 1. Bone marrow micro-environment.

Pathways	Consequences of activation of pathways
Raf/MEK/P42/44 MAPK*	Proliferation
β-catenin*	Proliferation
PI-3 K/Akt**	Proliferation Anti-apoptosis Drug resistance
JAK/STAT3*	Proliferation Anti-apoptosis Drug resistance
NF-κB*	Proliferation Anti-apoptosis Drug resistance
Notch-1*	Anti-apoptosis Drug resistance
MEK/ERK/P27**	Proliferation Anti-apoptosis Drug resistance (Cytokine mediated)

*van de Donk et al. [80].
**Kizaki and Tabayashi [81].

Table 2. Intracellular signaling pathways in the pathogenesis of multiple myeloma.

that obtained from the blood [73]. So on relapse after receiving CAR T cells therapy, new type of antigen or protein are developed on tumor cell surface (similar to the antibiotic resistance) [73]. While MILs can identify a huge variety of proteins on tumor cells, problem of resistance is significantly lower [73].

Protein BMI-1	substance PTC-209	Preclinical studies
Inhibitor of microRNA genes	EZH2 inhibitor	Preclinical studies
Irreversibly inhibition of 20S proteasome, pan-proteasome inhibitor	Marizomib	Phase 1 clinical trials, relapsed/refractory. Trials ongoing for CNS involvement in myeloma
Oral 26S proteasome inhibitor	Oprozomib	Phase 1 studies relapsed/refractory
Anti-CD138 monoclonal antibody conjugated to DM4, inhibitor of the microtubule assembly	Indatuximab	Phase 1/2 clinical trials, relapsed/refractory
Monoclonal antibody to CD38	SAR (SAR650984)	Phase 1 clinical trials, relapsed/refractory
Histone deacetylase (HDAC) 6 inhibitor	Panobinostat	Phase 3 clinical trials
HDAC6-specific histone deacetylase inhibitor	Ricolinostat	Preclinical studies
Non-specific histone deacetylase inhibitor	Vorinostat	Phase 3 clinical trials
Alkylating agent	Bendamustine	Phase 1/2 trial PR rate of 52%, with very good PR achieved in 24%
AKT kinase inhibitor	Afuresertib (PKB115125)	Phase 1 studies ORR—50% in relapsed/refractory
Bcl-2 inhibitors	ABT 199	Preclinical studies
BTK inhibitors	Ibrutinib	Phase 2 dose escalation study, relapsed or refractory
Inhibitor of cyclin-dependent kinases (CDKs)	Dinaciclib	Phase 2 dose escalation study
IL-6 inhibitors	Siltuximab	Phase 2, newly diagnosed MM, VGPR rate was significantly improved but not CR rate
Kinesin spindle protein (KSP)	Filanesib (ARRY-520)	Phase 2 clinical trials, ORR was 58%, relapsed/refractory
Phosphoinositide 3-kinase (PI3K)	Idelalisib BAY80-6946 GDC-0941	Relapsed/refractory, preclinical investigation
Heat-shock protein 90 inhibitor	Tanespimycin	Phase 1 dose-escalation study

Source: Refs. [139, 140].

Table 3. Potential Target for Multiple Myeloma.

Adoptive T-cell therapy (ACT) has been assessed in trials, in which activated tumor-specific T cells has been used to activate antitumor immunity after myeloablative chemotherapy in patients with multiple myeloma (MM) [73]. But efficacy of this approach is limited by the tumor-non specific T cells [73]. In phase I study, Noonan and colleagues assess the safety, and efficacy of this approach in 25 patients in multiple myeloma patients [74]. MILs infused after autologous stem cell transplant in 22 patients and found complete remission/partial response/stable disease in six/seven/five patients [74]. Progression-free survival was correlated with greater than 90% reduction in tumor burden (25.1 vs. 11.8 months) [74]. Borrello and colleagues also showed that marrow-infiltrating T lymphocytes (MILs) can led to clinical antitumor immunity [73]. Results from small studies are encouraging but need confirmation in a larger trials [73].

5.9. PD-1/PD-L1

The PD-1 receptor is present on T, B cells, monocytes, and natural killer (NK) T cells when activated to certain antigen stimulus [75]. PD-L1 and PD-L2 are present on antigen presenting cells, i.e., dendritic cells and macrophages [75]. After contact of PD-1 to PD-L1 or PD-L2, this complex reduces secretion of Th1 cytokines, inhibits T-cell proliferation and inhibits CTL-mediated killing [75]. In the physiologic state, this pathway maintains immunologic equilibrium. While, in pathologic settings, e.g., in malignancy, over expression of this pathway leads to to activation and function of cancer related T-cell populations, which supports for immune escape and tumor proliferation [75]. PD-L1 expression is also documented in cells of the tumor microenvironment, i.e., myeloid-derived suppressor cells that helps in escape to natural body defense system [75]. To improve already decrease immunity in myeloma patients, strategies have been explored at molecular and cellular levels [76]. These are: passive immunotherapy with monoclonal antibodies that hit myeloma specific antigens; cancer vaccines; T-cell therapy and change immunosuppressive microenvironment of the bone marrow via immunomodulatory medicines or by inhibiting immune checkpoints [76]. There are studies under process for PD-1 receptor/PD-L1 and PD-L2 inhibitors in myeloma, i.e., Pembrolizumab in combination with IMiDs [77]. Preliminary results of a phase II trial with pembrolizumab with pomalidomide showed 50% objective response with near complete and very good partial responses in refractory patients [77].

5.10. Monoclonal antibodies

In 2015, two monoclonal antibodies were approved for the treatment of relapsed or refractory multiple myeloma (RRMM), elotuzumab and daratumumab [78]. CD38 is a type II cell membrane glycoprotein. It has multiple functions in cell to cell adhesion, enzymatic (cellular nucleic acid metabolism) activity [77]. It is present on a multiple hematopoietic and non-hematopoietic cell types. Cell that harbors this receptor are: medullary thymocytes, activated B and T lymphocytes, NK cells and dendritic cells [77].

Daratumumab is a fully humanized monoclonal IgG-κ antibody directed that works against CD38 of myeloma cells [77]. It exerts its effects like other monoclonal antibodies, i.e., antibody dependent cytotoxicity, complement mediated cytotoxicity and antibody dependent phagocytosis (ADCP), induction of autophagy/apoptosis [77].

Antibodies targeting CD38 are easily tolerated and showed partial response or better in approximately 30% of relapsed/refractory MM patients as single agent [79]. In future, deep responses and better progression-free survival can be obtained by combining them with immunomodulatory agent or proteasome inhibitors [79].

In phase I/II study recently published by Lokhorst et al., impressive clinical responses were seen in heavily pretreated patient population with 64% double refractory to PIs and IMiDs and had undergone ASCT in 76% [77]. Daratumumab as a single agent yielded 36% overall response rate in 16 mg/kg arm and remarkably, in the responder group, 65% remained progression free in 12 months [77].

Elotuzumab is a monoclonal IgG-κ antibody works against signaling lymphocytic activation molecule F7 (l surface receptor helps in activation of natural killer cell) [78]. This antibody induces cell death via antibody dependent cytotoxicity (ADCC) and inhibits CS1-mediated MM cell adhesion to bone marrow stem cells [79].

In phase III ELOQUENT-2 study, different regimens with this agent were tried in relapsed/refractory setting. It was found that 1-year PFS rate was higher in the ELO-LEN-DEX (-Elotuzumab-Lenalidomide-Dexamethasone) arm (68 vs. 57%), and this difference was slightly greater at 2 years (41 vs. 27%). Other targeted antigens on which trials are being conducted are: CD74, CD138, B-cell activating factor, interleukin-6 [79].

5.11. CART cells

CART cells, is made by fusing the variable fragment (scFv) of a monoclonal antibody (mAb) with intracellular signaling domain related to CD-19 related antigen [77]. The MHC-independency, in vivo expansion and memory cell growth make these cells more beneficial the antibodies [77]. Plasma cells do not have a strong CD-19 expression but Garfall et al. have observed a relatively more frequent expression than previously reported [77]. In 43 years old patients after nine lines of treatment this approach showed remission. This generates a hypothesis that there may be a role of this strategy even in minimally/weakly expressed antigens Currently, it remains unclear whether concurrent targeting of multiple antigens (such as CD38, CS1, BCMA, CD138, etc.) is helpful for achieving eradication of myeloma clone [77]. For CART cells, costimulatory molecules are required to prevent the immune system from eradication of these cells, but best costimulatory antigen is not known yet. Few costimulators are under study, these are: CD19, CD138, CD38, CD56, Lewis Y, CD44v6, CS1, and BCMA.

In new data from a Garfall pilot study, after anti-CD19 CAR and a salvage SCT, progression-free survival (PFS) was reported after first-line SCT in 3 of 10 study participants. In 2017, studies with chimeric antigen receptor (CAR)-T cells targeting B-cell maturation antigen (BCMA) have shown good response in relapsed/refractory myeloma patients. But this option is impeded by short half lived effector cells, acute toxicity, and host immune responses against CARs.

6. Pathways involved in multiple myeloma

6.1. Gene expression profile (GEP) and molecular variability in myeloma

The MM transcriptome has been evaluated in different groups [81–84]. Different genes have been explored between MM and normal plasma cells and also during different phases of disease. Impaired control of certain genes of the Cyclin D family (CCND1, CCND2 and CCND3) appeared to be a universal characteristic of MM cells, especially early MGUS (monoclonal gammopathy of undetermined significance) stage [43]. The mechanisms elaborate in Cyclin D mutation are multiple and comprised of 1—cyclin D amplifications, 2—translocation of CCND1 or CCND3 with the IgH gene in the t(11;14) and the t(6;14), 3—trisomies and other cytogenetics events that incidentally contribute to over-expression of CCND genes. In particular, CCND2 is overexpressed in certain group of patients that carry t(4;14) and t(14;16) MM [81, 82]. These observations allowed classification of MM in eight subgroups in the translocation cyclin D (TC) classification [43]. Additional studies have observed other molecular subgroups independent of Cyclin D involvement and linked with other clinical and phenotypical characteristics. For example, a Low-Bone subgroup, that includes MM patients with minimal or few bony lesions and minimal expression of Dickkopf WNT Signaling Pathway Inhibitor 1 (DKK1) or the proliferative subgroup which shows over expression of specific cell cycle- and proliferation-associated genes [83]. Overall, GEP emphasis an important molecular heterogeneity in this disease. Over 500 genes have a substantial difference between the different clinical subgroups [43]. Cytogenetic changes, mainly hyperdiploidy and translocations involving IgH are highly connected with certain molecular subcategories clusters. For example, t(4;14) which primes to the over-expression of the histone methyl transferase Multiple Myeloma SET Domain (MMSET) is linked with a specific gene expression profile secondary to MMSET activity [85]. More globally, HDMM and NHDMM can be observed by using GEP [86].

6.2. Definition of myeloma pathogenesis by using GEP

In order to explore the molecular basis of myeloma cell development, several studies have observed GEP at the different stages of the disease [87]. In these studies, normal plasma cell was compared with cells during different stages of MM i.e. MGUS cell, Myeloma, smoldering MM, newly-diagnosed symptomatic MM, relapsed MM and cells from patients with plasma cell leukemia (PCL) by using GEP [87]. In one study of 877 patients, authors concluded that MGUS plasma cells share similar features with MM and relapse MM but have different genes and pathways that are expressed lately during MM progression [87]. These activated pathways comprises of E2F activation, cMYC and chromosomal instability genes and these demonstrates a possibility of progression to MM if exist at MGUS or SMM stage [88]. Other groups have examined other different genes, i.e., antiapoptotic DNA repair, NF-kB and cytokines-signaling pathway related genes in established MM cells in comparison with premalignant MGUS cells [88]. Interestingly, influence of microenvironment on gene profile of the MM cells has been assessed that confirmed activation of crucial critical pathways such as Notch and Ras, NF-kB, and genes affecting proliferation, survival, cell cycle regulators/activation in MM cells [89].

6.3. Link of prognosis with GEP

Ability to explore complete transcriptomic expression profile of MM cell provided an unique opportunity to confirm predictive role of GEP on disease behavior. Clinical trials and long term follow-up of MM patients revealed the ability of GEP to predict prognosis in different cohorts. Many studies have identified gene expression signatures capable of predicting EFS and OS in MM by using different approaches. Most of these studies have shown GEP profile as an independent prognostic factor. Some studies have used a biological approach with respect to specific features of MM cells. Chromosome instability signature [90], centrosome index signature, and cell death profile [91] were explained based on instability of genomes, whereas a 7-gene prognostic expression profile was developed from MM cell lines study [92, 93]. Other prognostic signatures like the 15-gene prognostic signature or the proliferation signature have also been published in literature [94]. Other groups evaluated GEP signature correlation between GEP with overall survival of MM patients in separate cohorts. The HOVON-65/GMMG-HD4 clinical trial researchers [94], the Intergroup Francophone du Myeloma 99 clinical trial [84], and UAMS researchers [95] published reports on 92, 15 and 70 genes signature respectively [95]. Importantly, only minimal or no genes overlay between these signatures signifying that each signature does not encompass all high risk patients and also highpoints the dismissal in the system. In an attempt to streamline GEP use in clinical practice and to define a distinctive tool, amalgamation of existing prognostic signatures have been recently reported. That combination will define a single reliable signature that might be able to predict outcome in MM at diagnosis and relapse [96].

Interestingly, GEP signature has also shown significance in early stages of MM or in plasma cell leukemia patients. Investigators from UAMS have reported that 70-genes signature and its derivative are able to predict outcome in context of MGUS and SMM [97]. In the context of PCL, in a cohort of 21 patients, a 27 gene expression signature was identified as an independent prognostic factor [24].

6.4. Transcriptome modifiers profiling

The RNA-sequencing have been created and will be incorporated into GEP to enhance estimation of the outcome in the future [98]. Of these modifiers, non-coding RNA are mainly researched in MM since reports have already proved that micro-RNA contribute to myeloma formation and can be used to predict prognosis or response to auto-transplant [98]. MiR17 and miR886-5p have been observed as a strong prognostic indicator in a study of 163 newly diagnosed patients from the MRC Myeloma IX l trial [99]. Recent literature is now signifying importance of microRNAs MM and separate MM subgroups [100]. For example, miR-126 stimulates cMYC overexpression in t(4;14) MM [101], and miRs-192, -194, and -215 leads to impaired control of p53 and MDM2 in a subgroup of MM, causing poorer outcome [102, 103]. Very interestingly, overexpression of circulating microRNAs, which are easily access for investigations has been researched and may represent a decent prognostic biomarkers in MM [104]. Furthermore, management options that can reestablish miRNAs (Tumor suppressor miRNA) or impede miRNAs (Oncogene miRNA) are in process to be used as major therapeutic option in the future [105, 106]. Long noncoding RNAs (lnc RNA) are also being sensibly studied inMM. Samur et al. with others is currently identifying important changes in deregulation of lncRNAs over- or underexpression and its impact on clinical outcome [108].

In post-transcriptional event, alternate splicing is an important event that extremely increases the transcript collection affecting number of cell development process including cell growth and survival. It has been documented as important marker of malignant phenotype and the knowing the alternate splicing events will help in future to better predict prognosis in MM.

There is evidence that splicing events affect specific genes as hyaluronan synthase 1 (HAS1) [109] or deleted in colorectal carcinoma gene (DCC) occur repeatedly in MM [110], or that a targeted therapy that control the splicing of X-box binding protein 1 (XBP1) increases sensitivity of MM cells to proteasome inhibitor. Pilot investigations by Nagoshi et al. as well as and by some other researchers have identified important number of spliced isoforms in myeloma in comparison to normal plasma cells with regards to both functional concern as well as prognostic importance. Interestingly, the ability to depict mutations at the RNA level is becoming well recognized entity. DNA-based studies in MM, including mainly whole exome sequencing, have emphasized the mutational background of the disease, which includes few repeated mutations (NRAS, KRAS, TP53, DIS3, and FAM46C). NFkB and ERK trails are the most involved pathways, with mutations in 43 and 17% of MM cases respectively [111–114]. Although only specific mutations have a clear impact on prognosis (TP53, ATR, and ATM) until now. The capability to diagnose these mutations at the RNA level [114] can now be used to predict outcome that can be integrated in the future models expecting prognosis in MM. Finally, next generation sequencing helps us to perform single cell studies. This method, exemplified by the drop-seq technology [115], allows documentation of the variable clones as well as identification of the transcriptome in the reference of the microenvironment. The initial data regarding single cell transcriptome assessment depicts exciting applications [116] including amalgamation into a new GEP signature [117].

6.5. GEP and variability in clones

Intraclonal variability is an important characteristic of cancer that has been shown in MM [118, 119]. It refers to malignant cells having same genomic changes but with subtle differences in mutations, copy number abnormalities and chromosome changes including translocations among different clones. In MM cells, the evaluation of Ig gene rearrangement by next-generation sequencing is particularly helpful. Munshi NC et al. did deep sequencing of the IgH gene at time of diagnosis and relapse in a large series of patients emphasizing the complexity of the clonal and sub-clonal architecture of the disease [120]. However, only few reports have been published the evolution of in MM. Four patterns of this clonal changes have been observed [112, 121]. The modification in sub clonal copiousness will be correlated with changes in GEP. For example a linear development may not meaningfully influence on overall GEP, on the other hand branching evolution may reveal decrease in expression of genes representing clones The ability to assess transcriptome at a single cell level might be essential in order to define the true influence of intraclonal heterogeneity on GEP and to recognize potential marker of sensitivity or resistance to specific therapeutic drugs [116, 122].

6.6. Significance of GEP in combination with ISS

A recent study reported GEP in combination with clinical prognostic marker in MM comprising cytogenetic alterations and ISS score. This study used different GEP signature and revealed that the combination of GEP with ISS is a useful and better prognostic tool that significantly improves risk stratification then alone ISS [123]. Recognizing high risk patients remains an important task to try and modify treatment in future discussed by Landgren and Rajkumar in this CCR Focus section [124]. Currently, no specific targeted agent therapy is indicated especially for the high-risk patients in upfront setting, there is increasing emphasis on including multi-agent therapy as consolidation followed by transplant and post-transplant maintenance in transplant eligible patients. High dose melphalan followed by autologous stem cell transplant (ASCT) appears to be the best consolidation therapy to date in multiple studies [125].

6.7. Response to treatment prediction by using GEP

GEP has also been assessed to forecast complete response (CR) to different treatment as well. CR is an independent factor to not only tell progression free survival but also an indirect marker of overall survival [126]. A precise GEP signature has been identified with reference to upfront three drug combinations (VTD) in newly diagnosed MM, high dose therapy (54 IMiDs/dexamethasone, tandem auto-transplant at relapse and the bortezomib-based regimen [129]. However, a prediction model research that compared different dataset has shown that GEP alone is not well-organized to predict CR in different datasets [127–130].

In this study, various methods have been used to develop a response predictive model; even with the best GEP-based CR predictive model, precision was between 56 and 78% that was found in different datasets. The ability to predict CR was not affected by different methods used measure GEP, or treatment regimens used or in newly-diagnosed or at time of relapsed patients. This study signifies the fact that it may be necessary to combine multiple other genomic parameters in response predicting model in future.

6.8. Personalized therapy assortment

Based on GEP, the derangements in certain pathways can be controlled and offer an important information to guide treatment therapy. For example, the presence of high DKK1 level, that shows bone involvement can be explored for the use of anti-DKK1 drug [131, 132] or the assessment of the ratio between BCL2/MCL1 level can point out the sensitivity to BH3 mimetic drugs [133]. On the other side, combining the information of gene expression with mutation expression helps to select treatment options as personalized medicine [134]. The detection of precise mutations such as BRAF V600E can direct for use of BRAF inhibitor such as vemurafenib [135, 136], or mutations triggering the MAPK pathway can give us rationale for the use of MEK inhibitors such as trametinib [137]. Other targetable mutations such as SF3B1, FGFR3, ATM/ATR, IDH1/2, and CCND1 as well as RAS/RAF, NFkB pathway-linked genes have been described in myeloma. These mutations can be controlled by appropriate inhibitors.

Some mutations can also be assessed to predict drug sensitivity. Initial data of one study, revealed that the presence of NRAS mutations in relapsed cases is associated with inferior response to bortezomib [138] or in contrast, that the occurrence of IRF4 mutations is related with higher sensitivity to immuno-modulatory agents [111]. These data needs confirmation in further clinical trials but it is hypothesis generating study.

The documentation of specific micro-RNA expression profile can also be exploited to guide therapy. Several microRNAs are being researched as treatment targets with hopes for development of small molecules that target these micro-RNA function.

Similarly, GEP has been employed to predict resistance to antimyeloma drugs with an interpretation that harmful agents are avoided that are not helpful. With the help of number of B-cell lines including multiple myeloma cell lines, a microarray-based GEP signature was established to predict resistance of melphalan. Although the expression profile was able to predict sensitivity vs. resistance in cell lines, its practical application needs further studies to be done [102, 103]. Interestingly, a pharmacogenomic study of global GEP of myeloma cells recovered from myeloma patients and specific time after administration of different drugs have been assessed [104, 105]. Prognostic information was acquired from GEP of refined plasma cells 2 days after providing thalidomide and dexamethasone or bortezomib to newly-diagnosed myeloma patients. An 80-gene signature was recognized following bortezomib administration that will guide us in future for better patients' risk stratification [105].

From treatment as well as prognostic points, it is also important to consider persistent changes in genome which occurs without stimulus or as well as under the influence of microenvironment, epigenomic changes or therapy. Therefore, assessment by GEP at a single time point may not be meaningful. The advancement of GEP from diagnosis, response and relapse should be interpreted intelligently to have an answer for proper selection of the most appropriate therapy.

7. Potential target for multiple myeloma

7.1. Constraint of GEP in existing clinical practice

Important impediments still present to prevent application of this important investigation in general clinical practice. Although many specific GEP signatures have been recognized and a recent study has joint some of these signatures to create a unique signature [32] but no consensus have been accepted to date for universal use for every MM patients. GEP remains a research tool and is not yet authenticated by the FDA. For clinician point of view, the GEP data have been created generally in a setting of certain treatments that includes thalidomide, lenalidomide and bortezomib with or without auto-transplant. Since the therapeutic landscape is largely progressing in MM, re-assessments are required for each novel drug and/or combination. In particular the arrival of new therapeutic classes such as antibody drug conjugates, targeted agents (Elotuzumab, Daratumumab) and new IMiDs and proteasome inhibitors [106, 107] markedly improve the prognosis and may need different GEP studies and signatures [107, 114]. GEP has been utilized to date in few myeloma centers and mostly for investigational purposes. The development of investigators friendly and quicker methods should be considered. Simple quantitative PCR has been assessed in a group of 157 newly diagnosed patients proved good acceptable results [115]. However, a final conclusion about this test is still pending. Most importantly an integrated approach that includes gene signatures, mutational profile and microRNA expression will be requisite to allow a wider application of genomic information to direct for treatment selection as well as prognostication. Taking the current understanding of these landscape genetic assessment to the next level, it will be essential to understand the clinical influence of clonal content and advancement along with identification of sub-clonal variants and molecular alterations on disease outcome [141]. The current information about mutational load that predicts outcome will need to be re-investigated for treatment purpose. These algorithms will be amended with the arrival of immunotherapeutic strategies which may have great achievement in malignancies with high mutational load. Again, as demonstrated by Rashid NU et al. with other colleagues Mutations must be studies further as predictive markers for treatment decisions [97].

8. Future trend

There is tremendous progress has reported so far, newer high-throughput technologies are being added with clinical parameters [142]. Array-based methodologies, sequencing-based method, and newer bio-informatics methodologies are in process of development. Furthermore, integrative oncogenomic work are merging new markers such as mutations, splicing events, noncoding RNA, miRs with older ones to help in better prognostication [143]. The personalized medicine depends on the assortment of a targeted therapy guided by the specific mutation or GEP signature is attractive tool treatment option. However, in future, in MM patients, treatment option selection depends on coexistence of sub-clones, dynamic evolution of the disease and triggering mutations in pathway, i.e., KRAS and BRAF for the ERK pathways [144].

To conclude, gene expression profile studies provide important knowledge regarding MM pathogenesis, and establish a powerful tool for prediction of outcome and to direct clinicians for selection of therapy [145]. The grouping of mutational profile, gene expression and splicing events with ISS and cytogenetic may become a standard of care in MM care [97].

Author details

Zeeshan Ansar Ahmed[1]*, Ashgar Nasir[1], Muhammad Shariq Shaikh[1], Tariq Moatter[1] and Afshan Asghar Rasheed[2]

*Address all correspondence to: zeeshan.ansar@aku.edu

1 Aga Khan University, Karachi, Pakistan

2 Sindh Institute of Urology and Transplantation, Karachi, Pakistan

References

[1] Rajkumar SV, Dimopoulos MA, Palumbo A, et al. International myeloma working group updated criteria for the diagnosis of multiple myeloma. The Lancet Oncology. 2014;**15**: e538-e548

[2] Rajkumar SV. Multiple myeloma: 2014 update on diagnosis, risk-stratification, and management. American Journal of Hematology. 2014;**89**:998-1009

[3] Siegel RL, Miller KD, Jemal A. Cancer statistics, 2016. CA: A Cancer Journal for Clinicians. 2016;**66**:7-30

[4] Kyle RA, Therneau TM, Rajkumar SV, Larson DR, Plevak MF, Melton LJ 3rd. Incidence of multiple myeloma in Olmsted County, Minnesota: Trend over 6 decades. Cancer. 2004; **101**:2667-2674

[5] Landgren O, Weiss BM. Patterns of monoclonal gammopathy of undetermined significance and multiple myeloma in various ethnic/racial groups: Support for genetic factors in pathogenesis. Leukemia. 2009;**23**:1691-1697

[6] Kyle RA, Gertz MA, Witzig TE, et al. Review of 1,027 patients with newly diagnosed multiple myeloma. Mayo Clinic Proceedings. 2003;**78**:21-33

[7] Roodman GD. Pathogenesis of myeloma bone disease. Leukemia. 2009;**23**:435-441

[8] Regelink JC, Minnema MC, Terpos E, et al. Comparison of modern and conventional imaging techniques in establishing multiple myeloma-related bone disease: A systematic review. British Journal of Haematology. 2013;**162**:50-61

[9] Short KD, Rajkumar SV, Larson D, et al. Incidence of extramedullary disease in patients with multiple myeloma in the era of novel therapy, and the activity of pomalidomide on extramedullary myeloma. Leukemia. 2011;**25**:906-908

[10] Landgren O, Kyle RA, Pfeiffer RM, et al. Monoclonal gammopathy of undetermined significance (MGUS) consistently precedes multiple myeloma: A prospective study. Blood. 2009;**113**:5412-5417

[11] Weiss BM, Abadie J, Verma P, Howard RS, Kuehl WM. A monoclonal gammopathy precedes multiple myeloma in most patients. Blood. 2009;**113**:5418-5422

[12] Kyle RA, Therneau TM, Rajkumar SV, et al. A long-term study of prognosis of monoclonal gammopathy of undetermined significance. The New England Journal of Medicine. 2002;**346**:564-569

[13] Kyle RA, Therneau TM, Rajkumar SV, et al. Prevalence of monoclonal gammopathy of undetermined significance. The New England Journal of Medicine. 2006;**354**:1362-1369

[14] Dispenzieri A, Katzmann JA, Kyle RA, et al. Prevalence and risk of progression of light-chain monoclonal gammopathy of undetermined significance: A retrospective population-based cohort study. Lancet. 2010;**375**:1721-1728

[15] Landgren O, Graubard BI, Katzmann JA, et al. Racial disparities in the prevalence of monoclonal gammopathies: A population-based study of 12 482 persons from the national health and nutritional examination survey. Leukemia. 2014;**28**:1537-1542

[16] Therneau TM, Kyle RA, Melton LJ III, et al. Incidence of monoclonal gammopathy of undetermined significance and estimation of duration before first clinical recognition. Mayo Clinic Proceedings. 2012;**87**:1071-1079

[17] Kyle RA, Remstein ED, Therneau TM, et al. Clinical course and prognosis of smoldering (asymptomatic) multiple myeloma. The New England Journal of Medicine. 2007;**356**: 2582-2590

[18] Rajkumar SV, Gupta V, Fonseca R, et al. Impact of primary molecular cytogenetic abnormalities and risk of progression in smoldering multiple myeloma. Leukemia. 2013;**27**: 1738-1744

[19] Neben K, Jauch A, Hielscher T, et al. Progression in smoldering myeloma is independently determined by the chromosomal abnormalities del(17p), t(4;14), gain 1q, hyperdiploidy, and tumor load. Journal of Clinical Oncology: Official Journal of the American Society of Clinical Oncology. 2013;**31**:4325-4332

[20] Katzmann JA, Dispenzieri A, Kyle R, et al. Elimination of the need for urine studies in the screening algorithm for monoclonal gammopathies by using serum immunofixation and free light chain assays. Mayo Clinic Proceedings. 2006;**81**:1575-1578

[21] Kumar SK, Mikhael JR, Buadi FK, et al. Management of newly diagnosed symptomatic multiple myeloma: Updated mayo stratification of myeloma and risk-adapted therapy (mSMART) consensus guidelines. Mayo Clinic Proceedings. 2009;**84**:1095-1110

[22] Zhou Y, Barlogie B, Shaughnessy JD Jr. The molecular characterization and clinical management of multiple myeloma in the post-genome era. Leukemia. 2009;**23**:1941-1956

[23] Dizdar O, Barista I, Kalyoncu U, et al. Biochemical markers of bone turnover in diagnosis of myeloma bone disease. American Journal of Hematology. 2007;**82**:185-191

[24] Silvestris F, Lombardi L, De Matteo M, Bruno A, Dammacco F. Myeloma bone disease: Pathogenetic mechanisms and clinical assessment. Leukemia Research. 2007;**31**:129-138

[25] Dimopoulos M, Terpos E, Comenzo RL, et al. International myeloma working group consensus statement and guidelines regarding the current role of imaging techniques in the diagnosis and monitoring of multiple myeloma. Leukemia. 2009;**23**:1545-1556

[26] Dispenzieri A, Kyle R, Merlini G, et al. International Myeloma Working Group guidelines for serum-free light chain analysis in multiple myeloma and related disorders. Leukemia. 2009;**23**:215-224

[27] Durie BGM, Harousseau J-L, Miguel JS, et al. International uniform response criteria for multiple myeloma. Leukemia. 2006;**20**:1467-1473

[28] Rajkumar SV, Harousseau JL, Durie B, et al. Consensus recommendations for the uniform reporting of clinical trials: Report of the international Myeloma Workshop Consensus Panel 1. Blood. 2011;**117**:4691-4465

[29] Kumar S, Fonseca R, Ketterling RP, et al. Trisomies in multiple myeloma: Impact on survival in patients with high-risk cytogenetics. Blood. 2012;**119**:2100-2105

[30] Rajan AM, Rajkumar SV. Interpretation of cytogenetic results in multiple myeloma for clinical practice. Blood Cancer Journal. 2015;**5**:e365

[31] Kuehl WM, Bergsagel PL. Multiple myeloma: Evolving genetic events and host interactions. Nature Reviews Cancer. 2002;**2**:175-187

[32] Bergsagel PL, Kuehl WM. Chromosome translocations in multiple myeloma. Oncogene. 2001;**20**:5611-5622

[33] Fonseca R, Bailey RJ, Ahmann GJ, et al. Genomic abnormalities in monoclonal gammopathy of undetermined significance. Blood. 2002;**100**:1417-1424

[34] Seidl S, Kaufmann H, Drach J. New insights into the pathophysiology of multiple myeloma. Lancet Oncology. 2003;**4**:557-564

[35] Russell SJ, Rajkumar SV. Multiple myeloma and the road to personalised medicine. The Lancet Oncology. 2011;**12**:617-619

[36] Vu T, Gonsalves W, Kumar S, et al. Characteristics of exceptional responders to lenalidomide-based therapy in multiple myeloma. Blood Cancer Journal. 2015;**5**:e363

[37] Durie BG, Salmon SE. A clinical staging system for multiple myeloma. Correlation of measured myeloma cell mass with presenting clinical features, response to treatment, and survival. Cancer. 1975;**36**:842-854

[38] Greipp PR, San Miguel JF, Durie BG, et al. International staging system for multiple myeloma. Journal of Clinical Oncology. 2005;**23**:3412-3420

[39] Hari PN, Zhang MJ, Roy V, et al. Is the international staging system superior to the Durie-Salmon staging system? A comparison in multiple myeloma patients undergoing autologous transplant. Leukemia. 2009;**23**:1528-1534

[40] Palumbo A, Avet-Loiseau H, Oliva S, et al. Revised international staging system for multiple myeloma: A report from International Myeloma Working Group. Journal of Clinical Oncology: Official Journal of the American Society of Clinical Oncology. 2015; **33**:2863-2869

[41] Mikhael JR, Dingli D, Roy V, et al. Management of newly diagnosed symptomatic multiple myeloma: Updated mayo stratification of myeloma and risk-adapted therapy (mSMART) consensus guidelines 2013. Mayo Clinic Proceedings. 2013;**88**:360-376

[42] Rajkumar SV. Treatment of multiple myeloma. Nature Reviews Clinical Oncology. 2011; **8**:479-491

[43] Bergsagel PL, Kuehl WM. Molecular pathogenesis and a consequent classification of multiple myeloma. Journal of Clinical Oncology. 2005;**23**(26):6333-6338

[44] Han K, Xu X, Chen G, Zeng Y, Zhu J, et al. Identification of a promising PI3K inhibitor for the treatment of multiple myeloma through the structural optimization. Journal of Hematology & Oncology. 2014;**7**:9

[45] Linda Wu Y, Maachani UB, Schweitzer M, Singh R, Wang M, et al. Dual inhibition of PI3K/AKT and MEK/ERK pathways induces synergistic antitumor effects in diffuse intrinsic pontine glioma cells. Translational Oncology. 2017;**10**:221-228

[46] Chang-Yew Leow C, Gerondakis S, Spencer A. MEK inhibitors as a chemotherapeutic intervention in multiple myeloma. Blood Cancer Journal. 2013;**3**:e105. DOI: 10.1038/bcj.2013.1

[47] Hsu JH, Shi Y, Hu L, Fisher M, Franke TF, et al. Role of the AKT kinase in expansion of multiple myeloma clones: Effects on cytokine-dependent proliferative and survival responses. Oncogene. 2002;**21**:1391-1400

[48] Chenard-Poirier M, et al. Results from the biomarker-driven basket trial of RO5126766 (CH5127566), a potent RAF/MEK inhibitor, in RAS-or RAF-mutated malignancies including multiple myeloma. 2017:2506-2506

[49] Liu Y, Zhou G, Zhang B, Liu Y. Bruton's tyrosine kinase: Structure and functions, expression and mutations. Gene Technology. 2013;**2**:106. DOI: 10.4172/2329-6682.1000106

[50] Rushworth SA, Murray MY, Zaitseva L, Bowles KM, MacEwan DJ. Identification of Bruton's tyrosine kinase as a therapeutic target in acute myeloid leukemia. Blood. 2014; **123**(8)

[51] Bam R, Venkateshaiah SU, Khan S, Ling W, Randal SS, et al. Role of Bruton's tyrosine kinase (BTK) in growth and and metastasis of INA6 myeloma cells. Blood Cancer Journal. 2014;**4**:e234. DOI: 10.1038/bcj.2014.54

[52] Chunyan G, Peng H, Lu Y, Yang H, Tian Z, et al. BTK suppresses myeloma cellular senescence through activating AKT/P27/Rb signaling. Oncotarget. 2017;**8**(34):56858-56867

[53] Tai Y-T, Anderson KC. Bruton's tyrosine kinase: Oncotarget in myeloma. Oncotarget. 2012;**3**:913-914

[54] Eugênio AIP, Fook-Alves VL, de Oliveira MB, Fernando RC, et al. Proteasome and heat shock protein 70 (HSP70) inhibitors as therapeutic alternative in multiple myeloma. Oncotarget. 2017;**8**(70):114698-114709

[55] Khong T, Spencer A. Targeting HSP 90 induces apoptosis and inhibits critical survival and proliferation pathways in multiple myeloma. Molecular Cancer Therapeutics. 2011; **10**(10):1909-1917

[56] Zhang L, Fok JHL, Davies FE. Heat shock proteins in multiple myeloma. Oncotarget. 2014;**5**(5)

[57] Shah SP, Nooka AK, Jaye DL, Bahlis NJ, Lonial S, Boise LH, et al. Bortezomib-induced heat shock response protects multiple myeloma cells and is activated by heat shock factor 1 serine 326 phosphorylation. Oncotarget. 2016;**7**(37)

[58] Richardson PG, Chanan-Khan AA, Lonial S, Krishnan AY, Carroll MP, Alsina M, et al. Tanespimycin and bortezomib combination treatment in patients with relapsed or relapsed and refractory multiple myeloma: Results of a phase 1/2 study. British Journal of Haematology. 2011;**153**(6):729-740. DOI: 10.1111/j.1365-2141.2011.08664.x (Epub Apr 28, 2011)

[59] Bustany S, Cahu J, Descamps G, Pellat-Deceunynck C, Sola B. Heat shock factor 1 is a potent therapeutic target for enhancing the efficacy of treatments for multiple myeloma with adverse prognosis. Journal of Hematology & Oncology. 2015;**8**:40. DOI: 10.1186/s13045-015-0135-3

[60] Bong IPN, Ng CC, Baharuddin P, Zakaria Z. MicroRNA expression patterns and target prediction in multiple myeloma development and malignancy. Genes & Genomics. 2017; **39**:533-540. DOI: 10.1007/s13258-017-0518-7

[61] Abdi J, Jian H, Chang H. Role of micro-RNAs in drug resistance of multiple myeloma. Oncotarget. 2016;**7**(37)

[62] Rossi M, Tagliaferri P, Tassone P. MicroRNAs in multiple myeloma and related bone disease. Annals of Translational Medicine. 2015;**3**(21):334

[63] Roccaro AM, Sacco A, Thompson B, Leleu X, Azab AK, et al. Ghobrial MicroRNAs 15a and 16 regulate tumor proliferation in multiple myeloma. Blood. 2009;**113**(26)

[64] Anderson KC. The 39th David A. Karnofsky lecture: Bench-to-bedside translation of targeted therapies in multiple myeloma. Journal of Clinical Oncology. 2012;**30**:445-452

[65] Kikuchi J, Wada T, Shimizu R, Izumi T, Akutsu M, et al. Histone deacetylases are critical targets of bortezomib-induced cytotoxicity in multiple myeloma. Blood. 2010;**116**(3)

[66] Deleu S, Menu E, Van Valckenborgh E, Van Camp B, Fraczek J, et al. Histone deacetylase inhibitors in multiple myeloma. Hematology Reviews. 2009;**1**:e9

[67] Mitsiades CS, Mitsiades NS, McMullan CJ, Poulaki V, Shringarpure R, Hideshima T, et al. Transcriptional signature of histone deacetylase inhibition in multiple myeloma: Biological and clinical implications. Proceedings of the National Academy of Sciences of the United States of America. 2004;**101**(2)

[68] Stakiw J, Bosch M, Goubran H. A closer look at the bone marrow microenvironment in multiple myeloma. Tumor and Microenvironment. 2018;**1**:1-8

[69] Masahiro ABE. Microenvironment for myeloma growth and drug resistance. International Journal of Myeloma. 2013;**3**(1):2-11

[70] Noonan K, Borrello I. The immune microenvironment of myeloma. Cancer Microenvironment. 2011;**4**:313-323. DOI: 10.1007/s12307-011-0086-3

[71] Mondello P, Cuzzocrea S, Navarra M, Mian M. Bone marrow micro-environment is a crucial player for myelomagenesis and disease progression. Oncotarget. 2017;**8**(12): 20394-20409

[72] Borrello I, Noonan KA. Marrow-infiltrating lymphocytes—Role in biology and cancer therapy. Frontiers in Immunology. 2016;**7** (Article 112)

[73] Noonan KA, Huff CA, Davis J, Lemas MV, Fiorino S, Bitzan J, et al. Adoptive transfer of activated marrow-infiltrating lymphocytes induces measurable antitumor immunity in the bone marrow in multiple myeloma. Science Translational Medicine. 2015;**7**:288ra78

[74] Rosenblatt J, Avigan D. Targeting the PD-1/PD-L1 axis in multiple myeloma: A dream or a reality? Blood. 2017;**129**(3):275

[75] Katarina Luptakova MD, David Avigan MD. Immune therapy in multiple myeloma. Clinical Advances in Hematology & Oncology. 2015;**13**(11)

[76] Kocoglu M, Badros A. The role of immunotherapy in multiple myeloma. Pharmaceuticals. 2016;**9**:3. DOI: 10.3390/ph9010003

[77] Sherbenou DW, Mark TM, Forsberg P. Monoclonal antibodies in multiple myeloma: A new wave of the future. Clinical Lymphoma, Myeloma & Leukemia. 2017;**17**(9):545-554. DOI: 10.1016/j.clml.2017.06.030 (Epub Jun 27, 2017)

[78] van de Donk NWCJ, Richardson PG, Malavasi F. CD38 antibodies in multiple myeloma: Back to the future. Blood. 2018;**131**:13-29. DOI: 10.1182/blood-2017-06-740944

[79] Lonial S, Durie B, Palumbo A, San-Miguel J. Monoclonal antibodies in the treatment of multiple myeloma: Current status and future perspectives. Leukemia. 2016;**30**:526-535

[80] van de Donk NWCJ, Lokhorst HM, Bloem AC. Growth factors and antiapoptotic signaling pathways in multiple myeloma. Leukemia. 2005;**19**:2177-2185

[81] Kizaki M, Tabayashi T. The role of intracellular signaling pathways in the pathogenesis of multiple myeloma and novel therapeutic approaches. Journal of Clinical and Experimental Hematopathology. 2016;**56**(1)

[82] Bergsagel PL, Kuehl WM, Zhan F, Sawyer J, Barlogie B, Shaughnessy J Jr. Cyclin D dysregulation: An early and unifying pathogenic event in multiple myeloma. Blood. 2005;**106**(1):296-303

[83] Broyl A, Hose D, Lokhorst H, de Knegt Y, Peeters J, Jauch A, et al. Gene expression profiling for molecular classification of multiple myeloma in newly diagnosed patients. Blood. 2010;**116**(14):2543-2553

[84] Zhan F, Huang Y, Colla S, Stewart JP, Hanamura I, Gupta S, et al. The molecular classification of multiple myeloma. Blood. 2006;**108**(6):2020-2028

[85] Decaux O, Lode L, Magrangeas F, Charbonnel C, Gouraud W, Jezequel P, et al. Prediction of survival in multiple myeloma based on gene expression profiles reveals cell cycle and chromosomal instability signatures in high-risk patients and hyperdiploid signatures in low-risk patients: A study of the Intergroupe francophone du Myelome. Journal of Clinical Oncology. 2008;**26**(29):4798-4805

[86] Dring AM, Davies FE, Fenton JA, Roddam PL, Scott K, Gonzalez D, et al. A global expression-based analysis of the consequences of the t(4,14) translocation in myeloma. Clinical Cancer Research. 2004;**10**(17):5692-5701

[87] Li Y, Wang X, Zheng H, Wang C, Minvielle S, Magrangeas F, et al. Classify hyperdiploidy status of multiple myeloma patients using gene expression profiles. PLoS One. 2013;**8**(3): e58809

[88] Anguiano A, Tuchman SA, Acharya C, Salter K, Gasparetto C, Zhan F, et al. Gene expression profiles of tumor biology provide a novel approach to prognosis and may guide the selection of therapeutic targets in multiple myeloma. Journal of Clinical Oncology. 2009;**27**(25):4197-4203

[89] Lopez-Corral L, Corchete LA, Sarasquete ME, Mateos MV, Garcia-Sanz R, Ferminan E, et al. Transcriptome analysis reveals molecular profiles associated with evolving steps of monoclonal gammopathies. Haematologica. 2014;**99**(8):1365-1372

[90] McMillin DW, Delmore J, Weisberg E, Negri JM, Geer DC, Klippel S, et al. Tumor cell-specific bioluminescence platform to identify stroma-induced changes to anticancer drug activity. Nature Medicine. 2010;**16**(4):483-489. DOI: 10.1038/nm.2112

[91] Chung TH, Mulligan G, Fonseca R, Chng WJ. A novel measure of chromosome instability can account for prognostic difference in multiple myeloma. PLoS One. 2013;**8**(6): e66361

[92] Chng WJ, Braggio E, Mulligan G, Bryant B, Remstein E, Valdez R, et al. The centrosome index is a powerful prognostic marker in myeloma and identifies a cohort of patients that might benefit from aurora kinase inhibition. Blood. 2008;**111**(3):1603-1609

[93] Moreaux J, Klein B, Bataille R, Descamps G, Maiga S, Hose D, et al. A high-risk signature for patients with multiple myeloma established from the molecular classification of human myeloma cell lines. Haematologica. 2011;**96**(4):574-582

[94] Hose D, Reme T, Hielscher T, Moreaux J, Messner T, Seckinger A, et al. Proliferation is a central independent prognostic factor and target for personalized and risk-adapted treatment in multiple myeloma. Haematologica. 2011;**96**(1):87-95

[95] Kuiper R, Broyl A, de Knegt Y, van Vliet MH, van Beers EH, van der Holt B, et al. A gene expression signature for high-risk multiple myeloma. Leukemia. 2012;**26**(11):2406-2413

[96] Shaughnessy JD Jr, Zhan F, Burington BE, Huang Y, Colla S, Hanamura I, et al. A validated gene expression model of high-risk multiple myeloma is defined by deregulated expression of genes mapping to chromosome 1. Blood. 2007;**109**(6):2276-2284

[97] Chng WJ, Chung TH, Kumar S, Usmani S, Munshi N, Avet-Loiseau H, et al. Gene signature combinations improve prognostic stratification of multiple myeloma patients. Leukemia. 2016;**30**(5):1071-1078

[98] Khan R, Dhodapkar M, Rosenthal A, Heuck C, Papanikolaou X, Qu P, et al. Four genes predict high risk of progression from smoldering to symptomatic multiple myeloma (SWOG S0120). Haematologica. 2015;**100**(9):1214-1221

[99] Todoerti K, Agnelli L, Fabris S, Lionetti M, Tuana G, Mosca L, et al. Transcriptional characterization of a prospective series of primary plasma cell leukemia revealed signatures associated with tumor progression and poorer outcome. Clinical Cancer Research. 2013;**19**(12):3247-3258

[100] Wu P, Agnelli L, Walker BA, Todoerti K, Lionetti M, Johnson DC, et al. Improved risk stratification in myeloma using a microRNA-based classifier. British Journal of Haematology. 2013;**162**(3):348-359

[101] Corthals SL, Sun SM, Kuiper R, de Knegt Y, Broyl A, van der Holt B, et al. MicroRNA signatures characterize multiple myeloma patients. Leukemia. 2011;**25**(11):1784-1789

[102] Min DJ, Ezponda T, Kim MK, Will CM, Martinez-Garcia E, Popovic R, et al. MMSET stimulates myeloma cell growth through microRNA-mediated modulation of c-MYC. Leukemia. 2013;**27**(3):686-694

[103] Pichiorri F, Suh SS, Rocci A, De Luca L, Taccioli C, Santhanam R, et al. Downregulation of p53-inducible microRNAs 192, 194, and 215 impairs the p53/MDM2 autoregulatory loop in multiple myeloma development. Cancer Cell. 2010;**18**(4):367-381

[104] Pichiorri F, Suh SS, Ladetto M, Kuehl M, Palumbo T, Drandi D, et al. MicroRNAs regulate critical genes associated with multiple myeloma pathogenesis. Proceedings of the National Academy of Sciences of the United States of America. 2008;**105**(35):12885-12890

[105] Rocci A, Hofmeister CC, Geyer S, Stiff A, Gambella M, Cascione L, et al. Circulating miRNA markers show promise as new prognosticators for multiple myeloma. Leukemia. 2014;**28**(9):1922-1926

[106] Di Martino MT, Leone E, Amodio N, Foresta U, Lionetti M, Pitari MR, et al. Synthetic miR-34a mimics as a novel therapeutic agent for multiple myeloma: In vitro and in vivo evidence. Clinical Cancer Research. 2012;**18**(22):6260-6270

[107] Ahmad N, Haider S, Jagannathan S, Anaissie E, Driscoll JJ. MicroRNA theragnostics for the clinical management of multiple myeloma. Leukemia. 2014;**28**(4):732-738

[108] Samur M, Gulla A, Cleynen A, Magrangeas F, Minvielle S, Anderson KC, et al. Differentially expressed and prognostically significant lincrnas may impact immune system and tumor progression in multiple myeloma (MM). Blood. 2015;**126**:2989

[109] Adamia S, Reichert AA, Kuppusamy H, Kriangkum J, Ghosh A, Hodges JJ, et al. Inherited and acquired variations in the hyaluronan synthase 1 (HAS1) gene may contribute to

disease progression in multiple myeloma and Waldenstrom macroglobulinemia. Blood. 2008;**112**(13):5111-5121

[110] Adamia S, Reiman T, Crainie M, Mant MJ, Belch AR, Pilarski LM. Intronic splicing of hyaluronan synthase 1 (HAS1): A biologically relevant indicator of poor outcome in multiple myeloma. Blood. 2005;**105**(12):4836-4844

[111] Nagoshi H, Taki T, Chinen Y, Tatekawa S, Tsukamoto T, Maegawa S, et al. Transcriptional dysregulation of the deleted in colorectal carcinoma gene in multiple myeloma and monoclonal gammopathy of undetermined significance. Genes, Chromosomes & Cancer. 2015;**54**(12):788-795

[112] Walker BA, Boyle EM, Wardell CP, Murison A, Begum DB, Dahir NM, et al. Mutational spectrum, copy number changes, and outcome: Results of a sequencing study of patients with newly diagnosed myeloma. Journal of Clinical Oncology. 2015;**33**(33):3911-3920

[113] Bolli N, Avet-Loiseau H, Wedge DC, Van Loo P, Alexandrov LB, Martincorena I, et al. Heterogeneity of genomic evolution and mutational profiles in multiple myeloma. Nature Communications. 2014;**5**:2997

[114] Lohr JG, Stojanov P, Carter SL, Cruz-Gordillo P, Lawrence MS, Auclair D, et al. Widespread genetic heterogeneity in multiple myeloma: Implications for targeted therapy. Cancer Cell. 2014;**25**(1):91-101

[115] Mosen-Ansorena D, Bolli N, Samur MK, Magrangeas F, Minvielle S, Anderson KC, et al. Redefining mutational profiling using RNA-Seq: Insight into the functional mutational landscape of multiple myeloma. Blood. 2015;**126**(23):837

[116] Macosko EZ, Basu A, Satija R, Nemesh J, Shekhar K, Goldman M, et al. Highly parallel genome-wide expression profiling of individual cells using nanoliter droplets. Cell. 2015; **161**(5):1202-1214

[117] Mitra AK, Mukherjee UK, Harding T, Jang JS, Stessman H, Li Y, et al. Single-cell analysis of targeted transcriptome predicts drug sensitivity of single cells within human myeloma tumors. Leukemia. 2016;**30**(5):1094-1102 [PubMed: 26710886]

[118] Rashid N, Minvielle S, Magrangeas F, Samur MK, Cleynen A, Sperling A, et al. Alternative splicing is a frequent event and impacts clinical outcome in myeloma: A large RNA-Seq data analysis of newly-diagnosed myeloma patients. Blood. 2014;**124**:638

[119] Walker BA, Wardell CP, Melchor L, Hulkki S, Potter NE, Johnson DC, et al. Intraclonal heterogeneity and distinct molecular mechanisms characterize the development of t(4;14) and t(11;14) myeloma. Blood. 2012;**120**(5):1077-1086

[120] Walker BA, Wardell CP, Melchor L, Brioli A, Johnson DC, Kaiser MF, et al. Intraclonal heterogeneity is a critical early event in the development of myeloma and precedes the development of clinical symptoms. Leukemia. 2014;**28**(2):384-390

[121] Munshi NC, Minvielle S, Tai Y-T, Fulciniti M, Samur MK, Richardson PG, et al. Deep Igh sequencing identifies an ongoing somatic hypermutation process with complex and evolving clonal architecture in myeloma. Blood. 2015;**126**(23):21

[122] Weinhold N, Ashby C, Rasche L, Chavan SS, Stein C, Stephens OW, et al. Clonal selection and double hit events involving tumor suppressor genes underlie relapse from chemotherapy: Myeloma as a model. Blood. 2016 (Epub ahead of print)

[123] Melchor L, Brioli A, Wardell CP, Murison A, Potter NE, Kaiser MF, et al. Single-cell genetic analysis reveals the composition of initiating clones and phylogenetic patterns of branching and parallel evolution in myeloma. Leukemia. 2014;**28**(8):1705-1715

[124] Kuiper R, van Duin M, van Vliet MH, Broijl A, van der Holt B, El Jarari L, et al. Prediction of high- and low-risk multiple myeloma based on gene expression and the international staging system. Blood. 2015;**126**(17):1996-2004

[125] Landgren O, Rajkumar SV. New developments in diagnosis, prognosis, and assessment of response in multiple myeloma. Clinical Cancer Research. 2016;**22**

[126] Attal M, Lauwers-Cances V, Hulin C, Facon T, Caillot D, Escoffre M, et al. Autologous transplantation for multiple myeloma in the era of new drugs: A phase III study of the Intergroupe francophone Du Myelome (IFM/DFCI 2009 trial). Blood. 2015;**126**(23):391

[127] Harousseau JL, Attal M, Avet-Loiseau H. The role of complete response in multiple myeloma. Blood. 2009;**114**(15):3139-3146

[128] Terragna C, Remondini D, Martello M, Zamagni E, Pantani L, Patriarca F, et al. The genetic and genomic background of multiple myeloma patients achieving complete response after induction therapy with bortezomib, thalidomide and dexamethasone (VTD). Oncotarget. 2016;**7**(9):9666-9679

[129] Wu P, Walker BA, Broyl A, Kaiser M, Johnson DC, Kuiper R, et al. A gene expression based predictor for high risk myeloma treated with intensive therapy and autologous stem cell rescue. Leukemia & Lymphoma. 2015;**56**(3):594-601

[130] Terragna C, Renzulli M, Remondini D, Tagliafico E, Di Raimondo F, Patriarca F, et al. Correlation between eight-gene expression profiling and response to therapy of newly diagnosed multiple myeloma patients treated with thalidomide-dexamethasone incorporated into double autologous transplantation. Annals of Hematology. 2013;**92**(9): 1271-1280

[131] Zhan F, Barlogie B, Mulligan G, Shaughnessy JD Jr, Bryant B. High-risk myeloma: A gene expression based risk-stratification model for newly diagnosed multiple myeloma treated with high-dose therapy is predictive of outcome in relapsed disease treated with single-agent bortezomib or high-dose dexamethasone. Blood. 2008; **111**(2):968-969

[132] Amin SB, Yip WK, Minvielle S, Broyl A, Li Y, Hanlon B, et al. Gene expression profile alone is inadequate in predicting complete response in multiple myeloma. Leukemia. 2014;**28**(11):2229-2234

[133] Tian E, Zhan F, Walker R, Rasmussen E, Ma Y, Barlogie B, et al. The role of the Wnt-signaling antagonist DKK1 in the development of osteolytic lesions in multiple myeloma. The New England Journal of Medicine. 2003;**349**(26):2483-2494

[134] Fulciniti M, Tassone P, Hideshima T, Vallet S, Nanjappa P, Ettenberg SA, et al. Anti-DKK1 mAb (BHQ880) as a potential therapeutic agent for multiple myeloma. Blood. 2009;**114**(2):371-379

[135] Touzeau C, Dousset C, Le Gouill S, Sampath D, Leverson JD, Souers AJ, et al. The Bcl-2 specific BH3 mimetic ABT-199: A promising targeted therapy for t(11;14) multiple myeloma. Leukemia. 2014;**28**(1):210-212

[136] Rashid NU, Sperling AS, Bolli N, Wedge DC, Van Loo P, Tai YT, et al. Differential and limited expression of mutant alleles in multiple myeloma. Blood. 2014;**124**(20):3110-3117

[137] Sharman JP, Chmielecki J, Morosini D, Palmer GA, Ross JS, Stephens PJ, et al. Vemurafenib response in 2 patients with posttransplant refractory BRAF V600E-mutated multiple myeloma. Clinical Lymphoma, Myeloma & Leukemia. 2014;**14**(5):e161-e163

[138] Andrulis M, Lehners N, Capper D, Penzel R, Heining C, Huellein J, et al. Targeting the BRAF V600E mutation in multiple myeloma. Cancer Discovery. 2013;**3**(8):862-869

[139] Heuck CJ, Jethava Y, Khan R, van Rhee F, Zangari M, Chavan S, et al. Inhibiting MEK in MAPK pathway-activated myeloma. Leukemia. 2016;**30**(4):976-980

[140] Alzrigat M, Atienza Párraga A, Mamun Majumder M, Ma A, Jin J, et al. The polycomb group protein BMI-1 inhibitor PTC-209 is a potent anti-myeloma agent alone or in combination with epigenetic inhibitors targeting EZH2 and the BET bromodomains. Oncotarget. 2017;**8**(61):103731-103743 (Published online Oct 20, 2017). DOI: 10.18632/oncotarget.21909

[141] Mulligan G, Lichter DI, Di Bacco A, Blakemore SJ, Berger A, Koenig E, et al. Mutation of NRAS but not KRAS significantly reduces myeloma sensitivity to single-agent bortezomib therapy. Blood. 2014;**123**(5):632-639

[142] Boegsted M, Holst JM, Fogd K, Falgreen S, Sorensen S, Schmitz A, et al. Generation of a predictive melphalan resistance index by drug screen of B-cell cancer cell lines. PLoS One. 2011;**6**(4):e19322

[143] Bogsted M, Bilgrau AE, Wardell CP, Bertsch U, Schmitz A, Bodker JS, et al. Proof of the concept to use a malignant B cell line drug screen strategy for identification and weight of melphalan resistance genes in multiple myeloma. PLoS One. 2013;**8**(12):e83252

[144] Burington B, Barlogie B, Zhan F, Crowley J, Shaughnessy JD Jr. Tumor cell gene expression changes following short-term in vivo exposure to single agent chemotherapeutics are related to survival in multiple myeloma. Clinical Cancer Research. 2008;**14**(15):4821-4829

[145] Shaughnessy JD Jr, Qu P, Usmani S, Heuck CJ, Zhang Q, Zhou Y, et al. Pharmacogenomics of bortezomib test-dosing identifies hyperexpression of proteasome genes, especially PSMD4, as novel high-risk feature in myeloma treated with total therapy 3. Blood. 2011;**118**(13):3512-3524

Chapter 4

Resistance Mechanisms to Novel Therapies in Myeloma

Craig T. Wallington-Beddoe and
Douglas W. Coghlan

Additional information is available at the end of the chapter

http://dx.doi.org/10.5772/intechopen.77004

Abstract

The number of novel therapies for the treatment of multiple myeloma (MM) is rapidly increasing with proteasome inhibitors, immunomodulatory agents and monoclonal antibodies being the most well-known therapeutic classes whilst histone deacetylase inhibitors, selective inhibitors of nuclear export and CAR-T cells amongst others also being actively investigated. However, in parallel with the development and application of these novel myeloma therapies is the emergence of novel mechanisms of resistance, many of which remain elusive, particularly for more recently developed agents. Whilst resistance mechanisms have been best studied for proteasome inhibitors, particularly Bortezomib, class effects do not universally apply to all proteasome inhibitors, and within-class differences in efficacy, toxicity and resistance mechanisms have been observed. Immunomodulatory agents share the common cellular target cereblon and thus resistance patterns relate to cereblon expression and its pathway components. However, the cell surface antigens to which monoclonal antibodies are directed means these agents frequently exhibit unique within-class differences in clinical efficacy and resistance patterns. Despite the progressive biological elucidation of resistance mechanisms to these novel therapies, attempts to specifically exploit these processes lag considerably behind and until such approaches become available, resistance to these therapies will remain a concern.

Keywords: myeloma, novel therapy, drug resistance, proteasome inhibitor, immunomodulatory agent, monoclonal antibody

1. Introduction

There has recently been an explosion of novel agents for the treatment of MM that have dramatically improved overall response rates (ORR), progression-free survival (PFS) and overall survival (OS) by targeting the malignant plasma cell and bone marrow microenvironment in unique ways. The main classes of novel agents are proteasome inhibitors, immunomodulatory agents and monoclonal antibodies, however several other classes of novel agents are emerging, including histone deacetylase inhibitors, BH3 mimetics, checkpoint inhibitors and selective inhibitors of nuclear export, as are alternative approaches, such as chimeric antigen receptor T-cells (CAR-T) with MM cell specificity. Whilst CAR-T technology in MM remains in pre-clinical and early clinical trial stages of development, this immunological approach is rapidly gaining momentum with several groups developing CAR-T cells for therapeutic use [1]. Despite these therapeutic advances, many MM patients develop disease relapse suggesting the development of drug resistance whilst some are primary refractory. In this chapter, for the three major classes of novel agents, we present a discussion on known biological mechanisms of resistance together with clinical trial efforts, if any, to overcome these. Of all therapeutic classes of novel agents, mechanisms of resistance to proteasome inhibitors have been studied in greatest detail and are the focus of this chapter.

2. Proteasome inhibitors

Plasma cells secrete immunoglobulin in response to infection and a range of other stimuli which requires folding in the endoplasmic reticulum (ER) lumen prior to secretion from the cell, resulting in a degree of ER stress due to misfolded protein [2]. ER stress is heightened in MM due to the high, sustained production of monoclonal immunoglobulin and a build-up of misfolded protein within the ER lumen. This ER stress activates three ER membrane stress sensors, protein kinase RNA-like ER kinase (PERK), inositol-requiring enzyme 1 (IRE1) and activating transcription factor 6 (ATF6) in a homeostatic process termed the Unfolded Protein Response (UPR) [2]. Activation of the UPR results in a global reduction in protein translation and the upregulation of ER chaperones and folding machinery to cope with the misfolded protein load, thereby rectifying the high ER stress levels that initiated the process. However, high sustained levels of ER stress can overwhelm the corrective capacity of the UPR which turns from a pro-survival, homeostatic mechanism to one that commits the MM cell to apoptosis. By inhibiting the 26S proteasome and preventing the degradation of misfolded proteins, proteasome inhibitors induce ER stress and a terminal UPR [2]. However, there are other mechanisms through which these agents exert their activity. Indeed, proteasome inhibitors are able to modulate a diverse array of cell signalling pathways whilst rendering the microenvironment less supportive of MM cell growth [3]. Perhaps due to the significant clinical impact the first-in-class proteasome inhibitor Bortezomib has made, resistance mechanisms to this agent have been studied in greatest detail compared to other proteasome inhibitors (**Table 1** and **Figure 1A**).

2.1. The ubiquitin-proteasome pathway

The ubiquitination and proteasome degradation pathway is a multistep enzymatic cascade in eukaryotes through which the cell removes excess and misfolded proteins and regulates

Resistance type	Resistance mediator(s)	Resistance mechanism
Proteasome inhibitors		
Mutations	*PSMB5* mutations encoding the β5 proteasome subunit	Impaired ability of proteasome inhibitors to bind to the catalytically active *N*-terminal threonine in proteasome subunits
Aberrant expression of ubiquitin-proteasome pathway components	β5 and other proteasome subunits	Increased or decreased numbers of binding sites for proteasome inhibitors, altering their ability to inhibit proteolysis
Activation of the aggresome-autophagy pathway	HDAC6 and autophagic machinery	Sequestration of toxic proteins in aggresomes and their removal by autophagy-mediated degradation
Heat shock protein induction	Grp78, Hsp90 and other family members including Hsp70 and Hsp8	Increased protein chaperoning resulting in greater ability to deal with misfolded and other toxic proteins
Drug efflux activity	P-glycoprotein and other ATP-binding cassette (ABC) superfamily members	Cellular efflux of proteasome inhibitors thereby reducing their ability to interact with proteasome subunits and other intracellular processes
Antioxidant response pathway induction	Over-expression of nuclear factor, erythroid 2 like 2 (*NFE2L2*)	Assists proteasome assembly by inducing expression of proteasome maturation protein (POMP)
Plasma cell differentiation	Reduced expression of Xbp1	Correlates with reduced immunoglobulin synthesis and ER stress/proteasome load therefore reduced sensitivity to proteasome inhibitors
Bone marrow microenvironment	Adhesion molecules on MM cells and bone marrow stromal cells (e.g. CD138, CD44, VCAM-1, LFA-1, MUC-1, ICAM-1 etc.)	Microenvironmental protection from proteasome inhibitors and other anti-MM therapies by increased MM cell migration, homing and adhesion to the bone marrow and activation of survival and proliferative intracellular signalling pathways
Survival signalling pathways	IL-6, VEGF, HGF, c-MET, NF-κB, PI3K/AKT, IGF-1/IGF-1R, tight junction protein 1 (TJP1) and EGFR/JAK/STAT signalling	Proliferation and cell survival signalling reducing the efficacy of proteasome inhibitors. Increased angiogenesis and MM cell migration. Induction of EGFR/JAK/STAT signalling associated with increased expression of proteasome subunits
Immunomodulatory agents		
Cereblon pathway abnormalities	Reduced cereblon expression	Less available target for IMiD binding
	Cereblon and other pathway component mutations	Reduced ability for IMiDs to bind to cereblon and other pathway components
Ras/Raf pathway activation	KRAS G12D and BRAF V600E mutations	Ras/Raf pathway activating mutations result in MM cell proliferation and resistance to IMiDs
Adhesion to bone marrow stroma	CD44 (Wnt/β-catenin signalling)	Greater adhesion to bone marrow stromal cells protecting MM cells from IMiDs
Monoclonal antibodies		
Target antigen expression	Reduced expression of CD38, SLAM7 and other cell surface proteins	Less available target for mAb binding through various mechanisms including trogocytosis

Resistance type	Resistance mediator(s)	Resistance mechanism
Resistance to complement-dependent cytotoxicity (CDC)	Increased expression of CD46, CD55 and CD59	Reduced ability for mAbs to activate CDC
Soluble antigen	Extracellular CD38 and SLAM7	Extracellular binding of mAbs to target antigen resulting in reduced mAb binding to cell surface antigen
Development of neutralising antibodies	Anti-mAb antibodies	Host derived anti-mAb antibodies neutralise therapeutic mAbs before reaching their cellular targets

Table 1. Mechanisms of resistance to the main classes of novel agents for multiple myeloma [143].

cellular processes including cell proliferation and survival [4]. The process involves the conjugation of ubiquitin via a lysine residue at position 48. Proteins tagged with lysine 48-linked chains of ubiquitin are marked for degradation in the proteasome enzyme complex [5, 6]. Eukaryotic cells contain the 26S proteasome which consists of a 20S core particle that is bound to two 19S regulatory particles [7, 8]. The 19S regulatory particle is responsible for substrate recognition, deubiquitination, unfolding and translocation into the 20S core particle which contains the active sites that hydrolyze substrate peptide bonds [9]. The 20S core particle is composed of four rings that are composed of seven α (α1–α7) subunits or seven β subunits (β1–β7), that are stacked in a specific order ($\alpha_7\beta_7\beta_7\alpha_7$). These rings generate three interconnected chambers: two outer chambers that are formed by the adjacent α and β rings and a catalytic chamber that is formed by the two adjacent β rings. Only the β1, β2 and β5 subunits are catalytically active proteases [10, 11]. Near the β subunit's active site lies a substrate specificity pocket which binds to 10 amino acid stretches in the substrate that flank the peptide bond that is cleaved and thereby determines the cleaving preferences of each β subunit [12, 13]. In particular, the β1 subunit has caspase-like activity (cleaving after acidic residues), β2 exhibits trypsin-like activity (cleaving after basic residues), and β5 has chymotrypsin-like activity (cleaving after hydrophobic residues) [14, 15].

Proteins that are targeted for proteasomal degradation must cross the 19S regulatory subunit in order to reach the proteolytic 20S core where they are degraded into peptides that vary from 3 to 25 amino acids in length [16, 17]. Each substrate is cleaved in multiple locations without release of partially hydrolyzed substrates from the core particle and the mechanism of degradation is conserved for all catalytically active β subunits [16, 18]. In eukaryotes, the 20S core particle components can change in response to biological stimuli. For example, stimulation of cells with interferon gamma induces the expression of all three catalytically active β subunits. These subunits, along with a unique 11S regulatory particle, form a complex called the immunoproteasome which is involved in generating peptides for presentation to major histocompatibility complex class I molecules, but also has classic proteolytic activity [19–21]. Increased expression of the immunoproteasome complex has been reported in MM, where it may represent the predominant form of the proteasome [22–25]. It is also noteworthy that relapsed MM may be associated with lower levels of the immunoproteasome and increased levels of the constitutive proteasome [25].

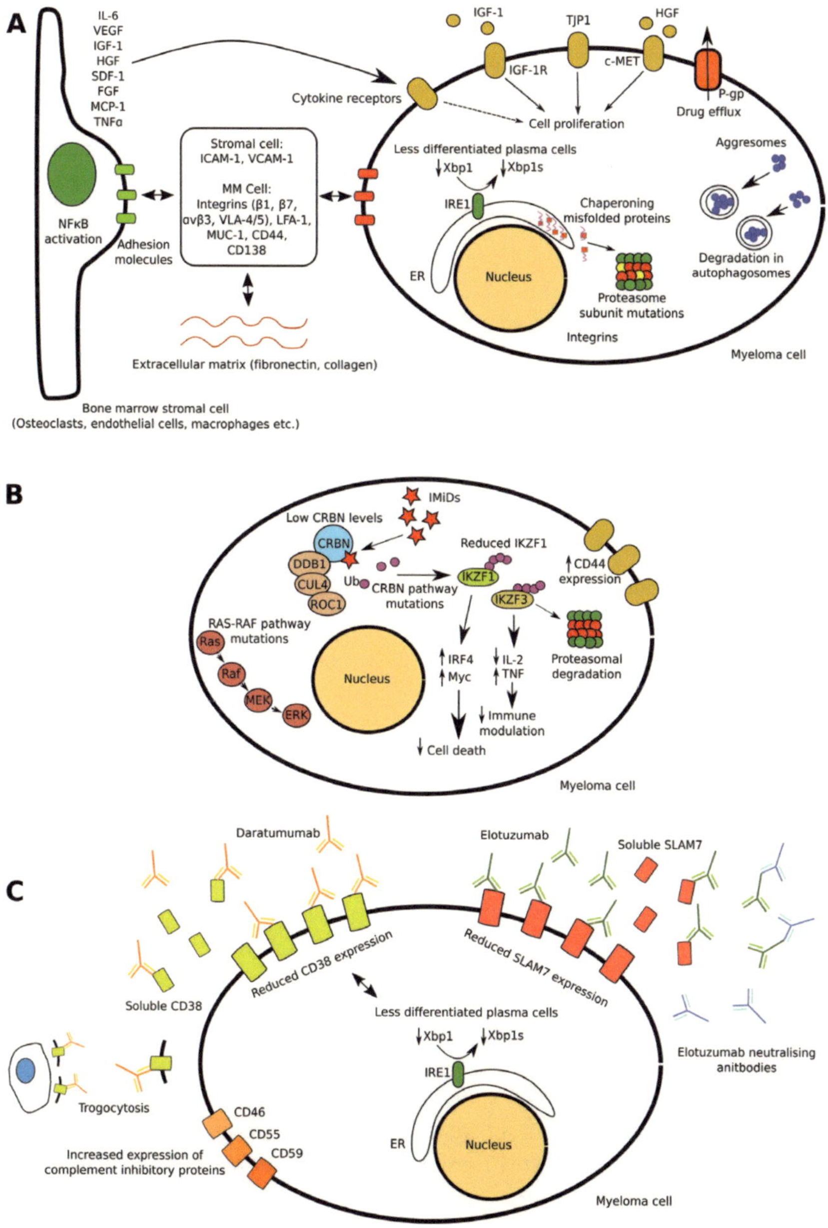

Figure 1. Known resistance mechanisms for the main classes of novel MM therapies [143]. (A) Proteasome inhibitors. (B) Immunomodulatory agents (IMiDs). (C) Monoclonal antibodies. See text for details. c-MET, hepatocyte growth factor receptor; FGF, fibroblast growth factor; HGF, hepatocyte growth factor; IGF-1, insulin-like growth factor; IL-6, Interleukin-6; ICAM-1, intercellular adhesion molecule-1; LFA-1, lymphocyte function-associated antigen-1; MCP-1, monocyte chemotactic protein 1; MUC-1, Mucin-1 antigen; P-gp, P-glycoprotein; SDF-1, stromal cell-derived factor; TNFα, tumour necrosis factor alpha; VCAM-1, vascular cell adhesion molecule-1; VEGF, vascular endothelial growth factor; VLA-4/5, very late antigen 4/5; Xpb1, X-box binding protein 1; ZO-1, Zonula occludens-1; CRBN, cereblon; Cul4, Cullin-4; DDB1, DNA damage-binding protein 1; Erk, extracellular signal-regulated kinases; IKZF, IKAROS family zinc finger; IL-2, Interleukin-2; IRF4, interferon regulatory factor 4; Mek, mitogen-activated protein kinase kinase; MYC, MYC proto-oncogene; Raf, rapidly accelerated fibrosarcoma; ROC1, regulator of cullins 1; Ub, ubiquitin; SLAM7, signalling lymphocytic activation molecule family member 7.

2.2. Proteasome inhibitors used to treat myeloma

Proteasome inhibitors are potent anti-MM agents which inhibit one or more proteolytic subunits of the 20S proteasome. Their efficacy is attributed to a number of factors including inhibition of NF-κB signalling, although this has recently come under question, induction of ER stress with the activation of a terminal UPR, and modification of the bone marrow microenvironment, amongst others [26, 27]. Several generations of proteasome inhibitors have been developed with Bortezomib, Carfilzomib and Ixazomib approved for clinical use in a number of countries. The proteasome inhibitors differ in their relative selectivity for β catalytic subunits, and half-life and reversibility of β subunit inhibition, that translates into differential anti-MM efficacy and toxicity profiles [26]. Thus, the individual proteasome inhibitors demonstrate significant within-class pharmacokinetic and pharmacodynamic variation and resistance to one proteasome inhibitor does not necessarily suggest resistance to another.

The first-in-class proteasome inhibitor Bortezomib (N-acyl-pseudo dipeptidyl boronic acid) is a dipeptide that binds *reversibly* to the chymotrypsin-like β5 subunit of the catalytic chamber of the 20S proteasome and to a lesser extent the β1 and β2 subunits [26]. Attempts to improve the efficacy and toxicity profiles of Bortezomib resulted in the development of the epoxyketone Carfilzomib, an *irreversible* 20S proteasome inhibitor that preferentially binds to and inhibits the chymotrypsin-like β5 subunit with demonstrated activity in Bortezomib-resistant MM patients (ASPIRE trial) [28, 29]. Like Bortezomib, Ixazomib is a *reversible* peptide boronate 20S proteasome inhibitor of the chymotrypsin-like β5 subunit also with activity in Bortezomib-resistant MM as demonstrated in the TOURMALINE phase III trial [30]. Unlike Bortezomib, however, Ixazomib is orally bioavailable and found to induce less toxicity in patients, possibly due to its much shorter β5 subunit dissociation half-life [31].

2.2.1. Later-generation proteasome inhibitors

There are ongoing attempts to expand and improve the repertoire of proteasome inhibitors. Marizomib *irreversibly* inhibits the three proteolytic sites of the 20S proteasome and pre-clinical studies have shown efficacy in Bortezomib-resistant MM cells [32]. A phase I study evaluating Marizomib, Pomalidomide and Dexamethasone in heavily pre-treated patients with relapsed/refractory MM demonstrated an impressive ORR of 53% and clinical benefit rate of 64% [33–35]. This new proteasome inhibitor will likely be examined in more advanced clinical trials in the near future, not only for its ability to re-sensitise patients to proteasome inhibition but for its activity in MM involving the central nervous system. Oprozomib is structurally similar to Carfilzomib with the advantage of being orally administered and has demonstrated pre-clinical efficacy in Bortezomib-resistant MM cells [36]. Whilst there are no clinical trial results at this time in relapsed/refractory MM, several early phase studies are currently active, including a phase Ib/II study of Oprozomib in combination with Dexamethasone (NCT01832727) and with Pomalidomide and Dexamethasone (NCT01999335 and NCT02939183).

2.3. Mechanisms of resistance to proteasome inhibitors

2.3.1. *Mutations and aberrant expression of ubiquitin-proteasome pathway components*

2.3.1.1. *Pre-clinical/clinical findings*

Several point mutations in proteasome subunits that render them insensitive to Bortezomib inhibition have been identified. A single point mutation in the Bortezomib binding pocket of the β5 subunit (*PSMB5* gene) resulting in substitution of Ala49 with Thr (A49T) was described in Bortezomib-resistant human myelomonocytic THP1 cells, generated by culturing cells in escalating concentrations of Bortezomib [37]. This mutation was also detected in Bortezomib-resistant Jurkat cells, as were other mutations including A49V and the combination of A49T with A50V [38, 39]. However, despite the A49T β5 subunit mutation being detected in Bortezomib-resistant KMS-11 and OPM-2 human MM cell lines, no such β5 mutations were detected in Bortezomib-resistant RPMI-8226 MM cells, suggesting other mechanisms of resistance were at play [40, 41]. There have been a number of other β5 mutations identified in pre-clinical studies which affect Bortezomib binding and until recently, no mutations in *PSMB5* have been detected in either newly-diagnosed MM patients or those with relapsed and/or refractory disease [42, 43]. However, the first report of *PSMB5* mutations in a patient resistant to Bortezomib has renewed interest in this area although the clinical significance of these mutations is yet to be determined [44].

Significantly increased protein expression of the β5 subunit and only modest increases in β1 and β2 subunits were observed in Bortezomib-resistant THP1 cells which were reversible upon withdrawal of Bortezomib from cell cultures [37]. Over-expression of β subunits has also been detected in some MM cell lines, as well as those of some other haematologic malignancies, however, studies in MM suggest that the induction of these proteins is at most modest with minimal contribution to resistance [45]. Furthermore, free β5 subunits are catalytically inactive by themselves and cannot generally bind proteasome inhibitors unless assembled into functional proteasomes [46]. The expression levels of tight junction protein 1 (TJP1/ZO-1) were shown to be strongly associated with Bortezomib sensitivity with the downstream mechanism being suppression of EGFR signalling, which decreased the levels of proteasome subunit synthesis in at STAT3-dependent manner [47]. High TJP1 expression in patient MM cells was associated with a significantly higher chance of responding to Bortezomib and a longer duration of response [47].

2.3.2. *Activation of the aggresome-autophagy pathway*

2.3.2.1. *Pre-clinical/clinical findings*

Cytosolic small protein aggregates form when misfolded proteins accumulate, which are then transported towards the microtubule organising centre into a structure called the aggresome. Acetylation of α-tubulin, which is reversed by histone deacetylase 6 (HDAC6), modulates the structure and function of the microtubule, thus playing a pivotal role in the movement of misfolded protein aggregates to the aggresome [48]. Cells that lack HDAC6 were found to be defective in the removal of protein aggregates and are not able to form large aggresomes [49]. Autophagy is predominantly a pro-survival homeostatic process whereby double-membrane vesicles known as autophagosomes sequester cytosolic proteins, including aggresomes, followed by fusion with lysosomes for degradation. Thus, misfolded proteins can be degraded via the ubiquitin-proteasome and/or aggresome-autophagy pathways and simultaneous blockade of both by combining Bortezomib and the HDAC inhibitor Panobinostat, respectively, showed synergistic anti-MM activity in pre-clinical models [50]. By inhibiting the proteasome, Bortezomib results in an increase in aggresome formation and also induction of autophagy, the latter a likely compensatory mechanism to eliminate misfolded proteins and other substrates of the ubiquitin-proteasome system which could be involved in resistance to proteasome inhibitors [51]. Thus, clinical studies combining a proteasome inhibitor with HDAC and/or autophagy inhibition have a sound biological basis for overcoming resistance to proteasome inhibitors.

2.3.2.2. Clinical studies to circumvent resistance

A large phase III study demonstrated a superior PFS when Panobinostat was combined with Bortezomib and Dexamethasone over Bortezomib and Dexamethasone alone in relapsed/refractory MM patients, leading FDA approval of Panobinostat in 2015 [52]. Despite this, no differences in OS or ORR were evident although the proportion of patients achieving a complete response (CR) was higher with Panobinostat. Given the activity of Carfilzomib in Bortezomib-resistant MM, early clinical studies are ongoing examining the combination of Panobinostat and Carfilzomib in relapsed/refractory MM and are expected to yield favourable results (NCT01496118). With regard to autophagy, a phase II trial evaluating the combination of Bortezomib and the autophagy inhibitor Chloroquine in patients with relapsed and/or refractory MM, supported by the finding of synergistic MM cell death in the pre-clinical setting, showed a clinical benefit rate of 40%, further cementing the role of the aggresome-autophagy pathway in proteasome inhibitor-resistant MM [53].

2.3.3. Heat shock protein induction

2.3.3.1. Pre-clinical/clinical findings

The heat shock response is part of the cell repair machinery that maintains homeostasis under stressful conditions such as infection, inflammation, starvation, hypoxia, and exposure to toxins, which is carried out by heat shock proteins (HSPs) [54]. HSPs assist in protein folding and preventing undesirable protein aggregation [54]. Blockade of proteasome-mediated protein degradation leads to the induction of HSPs and related chaperones, which have been shown to confer resistance to proteasome inhibitors [55]. Two well characterised HSPs in this setting are Grp78 (*HSPA5*; also known as Binding immunoglobulin protein, BiP) and Hsp90 (*HSP90AA1*).

Grp78 resides in the ER lumen where it is bound to the luminal domains of the three ER stress protein sensors, ATF6, PERK and IRE1 [2]. Upon accumulation of misfolded proteins in the ER, Grp78 (1) detaches from ATF6, PERK and IRE1 enabling activation of the homeostatic UPR and (2) chaperones the misfolded proteins for degradation by the 20S proteasome [2].

In MM, Grp78 was reported to play a role in resistance to proteasome inhibitors, and MM cells surviving proteasome inhibitor treatment showed increased Grp78 expression, which further increased with progressive disease [56]. However, this was not corroborated by others who could not demonstrate any significant differences in Grp78 expression in bone marrow plasma cells obtained from patients with MGUS, newly-diagnosed MM or relapsed/refractory MM [57]. Inhibition of Grp78 can induce MM cell death and pharmacological inhibition of Grp78 with Metformin, genetic ablation or mutational inactivation followed by Bortezomib treatment led to the accumulation of aggresomes, impaired autophagy and enhancement of the anti-MM effects of Bortezomib [58].

Hsp90 expression also increases with the accumulation of misfolded proteins in the ER lumen and has been investigated as a potential target to enhance the efficacy of Bortezomib [59]. Hsp90 was found to stabilise Grp78 at the post-transcriptional level, and treatment of Bortezomib-resistant mantle cell lymphoma cells with the Hsp90 inhibitor IPI-504 together with Grp78 knockdown led to synergistic cell death when combined with Bortezomib [60]. Other HSPs have also been shown to confer resistance to Bortezomib, including Hsp70 and small heat shock protein B8 (Hsp8) in MM and Hsp27 in lymphoma [61, 62].

2.3.3.2. Clinical studies to circumvent resistance

No advanced clinical trials employing Grp78 modulation in MM patients have been undertaken, although a study using an anti-Grp78 monoclonal antibody induced a PR in a heavily pre-treated patient when combined with Bortezomib and Lenalidomide [63]. Whilst early clinical trials have identified safe dose ranges for Hsp90 inhibitors, which have been tested either alone or in combination with Bortezomib and Dexamethasone in relapsed/refractory MM, results have been disappointing and to date no agents have progressed beyond the phase I/II stage [64].

2.3.4. Drug efflux

2.3.4.1. Pre-clinical/clinical findings

The efflux of drugs by members of the ATP-Binding Cassette (ABC) superfamily is a well-established mechanism by which tumours are able to acquire therapeutic resistance [65]. Whilst the multi-drug efflux transporter MDR1/P-glycoprotein (P-pg/ABCB1) has been shown to correlate with MM relapse and drug resistance [66, 67], its role in Bortezomib resistance has been controversial and it is generally thought that Bortezomib is a poor substrate [68]. P-gp was rarely detected in newly diagnosed MM patients [67], however, overexpression was associated with disease relapse and drug resistance, specifically to Vincristine, Doxorubicin, Etoposide and glucocorticoids [66, 67, 69]. Carfilzomib, on the other hand, is a *bona fide* P-gp substrate and patients treated with Carfilzomib show increased P-gp expression [70]. Upregulation of P-gp in MM cells confers resistance to Carfilzomib [71]. To date, there are no studies that relate P-gp to drug resistance to Ixazomib. Whilst Carfilzomib resistance in MM can be reversed *in vitro* by P-gp inhibition, for example using Verapamil or Vismodegib [72], this has not yet translated into clinical trials.

2.3.5. Antioxidant response pathway induction

2.3.5.1. Pre-clinical/clinical findings

Elevated levels of antioxidant-related pathway genes have been associated with drug resistance in other tumours, including resistance to Bortezomib in patients with mantle cell lymphoma [73]. Bortezomib resistance-related gene expression signatures revealed enrichment for Nuclear Factor, Erythroid 2 Like 2 (*NFE2L2*) which is activated as part of an antioxidant response pathway [74]. The downstream *NFE2L2* gene target *POMP* encodes the proteasome maturation protein proteassemblin, a chaperone responsible for the assembly of active proteasome particles from inactive precursor subunits [75]. Recently, *POMP* was found to be a mediator of the Bortezomib-resistant phenotype in MM cells [75], however, these findings have not been applied clinically.

2.3.6. Plasma cell differentiation

2.3.6.1. Pre-clinical/clinical findings

The transcription factor Xbp-1, a downstream component of the IRE1 arm of the UPR, is required for the differentiation of B-cells into plasma cells and more recently has been shown to be associated with Bortezomib sensitivity [76, 77]. Patient-derived bone marrow MM cells can be subdivided into populations based on their expression of Xbp-1, with plasma cells expressing low or absent Xbp-1 enriched in the bone marrow of patients who have relapsed after Bortezomib therapy or who have progressive disease [76]. These low or absent Xbp-1 expressing plasma cells were less differentiated with lower levels of immunoglobulin synthesis, reduced ER stress and less proteasome load. Conversely, at MM diagnosis, the majority of bone marrow plasma cells expressed higher Xbp-1 levels, conferring sensitivity to Bortezomib, although subpopulations of plasma cells with lower levels could be detected [76]. It is hypothesised that these subpopulations of plasma cells with low Xbp-1 expression are responsible for eventual relapse after induction therapy [76]. Interestingly, these findings would suggest that patients who are resistant to proteasome inhibitors should have non-secretory MM, however, only a small minority of these patients have this disease phenotype. To date, the degree of plasma cell differentiation has not been considered in clinical trials.

2.3.7. Bone marrow microenvironment and survival signalling pathways

2.3.7.1. Pre-clinical/clinical findings

The bone marrow microenvironment (BMME) includes (1) the non-cellular compartment formed by extracellular matrix (ECM) proteins (laminin, fibronectin and collagen) and soluble factors (cytokines, chemokines and growth factors) and (2) a cellular compartment comprising haemopoietic cells and non-haemopoietic cells (fibroblasts, osteoblasts, osteoclasts, endothelial cells, endothelial progenitor cells, pericytes, mesenchymal stem cells and mesenchymal stromal cells) which support MM cell survival and growth [78]. The interaction between ECM proteins and bone marrow stromal cells (BMSCs) with MM cells plays a crucial role in MM pathogenesis and drug resistance by secreting growth factors, cytokines and extracellular vesicles (exosomes) and by the expression of adhesion proteins [78].

Various soluble factors have been shown to confer resistance to Bortezomib and other therapeutic agents in MM. IL-6 enhances vascular endothelial growth factor (VEGF) secretion promoting angiogenesis which plays a role in MM cell migration [79]. Whilst Bortezomib can inhibit IL-6 and VEGF production, secretion of IL-6 by stromal cells and MM cells leads to Bortezomib resistance [80]. Hepatocyte growth factor (HGF) is upregulated during MM progression, enhancing the expression of its receptor, c-MET [81]. This signalling pathway is constitutively activated in MM cells and endothelial cells from patients with relapsed/refractory MM and mediates drug resistance [82]. Accordingly, an inhibitory effect on endothelial cells obtained from patients refractory to Bortezomib or Lenalidomide was demonstrated using the c-MET inhibitor SU11274 alone or in combination with Bortezomib or Lenalidomide, resulting in downregulation of angiogenic activity [83].

Constitutive activation of pro-survival signalling pathways (e.g. NF-κB and AKT) has been reported to reduce the sensitivity of MM cells to Bortezomib [84]. Insulin-like growth factor (IGF-1) is produced by plasma cells and is present in the BM microenvironment, where it promotes proliferation and drug resistance in MM cells through activation of MAPK and PI3K/AKT signalling cascades [85]. Over-expression of IGF-1/IGF-1R pathway components has been shown to be a potential mechanism for resistance to proteasome inhibitors with blockade of downstream IGF-1 effectors able to resensitise MM cell lines to Bortezomib [86]. Studies evaluating compounds that affect the IGF-1/IGF-1R interaction are ongoing with OSI-906, a small molecule inhibitor of IGF-1R, able to resensitise MM cells to Bortezomib [86]. A downstream target of IGF-1, AKT, increases in expression in response to proteasome inhibitors in pre-clinical MM studies and an early phase clinical trial suggests that AKT inhibition might overcome resistance to Bortezomib [87]. As previously discussed, reduced expression of tight junction protein 1 (TJP1/ZO-1) and downstream activation of EGFR signalling are strongly correlated with Bortezomib resistance [47].

Interactions between MM cells and the BM stroma and/or ECM components provide a mechanism whereby MM cells are protected from the cytotoxic effects of anti-MM therapies. Such interactions include those mediated by adhesion molecules of the integrin family, Syndecan-1 (CD138), CD44, vascular cell adhesion molecule-1 (VCAM-1), lymphocyte function-associated antigen-1 (LFA-1), Mucin-1 antigen (MUC-1) and intercellular adhesion molecule-1 (ICAM-1) [88]. The adhesion of MM cells to stromal cells triggers IL-6 secretion, NF-κB activation in stromal cells and activation of signalling pathways that result in MM cell survival and proliferation [88]. Such effects are seen with integrin β7 which increases MM cell adhesion, migration and homing into bone marrow and reduces Melphalan and Bortezomib-induced apoptosis [89]. Similar MM-promoting effects have been reported for the stromal cell-derived factor (SDF-1)/CXCR4 axis, however, clinical translation has not ensued [90].

Other important mechanisms of BMME-induced drug resistance are emerging. BMSCs can modulate certain miRNAs in MM cells [91]. The expression of miR-27a is associated with

Bortezomib resistance in MM patients [91] whilst suppression of miR-15a and -16 by BMSCs was shown to be responsible for the protection of MM cells from Bortezomib-induced apoptosis [91]. miR-29 acts as a tumour suppressor miRNA and is downregulated in patient MM cells and in MM cell lines with acquired resistance to Bortezomib, Carfilzomib and Ixazomib [91]. Finally, exosomes mediate local cell-cell signalling by transferring mRNAs, miRNAs and proteins. It has been shown that exosomes derived from BMSCs inhibited Bortezomib-induced cell death to protect MM cells from apoptosis [92].

2.3.7.2. Clinical studies to circumvent resistance

In a phase II study, the anti-IL-6 antibody Siltuximab was administered with Dexamethasone to patients with relapsed and/or refractory MM [93]. Although no responses to Siltuximab alone were observed, the addition of Dexamethasone resulted in ORR, PFS and OS of 23%, 3.7 months and 20.4 months, respectively. Despite these findings, this strategy has not progressed further. The c-MET inhibitor Tivantinib was examined as a single agent in a phase II study in relapsed/refractory MM patients [94]. Overall, 36% of patients showed stable disease as their best response with the authors concluding that Tivantinib did not show promise for unselected relapsed/refractory MM patients, however, the fact that a significant proportion did show disease stability suggests combining c-MET inhibition with other anti-MM therapy could be explored. There are a small number of phase I studies employing a monoclonal anti-IGF-1R antibody alone or in combination with Bortezomib in relapsed/refractory MM, however, the authors of one study conclude that due to low response rates, even in combination with Bortezomib, further development is not justified [95]. Note should be made that patient recruitment into this study was not performed based on evaluation of IGF-1R expression on patient MM cells. No small molecule inhibitors of IGF-1R have so far been tested clinically. A phase I clinical trial in relapsed/refractory MM patients suggests that AKT inhibition with Afuresertib might overcome resistance to Bortezomib [87]. In this study, the ORR was 8.8%, however, despite these potentially promising results in heavily pre-treated patients, more advanced clinical trials have not been undertaken.

3. Immunomodulatory agents

The immunomodulatory drugs (IMiDs), Thalidomide, Lenalidomide and Pomalidomide have also made a major impact in the management of MM. Despite a checkered history in the 1950s and 1960s due to teratogenicity, Thalidomide has high anti-MM activity and has been incorporated into many treatment regimens. The second generation IMiD Lenalidomide and third generation IMiD Pomalidomide represent sequential improvements in efficacy and toxicity profiles with demonstrable activity in patients who have developed resistance to an earlier generation IMiD [96]. With regard to Lenalidomide, the MM-009 [97] and MM-010 [98] phase III trials demonstrated the superiority of Lenalidomide and Dexamethasone over Dexamethasone in relapsed/refractory MM patients whilst the pivotal MM-003 study [99] demonstrated the efficacy of Pomalidomide and Dexamethasone in MM patients who were refractory to both Bortezomib and Lenalidomide.

http://dx.doi.org/10.5772/intechopen.77004

The anti-MM effects of IMiDs are related to their binding to the E3 ubiquitin ligase cereblon (CRBN) and subsequent ubiquitination and degradation of two B-cell transcription factors, Ikaros (IKZF1) and Aiolos (IKZF3) [96]. A landmark study identified CRBN as a primary target in Thalidomide teratogenicity, further demonstrating that Thalidomide binds to CRBN, disrupting the function of the E3 ubiquitin ligase complex, ultimately leading to the downregulation of fibroblast growth factor genes and the teratogenic effects associated with Thalidomide [100]. Subsequently, it was shown that the anti-MM efficacy of IMiDs is directly related to CRBN expression.

3.1. Mechanisms of resistance to immunomodulatory agents

3.1.1. Pre-clinical/clinical findings

Resistance mechanisms to IMiDs have been elucidated to a far lesser extent than have those for proteasome inhibitors (**Table 1** and **Figure 1B**) and mostly hinge on the presence of functional CRBN in MM cells [100]. MM patients exposed to and thought to be resistant to Lenalidomide had lower CRBN levels compared to paired samples before and after therapy [101]. Subsequently, it was shown that high expression of CRBN is associated with a favourable response to Thalidomide and Lenalidomide in newly-diagnosed MM patients [102, 103] and no IMiD response occurred in patients with very low CRBN levels [104]. Moreover, in MM patients refractory to Pomalidomide, CRBN levels predicted for differences in PFS (3 versus 8.9 months) and OS (9.1 versus 27.2 months) when comparing patients in the lowest CRBN expression quartile versus those with higher expression [104]. Notably, as CRBN expression decreases in MM patients who develop resistance to Lenalidomide therapy, this does not affect sensitivity to Bortezomib, Melphalan and Dexamethasone [101, 105]. Low levels of the CRBN binding protein IKZF1 and high levels of another CRBN binding protein Karyopherin Subunit Alpha 2 (KPNA2) also correlated with lack of response to Pomalidomide and/or OS [106]. Specifically, patients with low IKZF1 expression had a median OS of 7.3 months compared with 27.2 months in those with higher IKZF1 expression which was also correlated with a similar pattern of PFS (4.9 vs. 7.3 months) [106].

In relapsed/refractory MM patients, the majority (88%) of whom were refractory to an IMiD, an increased prevalence of mutations in the Ras pathway genes KRAS, NRAS and/or BRAF (72%), as well as TP53 (26%), CRBN (12%) and CRBN pathway genes (10%) were observed [107]. Notably, all CRBN-mutated patients and 91% of the CRBN pathway-mutated patients were unresponsive to IMiD based treatment. Moreover, three patients with CRBN mutations at the time of IMiD resistance did not possess these genetic aberrations at the time of IMiD sensitivity. Importantly, the introduction of these mutations in MM cells conferred Lenalidomide resistance *in vitro* [107]. Finally, a pre-clinical study has demonstrated that Lenalidomide resistant MM models over-express the hyaluronan (HA)-binding protein CD44, a downstream Wnt/β-catenin transcriptional target [108]. Consistent with this hypothesis, Lenalidomide resistant MM cell lines show greater adhesion to bone marrow stromal cells. Inhibition of CD44 by application of the humanised monoclonal anti-CD44 antibody RO5429083 induced a modest anti-proliferative effect whilst shRNA-mediated CD44 knockdown resulted in a marked re-sensitisation to Lenalidomide [108].

3.1.2. Clinical studies to circumvent resistance

Whilst the CRBN pathway has been shown to be pivotal in IMiD responsiveness, no clinical studies have eventuated that make use of this important biology as a strategy to overcome resistance to IMiDs and many questions remain such as how much functional CRBN is actually required to maintain IMiD sensitivity. Despite the controversies surrounding CRBN, activating mutations in Ras pathway components, such as KRAS G12D and BRAF V600E, could potentially be targeted with existing compounds in MM patients harbouring these mutations [109]. Such studies have not yet been conducted, although two patients with BRAF V600E positive relapsed/refractory MM achieved significant reductions in tumour burden when treated with the BRAF inhibitor Vemurafenib whilst a patient with highly resistant and rapidly progressive MM also harbouring the BRAF V600E mutation achieved a rapid and sustained response with dual BRAF and MEK inhibition [110].

4. Monoclonal antibodies

Binding of monoclonal antibody (mAb) to its target antigen on MM cells has been shown to induce cell death through several mechanisms including antibody-dependent cell-mediated cytotoxicity (ADCC), complement-dependent cytotoxicity (CDC), antibody-dependent cellular phagocytosis (ADCP), induction of apoptosis through FcγR-mediated crosslinking of tumour-bound antibodies and modulation of target antigen enzymatic activity after antibody binding [111]. Three mAbs, Daratumumab, Elotuzumab and Pembrolizumab have advanced to phase III clinical trials with Daratumumab the most successful of these.

CD38 is variably expressed on haemopoietic and some non-haemopoietic cells with surface expression depending on the differentiation and activation status of the cell. High cell surface expression occurs on benign and malignant plasma cells [111] with the fully-humanised anti-CD38 mAb Daratumumab demonstrating impressive outcomes when combined with Bortezomib (CASTOR) or Lenalidomide (POLLUX) in the relapsed/refractory MM setting [112, 113]. Other CD38 mAbs, such as Isatuximab (chimeric) and MOR202 (fully human), with differing biological activities from Daratumumab are currently being evaluated in clinical trials (Isatuximab: NCT03275285, NCT03319667, NCT02990338; MOR202: NCT01421186). Elotuzumab binds to signalling lymphocytic activation molecule family member 7 (SLAM7) reducing MM cell binding to bone marrow stroma and activating ADCC [114]. Interestingly, whilst no responses to Elotuzumab as a single agent were observed, the addition of Elotuzumab to Lenalidomide and Dexamethasone in relapsed/refractory MM patients (ELOQUENT-2 trial) resulted in improvements in ORR and PFS, and Elotuzumab is currently the subject of ongoing clinical trials (NCT01891643, NCT02495922, NCT01335399) [115]. Pembrolizumab targets the programmed death 1 (PD-1)/programmed cell death ligand 1 (PD-L1) pathway, a critical initiator of immune activation, playing a role in mediating tolerance [116]. However, two phase III trials KEYNOTE-183 and KEYNOTE-185 have recently been suspended by the US Food and Drug Administration due to more deaths being observed in the Pembrolizumab arms and further information on the use of Pembrolizumab in MM is pending.

4.1. Mechanisms of resistance to monoclonal antibodies

4.1.1. *Pre-clinical/clinical findings*

The relatively recent addition of mAbs to MM pharmacotherapy means there is a paucity of studies examining resistance mechanisms although these are now being explored with their increasing clinical use (**Table 1** and **Figure 1C**). Examination of CD38 expression on MM cells in 102 patients treated with Daratumumab monotherapy has been insightful [117]. With regard to the effect of Daratumumab on residual bone marrow plasma cells, two important points were clear from this analysis. Firstly, CD38 cell surface expression on plasma cells is highest before Daratumumab treatment and is significantly decreased during treatment. At the time of progressive disease, plasma cells isolated from the bone marrow of these patients exhibited low expression of CD38 suggesting Daratumumab therapy would be less effective, a finding corroborated previously [76]. Secondly, pre-treatment CD38 expression on the surface of MM cells was higher in patients who achieved at least a PR compared to those who did not. Recently, it was shown that Daratumumab-CD38 complexes and accompanying cell membrane are actively transferred from MM cells to monocytes and granulocytes in a process called trogocytosis that was also associated with reduced MM cell surface expression of CD49d, CD56 and CD138 [118]. However, Daratumumab-induced reductions in CD38 expression on MM cells occur in patients with deep and durable responses suggesting reductions in CD38 alone are not responsible for Daratumumab resistance [118]. Cell surface expression of the complement-inhibitory proteins, CD46, CD55 and CD59, was not associated with clinical response but significantly increased only at the time of disease progression. Furthermore, all-*trans* retinoic acid increased CD38 expression whilst decreasing expression of CD55 and CD59 on MM cells from patients who developed Daratumumab resistance to approximately pre-treatment levels, resulting in enhancement of Daratumumab-mediated CDC [117].

In addition to the cell surface expression of target antigens on MM cells, several other potential mechanisms of resistance to mAbs may be at play. Soluble forms of CD38 [119] and SLAM7 [120] may affect the efficacy of Daratumumab and Elotuzumab, respectively. Another potential mechanism of resistance is the development of neutralising antibodies to the therapeutic antibody. This phenomenon was noted in 39% of patients treated with single agent Elotuzumab resulting in more pronounced effects on serum Elotuzumab concentrations [121]. Furthermore, in the ELOQUENT-2 trial, 15% of patients developed anti-Elotuzumab antibodies on at least one occasion [115], however, antibodies directed against Daratumumab have to this day not been detected. Other factors that may contribute to the clinical efficacy of mAb therapy include the frequency and activity of effector immune cells [122], Fcγ receptor polymorphisms [123] and even KIR and HLA genotypes [124].

4.1.2. *Clinical studies to circumvent resistance*

Whilst the mechanisms of resistance to mAbs are being elucidated, clinical studies specifically designed to overcome these biological processes are largely lacking with the exception of an ongoing phase I/II trial of Daratumumab in combination with all-*trans* retinoic acid for patients with relapsed/refractory MM (NCT02751255).

5. Other factors potentially influencing resistance to myeloma therapies

5.1. Cytogenetics, mutation patterns and clonal evolution

Cytogenetic abnormalities in MM are broadly divided into copy number changes or translocations, most commonly involving the immunoglobulin heavy chain gene [125]. Various cytogenetic abnormalities were shown to be associated with the likelihood of durable responses to therapy but they do not directly explain mechanisms of drug resistance or disease progression [126]. High risk genetic features frequently result in the dysregulation of transcription factors or tumour suppressors and include t(4;14), t(14;16), t(16;20), del(17p) and copy number changes of chromosome 1, which are used for stratifying MM patients in clinical trials and are now becoming important in guiding therapy in routine practice [126]. For example, the EMN02/HO95 study demonstrated the benefit of double autologous stem cell transplantation in patient with high-risk genetics, essentially negating the adverse prognosis of high genetic risk MM [127]. Similarly, the addition of Bortezomib to induction regimens in patients receiving HDM/ASCT may partially overcome cytogenetically defined poor risk [128]. On the other hand, patients with trisomies may respond particularly well to lenalidomide based protocols [129]. Mutational events such as those involving p53 are associated with particularly poor PFS, however, the significant heterogeneity of point mutational events elucidated in whole exome sequencing studies means generalisations of such molecular changes are not possible [130].

The development of whole exome sequencing and copy number profiling was combined with cytogenetics in a landmark paper by a consortium of European and American groups [131]. This elegant paper demonstrated that the majority of MM patients had multiple sub-clones present at the time of diagnosis and that within sub-clones there could be differing mutational events potentially driving behaviour [131]. When serial MM samples were analysed, diverse patterns of clonal evolution were detected. In some cases, simple clonal selection could be observed following a linear pattern of clonal evolution [131]. Differential clonal responses could explain the clinical observation that a MM patient may respond to a treatment initially, lose this response, respond to another treatment and at the time of subsequent relapse respond again to the initial therapy [132]. Branching evolution was also observed in some progressing patients [131]. During disease evolution differing processes may contribute to the mutational repertoire and the relative contributions may vary over time in the same patient resulting in mutational heterogeneity, frequently with very few recurrent genes [131].

5.2. The myeloma stem cell

Identification of the multiple myeloma stem cell (MMSC) has been a challenge predominantly because an agreed phenotype with MM propagating potential has not been definitively established, in part due to differences in experimental techniques and assays. The dominant viewpoint is that clonotypic $CD138^{-}$ cells represent MMSCs, however, some researchers have also shown that clonotypic $CD138^{+}$ plasma cells have properties of cancer stem cells such as self-renewal, tumour-initiating potential and drug resistance [133, 134]. Controversy also exists as to whether the MMSC derives from a clonotypic B cell ($CD19^+CD138^-$) or clonotypic non-B cell ($CD19^-CD138^{+/-}$). Clonotypic B cells were found to be resistant to a range of anti-MM therapies including Bortezomib and Lenalidomide and possessed a high drug efflux capacity [135]. However, clonotypic non-B cells have also been shown in many studies to result in robust MM reconstitution in the absence of a $CD19^+$ population [136]. To shed some light on this dichotomy with respect to clonotypic non-B cells, there appears to be an interconversion between undifferentiated pre-plasma cells ($CD19^-CD138^-$) and differentiated plasma cells ($CD19^-CD138^+$) thus representing reversible, bi-directional phenotypic and functional states that share MMSC activity [137]. Furthermore, the pre-plasma cells were found to be more quiescent, primarily located at extramedullary sites, and up to 300-fold more drug resistant to agents including Bortezomib [137]. These informative findings imply phenotypic and functional plasticity between undifferentiated and differentiated clonotypic plasma cells which could explain why differentiated MM plasma cells possess clonogenic capacity and also reconciles inconsistencies surrounding the MMSC phenotype.

Several factors have been attributed to the MMSC that confer drug resistance. (1) Side population (SP) MM cells, which possess stem-like properties, show stronger activity of several ABC transporters when compared to main population (MP) cells [138]. (2) High levels of aldehyde dehydrogenase (ALDH) have been demonstrated in $CD138^-$ plasma cells compared to their $CD138^+$ counterparts rendering the $CD138^-$ population more resistant to certain chemotherapeutic agents which result in the generation of toxic aldehyde intermediates that are metabolised by ALDH1 [135]. In one study, forced expression of member A1 of the ALDH1 family of proteins resulted in resistance to Bortezomib [139]. (3) Increased expression of Bcl-2 family members in MMSCs expressing the retinoid acid receptor alpha 2 (RARα2) endowed these cells with increased drug resistance [140], and more recently, increased expression of Bruton's tyrosine kinase (BTK) in MMSCs also induced drug resistance [141]. (4) $CD19^-CD138^+$ plasma cells and $CD19^-CD138^-$ pre-plasma cells harbour MMSC activity but exhibit differential resistance to treatment since pre-plasma cells are more quiescent than plasma cells, shown by a lower proportion of these cells in S phase of the cell cycle [137]. Finally, (5) the Wingless (Wnt), Hedgehog and Notch signalling pathways are all highly active in MMSCs and may be responsible for maintaining stem cell properties, propagating MM and promoting therapeutic resistance together with a supportive and protective BMME [142].

6. Conclusion

Continued improvements in the efficacy and toxicity profiles of an ever-expanding number of novel MM therapies are challenging the current paradigm of high-dose therapy and autologous stem cell transplantation for newly-diagnosed MM. However, despite these advances, resistance to novel agents has been observed and will continue to be observed, requiring innovative ways to circumvent this problem. Changing therapy from one novel agent containing treatment regimen to a different one upon MM progression or relapse is reasonable, however, there is often little scientific basis for choosing the sequence of such regimens and the era of precision medicine for MM patients remains distant. Moreover, the inability to tailor treatment regimens for an individual patient based on the biology of their MM due to government mandated prescribing restrictions likely contributes to inadequate responses and drug resistance.

In addition to those discussed, there are other potential mechanisms through which resistance to novel therapies in MM may occur, such as the role miRNAs play in promoting MM, and this list is likely to increase. However, despite the varied resistance mechanisms reported to date, the survival of patients with MM continues to improve. Whilst genetic profiling has established a so-called high-risk group of MM patients, these genetic changes do not specifically explain why resistance to a particular novel agent develops. Thus, in this Chapter, an exposition of specific biological aberrations that have been linked to drug resistance has been presented.

Acknowledgements

We would like to thank the staff of the Haematology Department at Flinders Medical Centre, South Australia, for their ongoing support and encouragement to produce this Chapter.

Conflict of interest

The authors have no conflicts of interest to declare.

Author details

Craig T. Wallington-Beddoe[1,2,3,4]* and Douglas W. Coghlan[1,2]

*Address all correspondence to: craig.wallington-beddoe@sa.gov.au

1 Flinders Medical Centre, Bedford Park, South Australia

2 College of Medicine and Public Health, Flinders University, Bedford Park, South Australia

3 Centre for Cancer Biology, University of South Australia and SA Pathology, South Australia

4 Faculty of Health and Medical Sciences, University of Adelaide, South Australia

References

[1] Mikkilineni L, Kochenderfer JN. Chimeric antigen receptor t-cell therapies for multiple myeloma. Blood. 2017;**130**:2594-2602. DOI: 10.1182/blood-2017-06-793869

[2] Vincenz L, Jager R, O'Dwyer M, Samali A. Endoplasmic reticulum stress and the unfolded protein response: Targeting the achilles heel of multiple myeloma. Molecular Cancer Therapeutics. 2013;**12**:831-843. DOI: 10.1158/1535-7163.MCT-12-0782

[3] Accardi F, Toscani D, Bolzoni M, Dalla Palma B, Aversa F, Giuliani N. Mechanism of action of bortezomib and the new proteasome inhibitors on myeloma cells and the bone microenvironment: Impact on myeloma-induced alterations of bone remodeling. BioMed Research International. 2015;**2015**:172458. DOI: 10.1155/2015/172458

[4] Streich FC Jr, Lima CD. Structural and functional insights to ubiquitin-like protein conjugation. Annual Review of Biophysics. 2014;**43**:357-379. DOI: 10.1146/annurev-biophys-051013-022958

[5] Walden H, Podgorski MS, Schulman BA. Insights into the ubiquitin transfer cascade from the structure of the activating enzyme for nedd8. Nature. 2003;**422**:330-334. DOI: 10.1038/nature01456

[6] Ciechanover A. Proteolysis: From the lysosome to ubiquitin and the proteasome. Nature Reviews. Molecular Cell Biology. 2005;**6**:79-87. DOI: 10.1038/nrm1552

[7] Coux O, Tanaka K, Goldberg AL. Structure and functions of the 20s and 26s proteasomes. Annual Review of Biochemistry. 1996;**65**:801-847. DOI: 10.1146/annurev.bi.65.070196.004101

[8] Baumeister W, Walz J, Zuhl F, Seemuller E. The proteasome: Paradigm of a self-compartmentalizing protease. Cell. 1998;**92**:367-380

[9] Glickman MH, Rubin DM, Coux O, Wefes I, Pfeifer G, Cjeka Z, et al. A subcomplex of the proteasome regulatory particle required for ubiquitin-conjugate degradation and related to the cop9-signalosome and eif3. Cell. 1998;**94**:615-623

[10] Heinemeyer W, Fischer M, Krimmer T, Stachon U, Wolf DH. The active sites of the eukaryotic 20 s proteasome and their involvement in subunit precursor processing. The Journal of Biological Chemistry. 1997;**272**:25200-25209

[11] Chen P, Hochstrasser M. Autocatalytic subunit processing couples active site formation in the 20s proteasome to completion of assembly. Cell. 1996;**86**:961-972

[12] Ditzel L, Huber R, Mann K, Heinemeyer W, Wolf DH, Groll M. Conformational constraints for protein self-cleavage in the proteasome. Journal of Molecular Biology. 1998; **279**:1187-1191. DOI: 10.1006/jmbi.1998.1818

[13] Nussbaum AK, Dick TP, Keilholz W, Schirle M, Stevanovic S, Dietz K, et al. Cleavage motifs of the yeast 20s proteasome beta subunits deduced from digests of enolase 1. Proceedings of the National Academy of Sciences of the United States of America. 1998;**95**:12504-12509

[14] Arendt CS, Hochstrasser M. Identification of the yeast 20s proteasome catalytic centers and subunit interactions required for active-site formation. Proceedings of the National Academy of Sciences of the United States of America. 1997;**94**:7156-7161

[15] Dick TP, Nussbaum AK, Deeg M, Heinemeyer W, Groll M, Schirle M, et al. Contribution of proteasomal beta-subunits to the cleavage of peptide substrates analyzed with yeast mutants. The Journal of Biological Chemistry. 1998;**273**:25637-25646

[16] Akopian TN, Kisselev AF, Goldberg AL. Processive degradation of proteins and other catalytic properties of the proteasome from *Thermoplasma acidophilum*. The Journal of Biological Chemistry. 1997;**272**:1791-1798

[17] Kisselev AF, Akopian TN, Goldberg AL. Range of sizes of peptide products generated during degradation of different proteins by archaeal proteasomes. The Journal of Biological Chemistry. 1998;**273**:1982-1989

[18] Groll M, Heinemeyer W, Jager S, Ullrich T, Bochtler M, Wolf DH, et al. The catalytic sites of 20s proteasomes and their role in subunit maturation: A mutational and crystallographic study. Proceedings of the National Academy of Sciences of the United States of America. 1999;**96**:10976-10983

[19] Glynne R, Powis SH, Beck S, Kelly A, Kerr LA, Trowsdale J. A proteasome-related gene between the two abc transporter loci in the class ii region of the human mhc. Nature. 1991;**353**:357-360. DOI: 10.1038/353357a0

[20] Martinez CK, Monaco JJ. Homology of proteasome subunits to a major histocompatibility complex-linked lmp gene. Nature. 1991;**353**:664-667. DOI: 10.1038/353664a0

[21] Nandi D, Jiang H, Monaco JJ. Identification of mecl-1 (lmp-10) as the third IFN-gamma-inducible proteasome subunit. Journal of Immunology. 1996;**156**:2361-2364

[22] Altun M, Galardy PJ, Shringarpure R, Hideshima T, LeBlanc R, Anderson KC, et al. Effects of ps-341 on the activity and composition of proteasomes in multiple myeloma cells. Cancer Research. 2005;**65**:7896-7901. DOI: 10.1158/0008-5472.CAN-05-0506

[23] Busse A, Kraus M, Na IK, Rietz A, Scheibenbogen C, Driessen C, et al. Sensitivity of tumor cells to proteasome inhibitors is associated with expression levels and composition of proteasome subunits. Cancer. 2008;**112**:659-670. DOI: 10.1002/cncr.23224

[24] Kuhn DJ, Hunsucker SA, Chen Q, Voorhees PM, Orlowski M, Orlowski RZ. Targeted inhibition of the immunoproteasome is a potent strategy against models of multiple myeloma that overcomes resistance to conventional drugs and nonspecific proteasome inhibitors. Blood. 2009;**113**:4667-4676. DOI: 10.1182/blood-2008-07-171637

[25] Parlati F, Lee SJ, Aujay M, Suzuki E, Levitsky K, Lorens JB, et al. Carfilzomib can induce tumor cell death through selective inhibition of the chymotrypsin-like activity of the proteasome. Blood. 2009;**114**:3439-3447. DOI: 10.1182/blood-2009-05-223677

[26] Kubiczkova L, Pour L, Sedlarikova L, Hajek R, Sevcikova S. Proteasome inhibitors—Molecular basis and current perspectives in multiple myeloma. Journal of Cellular and Molecular Medicine. 2014;**18**:947-961. DOI: 10.1111/jcmm.12279

[27] Hideshima T, Ikeda H, Chauhan D, Okawa Y, Raje N, Podar K, et al. Bortezomib induces canonical nuclear factor-kappab activation in multiple myeloma cells. Blood. 2009;**114**:1046-1052. DOI: 10.1182/blood-2009-01-199604

[28] Kuhn DJ, Chen Q, Voorhees PM, Strader JS, Shenk KD, Sun CM, et al. Potent activity of carfilzomib, a novel, irreversible inhibitor of the ubiquitin-proteasome pathway, against

preclinical models of multiple myeloma. Blood. 2007;**110**:3281-3290. DOI: 10.1182/blood-2007-01-065888

[29] Stewart AK, Rajkumar SV, Dimopoulos MA, Masszi T, Spicka I, Oriol A, et al. Carfilzomib, lenalidomide, and dexamethasone for relapsed multiple myeloma. The New England Journal of Medicine. 2015;**372**:142-152. DOI: 10.1056/NEJMoa1411321

[30] Moreau P, Masszi T, Grzasko N, Bahlis NJ, Hansson M, Pour L, et al. Oral ixazomib, lenalidomide, and dexamethasone for multiple myeloma. The New England Journal of Medicine. 2016;**374**:1621-1634. DOI: 10.1056/NEJMoa1516282

[31] Bonnet A, Moreau P. Safety of ixazomib for the treatment of multiple myeloma. Expert Opinion on Drug Safety. 2017;**16**:973-980. DOI: 10.1080/14740338.2017.1344212

[32] Chauhan D, Catley L, Li G, Podar K, Hideshima T, Velankar M, et al. A novel orally active proteasome inhibitor induces apoptosis in multiple myeloma cells with mechanisms distinct from bortezomib. Cancer Cell. 2005;**8**:407-419. DOI: 10.1016/j.ccr.2005.10.013

[33] Richardson PG, Zimmerman TM, Hofmeister CC, Talpaz M, Chanan-Khan AA, Kaufman JL, et al. Phase 1 study of marizomib in relapsed or relapsed and refractory multiple myeloma: Npi-0052-101 part 1. Blood. 2016;**127**:2693-2700. DOI: 10.1182/blood-2015-12-686378

[34] Spencer A, Harrison S, Zonder J, Badros A, Laubach J, Bergin K, et al. A phase 1 clinical trial evaluating marizomib, pomalidomide and low-dose dexamethasone in relapsed and refractory multiple myeloma (npi-0052-107): Final study results. British Journal of Haematology. 2018;**180**:41-51. DOI: 10.1111/bjh.14987

[35] Badros A, Singh Z, Dhakal B, Kwok Y, MacLaren A, Richardson P, et al. Marizomib for central nervous system-multiple myeloma. British Journal of Haematology. 2017;**177**:221-225. DOI: 10.1111/bjh.14498

[36] Chauhan D, Singh AV, Aujay M, Kirk CJ, Bandi M, Ciccarelli B, et al. A novel orally active proteasome inhibitor onx 0912 triggers in vitro and in vivo cytotoxicity in multiple myeloma. Blood. 2010;**116**:4906-4915. DOI: 10.1182/blood-2010-04-276626

[37] Oerlemans R, Franke NE, Assaraf YG, Cloos J, van Zantwijk I, Berkers CR, et al. Molecular basis of bortezomib resistance: Proteasome subunit beta5 (psmb5) gene mutation and overexpression of psmb5 protein. Blood. 2008;**112**:2489-2499. DOI: 10.1182/blood-2007-08-104950

[38] Lu S, Chen Z, Yang J, Chen L, Gong S, Zhou H, et al. Overexpression of the psmb5 gene contributes to bortezomib resistance in t-lymphoblastic lymphoma/leukemia cells derived from jurkat line. Experimental Hematology. 2008;**36**:1278-1284. DOI: 10.1016/j.exphem.2008.04.013

[39] Lu S, Yang J, Song X, Gong S, Zhou H, Guo L, et al. Point mutation of the proteasome beta5 subunit gene is an important mechanism of bortezomib resistance in bortezomib-selected variants of jurkat t cell lymphoblastic lymphoma/leukemia line. The Journal of Pharmacology and Experimental Therapeutics. 2008;**326**:423-431. DOI: 10.1124/jpet.108.138131

[40] Balsas P, Galan-Malo P, Marzo I, Naval J. Bortezomib resistance in a myeloma cell line is associated to psmbeta5 overexpression and polyploidy. Leukemia Research. 2012;**36**:212-218. DOI: 10.1016/j.leukres.2011.09.011

[41] Ri M, Iida S, Nakashima T, Miyazaki H, Mori F, Ito A, et al. Bortezomib-resistant myeloma cell lines: A role for mutated psmb5 in preventing the accumulation of unfolded proteins and fatal ER stress. Leukemia. 2010;**24**:1506-1512. DOI: 10.1038/leu.2010.137

[42] Chapman MA, Lawrence MS, Keats JJ, Cibulskis K, Sougnez C, Schinzel AC, et al. Initial genome sequencing and analysis of multiple myeloma. Nature. 2011;**471**:467-472. DOI: 10.1038/nature09837

[43] Lichter DI, Danaee H, Pickard MD, Tayber O, Sintchak M, Shi HL, et al. Sequence analysis of beta-subunit genes of the 20s proteasome in patients with relapsed multiple myeloma treated with bortezomib or dexamethasone. Blood. 2012;**120**:4513-4516. DOI: 10.1182/blood-2012-05-426924

[44] Barrio S, Stühmer T, Teufel E, Barrio-Garcia C, Chatterjee M, Schreder M, et al. Parallel evolution of multiple *psmb5* mutations in a myeloma patient treated with bortezomib. Blood. 2016;**128**:3282-3282

[45] Fuchs D, Berges C, Opelz G, Daniel V, Naujokat C. Increased expression and altered subunit composition of proteasomes induced by continuous proteasome inhibition establish apoptosis resistance and hyperproliferation of Burkitt lymphoma cells. Journal of Cellular Biochemistry. 2008;**103**:270-283. DOI: 10.1002/jcb.21405

[46] Garcia-Mata R, Bebok Z, Sorscher EJ, Sztul ES. Characterization and dynamics of aggresome formation by a cytosolic GFP-chimera. The Journal of Cell Biology. 1999;**146**: 1239-1254

[47] Zhang XD, Baladandayuthapani V, Lin H, Mulligan G, Li B, Esseltine DW, et al. Tight junction protein 1 modulates proteasome capacity and proteasome inhibitor sensitivity in multiple myeloma via egfr/jak1/stat3 signaling. Cancer Cell. 2016;**29**:639-652. DOI: 10.1016/j.ccell.2016.03.026

[48] Kawaguchi Y, Kovacs JJ, McLaurin A, Vance JM, Ito A, Yao TP. The deacetylase hdac6 regulates aggresome formation and cell viability in response to misfolded protein stress. Cell. 2003;**115**:727-738

[49] McConkey DJ, White M, Yan W. Hdac inhibitor modulation of proteotoxicity as a therapeutic approach in cancer. Advances in Cancer Research. 2012;**116**:131-163. DOI: 10.1016/B978-0-12-394387-3.00004-5

[50] Hideshima T, Bradner JE, Wong J, Chauhan D, Richardson P, Schreiber SL, et al. Small-molecule inhibition of proteasome and aggresome function induces synergistic antitumor activity in multiple myeloma. Proceedings of the National Academy of Sciences of the United States of America. 2005;**102**:8567-8572. DOI: 10.1073/pnas.0503221102

[51] Catley L, Weisberg E, Kiziltepe T, Tai YT, Hideshima T, Neri P, et al. Aggresome induction by proteasome inhibitor bortezomib and alpha-tubulin hyperacetylation by tubulin

deacetylase (tdac) inhibitor lbh589 are synergistic in myeloma cells. Blood. 2006;**108**:3441-3449. DOI: 10.1182/blood-2006-04-016055

[52] San-Miguel JF, Hungria VT, Yoon SS, Beksac M, Dimopoulos MA, Elghandour A, et al. Panobinostat plus bortezomib and dexamethasone versus placebo plus bortezomib and dexamethasone in patients with relapsed or relapsed and refractory multiple myeloma: A multicentre, randomised, double-blind phase 3 trial. The Lancet Oncology. 2014;**15**:1195-1206. DOI: 10.1016/S1470-2045(14)70440-1

[53] Montanari F, Lu M, Marcus S, Saran A, Malankar A, Mazumder A. A phase ii trial of chloroquine in combination with bortezomib and cyclophosphamide in patients with relapsed and refractory multiple myeloma. Blood. 2014;**124**:5775

[54] Zhang L, Fok JH, Davies FE. Heat shock proteins in multiple myeloma. Oncotarget. 2014;**5**:1132-1148. DOI: 10.18632/oncotarget.1584

[55] Mitsiades N, Mitsiades CS, Poulaki V, Chauhan D, Fanourakis G, Gu X, et al. Molecular sequelae of proteasome inhibition in human multiple myeloma cells. Proceedings of the National Academy of Sciences of the United States of America. 2002;**99**:14374-14379. DOI: 10.1073/pnas.202445099

[56] Adomako A, Calvo V, Biran N, Osman K, Chari A, Paton JC, et al. Identification of markers that functionally define a quiescent multiple myeloma cell sub-population surviving bortezomib treatment. BMC Cancer. 2015;**15**:444. DOI: 10.1186/s12885-015-1460-1

[57] Steiner N, Borjan B, Hajek R, Johrer K, Gobel G, Willenbacher W, et al. Expression and release of glucose-regulated protein-78 (grp78) in multiple myeloma. Oncotarget. 2017;**8**: 56243-56254. DOI: 10.18632/oncotarget.17353

[58] Abdel Malek MA, Jagannathan S, Malek E, Sayed DM, Elgammal SA, Abd El-Azeem HG, et al. Molecular chaperone grp78 enhances aggresome delivery to autophagosomes to promote drug resistance in multiple myeloma. Oncotarget. 2015;**6**:3098-3110. DOI: 10.18632/oncotarget.3075

[59] Mitsiades CS, Mitsiades NS, McMullan CJ, Poulaki V, Kung AL, Davies FE, et al. Antimyeloma activity of heat shock protein-90 inhibition. Blood. 2006;**107**:1092-1100. DOI: 10.1182/blood-2005-03-1158

[60] Roue G, Perez-Galan P, Mozos A, Lopez-Guerra M, Xargay-Torrent S, Rosich L, et al. The hsp90 inhibitor ipi-504 overcomes bortezomib resistance in mantle cell lymphoma in vitro and in vivo by down-regulation of the prosurvival ER chaperone bip/grp78. Blood. 2011;**117**:1270-1279. DOI: 10.1182/blood-2010-04-278853

[61] Chauhan D, Li G, Shringarpure R, Podar K, Ohtake Y, Hideshima T, et al. Blockade of hsp27 overcomes bortezomib/proteasome inhibitor ps-341 resistance in lymphoma cells. Cancer Research. 2003;**63**:6174-6177

[62] Hamouda MA, Belhacene N, Puissant A, Colosetti P, Robert G, Jacquel A, et al. The small heat shock protein b8 (hspb8) confers resistance to bortezomib by promoting autophagic removal of misfolded proteins in multiple myeloma cells. Oncotarget. 2014;**5**:6252-6266. DOI: 10.18632/oncotarget.2193

[63] Rasche L, Menoret E, Dubljevic V, Menu E, Vanderkerken K, Lapa C, et al. A grp78-directed monoclonal antibody recaptures response in refractory multiple myeloma with extramedullary involvement. Clinical Cancer Research. 2016;**22**:4341-4349. DOI: 10.1158/1078-0432.CCR-15-3111

[64] Cavenagh J, Oakervee H, Baetiong-Caguioa P, Davies F, Gharibo M, Rabin N, et al. A phase i/ii study of kw-2478, an hsp90 inhibitor, in combination with bortezomib in patients with relapsed/refractory multiple myeloma. British Journal of Cancer. 2017;**117**: 1295-1302. DOI: 10.1038/bjc.2017.302

[65] Nigam SK. What do drug transporters really do? Nature Reviews. Drug Discovery. 2015;**14**:29-44. DOI: 10.1038/nrd4461

[66] Cornelissen JJ, Sonneveld P, Schoester M, Raaijmakers HG, Nieuwenhuis HK, Dekker AW, et al. Mdr-1 expression and response to vincristine, doxorubicin, and dexamethasone chemotherapy in multiple myeloma refractory to alkylating agents. Journal of Clinical Oncology. 1994;**12**:115-119. DOI: 10.1200/JCO.1994.12.1.115

[67] Grogan TM, Spier CM, Salmon SE, Matzner M, Rybski J, Weinstein RS, et al. P-glycoprotein expression in human plasma cell myeloma: Correlation with prior chemotherapy. Blood. 1993;**81**:490-495

[68] Lu S, Wang J. The resistance mechanisms of proteasome inhibitor bortezomib. Biomarker Research. 2013;**1**:13. DOI: 10.1186/2050-7771-1-13

[69] Dalton WS. Detection of multidrug resistance gene expression in multiple myeloma. Leukemia. 1997;**11**:1166-1169

[70] Verbrugge SE, Assaraf YG, Dijkmans BA, Scheffer GL, Al M, den Uyl D, et al. Inactivating psmb5 mutations and p-glycoprotein (multidrug resistance-associated protein/atp-binding cassette b1) mediate resistance to proteasome inhibitors: Ex vivo efficacy of (immuno) proteasome inhibitors in mononuclear blood cells from patients with rheumatoid arthritis. The Journal of Pharmacology and Experimental Therapeutics. 2012;**341**:174-182. DOI: 10.1124/jpet.111.187542

[71] Hawley TS, Riz I, Yang W, Wakabayashi Y, Depalma L, Chang YT, et al. Identification of an abcb1 (p-glycoprotein)-positive carfilzomib-resistant myeloma subpopulation by the pluripotent stem cell fluorescent dye cdy1. American Journal of Hematology. 2013;**88**:265-272. DOI: 10.1002/ajh.23387

[72] Besse A, Stolze SC, Rasche L, Weinhold N, Morgan GJ, Kraus M, et al. Carfilzomib resistance due to abcb1/mdr1 overexpression is overcome by nelfinavir and lopinavir in multiple myeloma. Leukemia. 2017;**32**:391-401. DOI: 10.1038/leu.2017.212

[73] Weniger MA, Rizzatti EG, Perez-Galan P, Liu D, Wang Q, Munson PJ, et al. Treatment-induced oxidative stress and cellular antioxidant capacity determine response to bortezomib in mantle cell lymphoma. Clinical Cancer Research. 2011;**17**:5101-5112. DOI: 10.1158/1078-0432.CCR-10-3367

[74] Stessman HA, Baughn LB, Sarver A, Xia T, Deshpande R, Mansoor A, et al. Profiling bortezomib resistance identifies secondary therapies in a mouse myeloma model. Molecular Cancer Therapeutics. 2013;**12**:1140-1150. DOI: 10.1158/1535-7163.MCT-12-1151

[75] Li B, Fu J, Chen P, Ge X, Li Y, Kuiatse I, et al. The nuclear factor (erythroid-derived 2)-like 2 and proteasome maturation protein axis mediate bortezomib resistance in multiple myeloma. The Journal of Biological Chemistry. 2015;**290**:29854-29868. DOI: 10.1074/jbc.M115.664953

[76] Leung-Hagesteijn C, Erdmann N, Cheung G, Keats JJ, Stewart AK, Reece DE, et al. Xbp1s-negative tumor b cells and pre-plasmablasts mediate therapeutic proteasome inhibitor resistance in multiple myeloma. Cancer Cell. 2013;**24**:289-304. DOI: 10.1016/j.ccr.2013.08.009

[77] Perez-Galan P, Mora-Jensen H, Weniger MA, Shaffer AL 3rd, Rizzatti EG, Chapman CM, et al. Bortezomib resistance in mantle cell lymphoma is associated with plasmacytic differentiation. Blood. 2011;**117**:542-552. DOI: 10.1182/blood-2010-02-269514

[78] Manier S, Sacco A, Leleu X, Ghobrial IM, Roccaro AM. Bone marrow microenvironment in multiple myeloma progression. Journal of Biomedicine & Biotechnology. 2012;**2012**:157496. DOI: 10.1155/2012/157496

[79] Vacca A, Ria R, Ribatti D, Semeraro F, Djonov V, Di Raimondo F, et al. A paracrine loop in the vascular endothelial growth factor pathway triggers tumor angiogenesis and growth in multiple myeloma. Haematologica. 2003;**88**:176-185

[80] Hao M, Zhang L, An G, Sui W, Yu Z, Zou D, et al. Suppressing mirna-15a/-16 expression by interleukin-6 enhances drug-resistance in myeloma cells. Journal of Hematology & Oncology. 2011;**4**:37. DOI: 10.1186/1756-8722-4-37

[81] Zhang YW, Su Y, Volpert OV, Vande Woude GF. Hepatocyte growth factor/scatter factor mediates angiogenesis through positive vegf and negative thrombospondin 1 regulation. Proceedings of the National Academy of Sciences of the United States of America. 2003;**100**:12718-12723. DOI: 10.1073/pnas.2135113100

[82] Moschetta M, Basile A, Ferrucci A, Frassanito MA, Rao L, Ria R, et al. Novel targeting of phospho-cmet overcomes drug resistance and induces antitumor activity in multiple myeloma. Clinical Cancer Research. 2013;**19**:4371-4382. DOI: 10.1158/1078-0432.CCR-13-0039

[83] Ferrucci A, Moschetta M, Frassanito MA, Berardi S, Catacchio I, Ria R, et al. A hgf/cmet autocrine loop is operative in multiple myeloma bone marrow endothelial cells and may represent a novel therapeutic target. Clinical Cancer Research. 2014;**20**:5796-5807. DOI: 10.1158/1078-0432.CCR-14-0847

[84] Markovina S, Callander NS, O'Connor SL, Kim J, Werndli JE, Raschko M, et al. Bortezomib-resistant nuclear factor-kappab activity in multiple myeloma cells. Molecular Cancer Research. 2008;**6**:1356-1364. DOI: 10.1158/1541-7786.MCR-08-0108

[85] Podar K, Chauhan D, Anderson KC. Bone marrow microenvironment and the identification of new targets for myeloma therapy. Leukemia. 2009;**23**:10-24. DOI: 10.1038/leu.2008.259

[86] Kuhn DJ, Berkova Z, Jones RJ, Woessner R, Bjorklund CC, Ma W, et al. Targeting the insulin-like growth factor-1 receptor to overcome bortezomib resistance in preclinical models of multiple myeloma. Blood. 2012;**120**:3260-3270. DOI: 10.1182/blood-2011-10-386789

[87] Spencer A, Yoon SS, Harrison SJ, Morris SR, Smith DA, Brigandi RA, et al. The novel akt inhibitor afuresertib shows favorable safety, pharmacokinetics, and clinical activity in multiple myeloma. Blood. 2014;**124**:2190-2195. DOI: 10.1182/blood-2014-03-559963

[88] Di Marzo L, Desantis V, Solimando AG, Ruggieri S, Annese T, Nico B, et al. Microenvironment drug resistance in multiple myeloma: Emerging new players. Oncotarget. 2016;**7**:60698-60711. DOI: 10.18632/oncotarget.10849

[89] Neri P, Ren L, Azab AK, Brentnall M, Gratton K, Klimowicz AC, et al. Integrin beta7-mediated regulation of multiple myeloma cell adhesion, migration, and invasion. Blood. 2011;**117**:6202-6213. DOI: 10.1182/blood-2010-06-292243

[90] Alsayed Y, Ngo H, Runnels J, Leleu X, Singha UK, Pitsillides CM, et al. Mechanisms of regulation of cxcr4/sdf-1 (cxcl12)-dependent migration and homing in multiple myeloma. Blood. 2007;**109**:2708-2717. DOI: 10.1182/blood-2006-07-035857

[91] Abdi J, Jian H, Chang H. Role of micro-RNAs in drug resistance of multiple myeloma. Oncotarget. 2016;**7**:60723-60735. DOI: 10.18632/oncotarget.11032

[92] Wang J, Hendrix A, Hernot S, Lemaire M, De Bruyne E, Van Valckenborgh E, et al. Bone marrow stromal cell-derived exosomes as communicators in drug resistance in multiple myeloma cells. Blood. 2014;**124**:555-566. DOI: 10.1182/blood-2014-03-562439

[93] Voorhees PM, Manges RF, Sonneveld P, Jagannath S, Somlo G, Krishnan A, et al. A phase 2 multicentre study of siltuximab, an anti-interleukin-6 monoclonal antibody, in patients with relapsed or refractory multiple myeloma. British Journal of Haematology. 2013;**161**:357-366. DOI: 10.1111/bjh.12266

[94] Baljevic M, Zaman S, Baladandayuthapani V, Lin YH, de Partovi CM, Berkova Z, et al. Phase ii study of the c-met inhibitor tivantinib (arq 197) in patients with relapsed or relapsed/refractory multiple myeloma. Annals of Hematology. 2017;**96**:977-985. DOI: 10.1007/s00277-017-2980-3

[95] Moreau P, Cavallo F, Leleu X, Hulin C, Amiot M, Descamps G, et al. Phase i study of the anti-insulin-like growth factor 1 receptor (igf-1r) monoclonal antibody, ave1642, as single agent and in combination with bortezomib in patients with relapsed multiple myeloma. Leukemia. 2011;**25**:872-874. DOI: 10.1038/leu.2011.4

[96] Holstein SA, McCarthy PL. Immunomodulatory drugs in multiple myeloma: Mechanisms of action and clinical experience. Drugs. 2017;**77**:505-520. DOI: 10.1007/s40265-017-0689-1

[97] Weber DM, Chen C, Niesvizky R, Wang M, Belch A, Stadtmauer EA, et al. Lenalidomide plus dexamethasone for relapsed multiple myeloma in north America. The New England Journal of Medicine. 2007;**357**:2133-2142. DOI: 10.1056/NEJMoa070596

[98] Dimopoulos M, Spencer A, Attal M, Prince HM, Harousseau JL, Dmoszynska A, et al. Lenalidomide plus dexamethasone for relapsed or refractory multiple myeloma. The New England Journal of Medicine. 2007;**357**:2123-2132. DOI: 10.1056/NEJMoa070594

[99] San Miguel J, Weisel K, Moreau P, Lacy M, Song K, Delforge M, et al. Pomalidomide plus low-dose dexamethasone versus high-dose dexamethasone alone for patients with relapsed and refractory multiple myeloma (mm-003): A randomised, open-label, phase 3 trial. The Lancet Oncology. 2013;**14**:1055-1066. DOI: 10.1016/S1470-2045(13)70380-2

[100] Ito T, Ando H, Suzuki T, Ogura T, Hotta K, Imamura Y, et al. Identification of a primary target of thalidomide teratogenicity. Science. 2010;**327**:1345-1350. DOI: 10.1126/science.1177319

[101] Zhu YX, Braggio E, Shi CX, Bruins LA, Schmidt JE, Van Wier S, et al. Cereblon expression is required for the antimyeloma activity of lenalidomide and pomalidomide. Blood. 2011;**118**:4771-4779. DOI: 10.1182/blood-2011-05-356063

[102] Bedewy AM, El-Maghraby SM. Do baseline cereblon gene expression and il-6 receptor expression determine the response to thalidomide-dexamethasone treatment in multiple myeloma patients? European Journal of Haematology. 2014;**92**:13-18. DOI: 10.1111/ejh.12207

[103] Heintel D, Rocci A, Ludwig H, Bolomsky A, Caltagirone S, Schreder M, et al. High expression of cereblon (crbn) is associated with improved clinical response in patients with multiple myeloma treated with lenalidomide and dexamethasone. British Journal of Haematology. 2013;**161**:695-700. DOI: 10.1111/bjh.12338

[104] Schuster SR, Kortuem KM, Zhu YX, Braggio E, Shi CX, Bruins LA, et al. The clinical significance of cereblon expression in multiple myeloma. Leukemia Research. 2014;**38**:23-28. DOI: 10.1016/j.leukres.2013.08.015

[105] Lopez-Girona A, Mendy D, Ito T, Miller K, Gandhi AK, Kang J, et al. Cereblon is a direct protein target for immunomodulatory and antiproliferative activities of lenalidomide and pomalidomide. Leukemia. 2012;**26**:2326-2335. DOI: 10.1038/leu.2012.119

[106] Zhu YX, Braggio E, Shi CX, Kortuem KM, Bruins LA, Schmidt JE, et al. Identification of cereblon-binding proteins and relationship with response and survival after imids in multiple myeloma. Blood. 2014;**124**:536-545. DOI: 10.1182/blood-2014-02-557819

[107] Kortum KM, Mai EK, Hanafiah NH, Shi CX, Zhu YX, Bruins L, et al. Targeted sequencing of refractory myeloma reveals a high incidence of mutations in crbn and ras pathway genes. Blood. 2016;**128**:1226-1233. DOI: 10.1182/blood-2016-02-698092

[108] Bjorklund CC, Baladandayuthapani V, Lin HY, Jones RJ, Kuiatse I, Wang H, et al. Evidence of a role for cd44 and cell adhesion in mediating resistance to lenalidomide in multiple myeloma: Therapeutic implications. Leukemia. 2014;**28**:373-383. DOI: 10.1038/leu.2013.174

[109] Xu J, Pfarr N, Endris V, Mai EK, Md Hanafiah NH, Lehners N, et al. Molecular signaling in multiple myeloma: Association of ras/raf mutations and mek/erk pathway activation. Oncogene. 2017;**6**:e337. DOI: 10.1038/oncsis.2017.36

[110] Mey UJM, Renner C, von Moos R. Vemurafenib in combination with cobimetinib in relapsed and refractory extramedullary multiple myeloma harboring the braf v600e mutation. Hematological Oncology. 2017;**35**:890-893. DOI: 10.1002/hon.2353

[111] van de Donk NW, Janmaat ML, Mutis T, Lammerts van Bueren JJ, Ahmadi T, Sasser AK, et al. Monoclonal antibodies targeting cd38 in hematological malignancies and beyond. Immunological Reviews. 2016;**270**:95-112. DOI: 10.1111/imr.12389

[112] Dimopoulos MA, Oriol A, Nahi H, San-Miguel J, Bahlis NJ, Usmani SZ, et al. Daratumumab, lenalidomide, and dexamethasone for multiple myeloma. The New England Journal of Medicine. 2016;**375**:1319-1331. DOI: 10.1056/NEJMoa1607751

[113] Palumbo A, Chanan-Khan A, Weisel K, Nooka AK, Masszi T, Beksac M, et al. Daratumumab, bortezomib, and dexamethasone for multiple myeloma. The New England Journal of Medicine. 2016;**375**:754-766. DOI: 10.1056/NEJMoa1606038

[114] Hsi ED, Steinle R, Balasa B, Szmania S, Draksharapu A, Shum BP, et al. Cs1, a potential new therapeutic antibody target for the treatment of multiple myeloma. Clinical Cancer Research. 2008;**14**:2775-2784. DOI: 10.1158/1078-0432.CCR-07-4246

[115] Lonial S, Dimopoulos M, Palumbo A, White D, Grosicki S, Spicka I, et al. Elotuzumab therapy for relapsed or refractory multiple myeloma. The New England Journal of Medicine. 2015;**373**:621-631. DOI: 10.1056/NEJMoa1505654

[116] Zhang T, Wang S, Lin T, Xie J, Zhao L, Liang Z, et al. Systematic review and meta-analysis of the efficacy and safety of novel monoclonal antibodies for treatment of relapsed/refractory multiple myeloma. Oncotarget. 2017;**8**:34001-34017. DOI: 10.18632/oncotarget.16987

[117] Nijhof IS, Casneuf T, van Velzen J, van Kessel B, Axel AE, Syed K, et al. Cd38 expression and complement inhibitors affect response and resistance to daratumumab therapy in myeloma. Blood. 2016;**128**:959-970. DOI: 10.1182/blood-2016-03-703439

[118] Krejcik J, Frerichs KA, Nijhof IS, van Kessel B, van Velzen JF, Bloem AC, et al. Monocytes and granulocytes reduce cd38 expression levels on myeloma cells in patients treated with daratumumab. Clinical Cancer Research. 2017;**23**:7498-7511. DOI: 10.1158/1078-0432.CCR-17-2027

[119] Funaro A, Horenstein AL, Calosso L, Morra M, Tarocco RP, Franco L, et al. Identification and characterization of an active soluble form of human cd38 in normal and pathological fluids. International Immunology. 1996;**8**:1643-1650

[120] Tai YT, Dillon M, Song W, Leiba M, Li XF, Burger P, et al. Anti-cs1 humanized monoclonal antibody huluc63 inhibits myeloma cell adhesion and induces antibody-dependent cellular cytotoxicity in the bone marrow milieu. Blood. 2008;**112**:1329-1337. DOI: 10.1182/blood-2007-08-107292

[121] Zonder JA, Mohrbacher AF, Singhal S, van Rhee F, Bensinger WI, Ding H, et al. A phase 1, multicenter, open-label, dose escalation study of elotuzumab in patients with advanced multiple myeloma. Blood. 2012;**120**:552-559. DOI: 10.1182/blood-2011-06-360552

[122] Nijhof IS, Groen RW, Lokhorst HM, van Kessel B, Bloem AC, van Velzen J, et al. Upregulation of cd38 expression on multiple myeloma cells by all-trans retinoic acid improves the efficacy of daratumumab. Leukemia. 2015;**29**:2039-2049. DOI: 10.1038/leu.2015.123

[123] van de Donk NW, Kamps S, Mutis T, Lokhorst HM. Monoclonal antibody-based therapy as a new treatment strategy in multiple myeloma. Leukemia. 2012;**26**:199-213. DOI: 10.1038/leu.2011.214

[124] Marra J, Du J, Hwang J, Wolf JL, Martin TG, Venstrom JM. Kir and hla genotypes influence clinical outcome in multiple myeloma patients treated with sar650984 (anti-cd38) in combination with lenalidomide and dexamethasone. Blood. 2014;**124**:2126

[125] Kuehl WM, Bergsagel PL. Multiple myeloma: Evolving genetic events and host interactions. Nature Reviews. Cancer. 2002;**2**:175-187. DOI: 10.1038/nrc746

[126] Rajan AM, Rajkumar SV. Interpretation of cytogenetic results in multiple myeloma for clinical practice. Blood Cancer Journal. 2015;**5**:e365. DOI: 10.1038/bcj.2015.92

[127] Cavo M, Petrucci MT, Di Raimondo F, Zamagni E, Gamberi B, Crippa C, et al. Upfront single versus double autologous stem cell transplantation for newly diagnosed multiple myeloma: An intergroup, multicenter, phase iii study of the European myeloma network (emn02/ho95 mm trial). Blood. 2016;**128**:991-991

[128] Sonneveld P, Schmidt-Wolf IG, van der Holt B, El Jarari L, Bertsch U, Salwender H, et al. Bortezomib induction and maintenance treatment in patients with newly diagnosed multiple myeloma: Results of the randomized phase iii hovon-65/ gmmg-hd4 trial. Journal of Clinical Oncology. 2012;**30**:2946-2955. DOI: 10.1200/JCO.2011.39.6820

[129] Rajkumar SV, Kapoor P, Ketterling RP, Lacy MQ, Gertz MA, Buadi F, et al. Impact of fish abnormalities on response to lenalidomide in patients with multiple myeloma. Blood. 2013;**122**:3210-3210

[130] Bolli N, Avet-Loiseau H, Wedge DC, Van Loo P, Alexandrov LB, Martincorena I, et al. Heterogeneity of genomic evolution and mutational profiles in multiple myeloma. Nature Communications. 2014;**5**:2997. DOI: 10.1038/ncomms3997

[131] Brioli A, Melchor L, Cavo M, Morgan GJ. The impact of intra-clonal heterogeneity on the treatment of multiple myeloma. British Journal of Haematology. 2014;**165**:441-454. DOI: 10.1111/bjh.12805

[132] Paino T, Paiva B, Sayagues JM, Mota I, Carvalheiro T, Corchete LA, et al. Phenotypic identification of subclones in multiple myeloma with different chemoresistant, cytogenetic and clonogenic potential. Leukemia. 2015;**29**:1186-1194. DOI: 10.1038/leu.2014.321

[133] Kim D, Park CY, Medeiros BC, Weissman IL. Cd19-cd45 low/− cd38 high/cd138+ plasma cells enrich for human tumorigenic myeloma cells. Leukemia. 2012;**26**:2530-2537. DOI: 10.1038/leu.2012.140

[134] Matsui W, Huff CA, Wang Q, Malehorn MT, Barber J, Tanhehco Y, et al. Characterization of clonogenic multiple myeloma cells. Blood. 2004;**103**:2332-2336. DOI: 10.1182/blood-2003-09-3064

[135] Matsui W, Wang Q, Barber JP, Brennan S, Smith BD, Borrello I, et al. Clonogenic multiple myeloma progenitors, stem cell properties, and drug resistance. Cancer Research. 2008;**68**:190-197. DOI: 10.1158/0008-5472.CAN-07-3096

[136] Hosen N, Matsuoka Y, Kishida S, Nakata J, Mizutani Y, Hasegawa K, et al. Cd138-negative clonogenic cells are plasma cells but not b cells in some multiple myeloma patients. Leukemia. 2012;**26**:2135-2141. DOI: 10.1038/leu.2012.80

[137] Chaidos A, Barnes CP, Cowan G, May PC, Melo V, Hatjiharissi E, et al. Clinical drug resistance linked to interconvertible phenotypic and functional states of tumor-propagating cells in multiple myeloma. Blood. 2013;**121**:318-328. DOI: 10.1182/blood-2012-06-436220

[138] Jakubikova J, Adamia S, Kost-Alimova M, Klippel S, Cervi D, Daley JF, et al. Lenalidomide targets clonogenic side population in multiple myeloma: Pathophysiologic and clinical implications. Blood. 2011;**117**:4409-4419. DOI: 10.1182/blood-2010-02-267344

[139] Yang Y, Zhou W, Xia J, Gu Z, Wendlandt E, Zhan X, et al. Nek2 mediates aldh1a1-dependent drug resistance in multiple myeloma. Oncotarget. 2014;**5**:11986-11997. DOI: 10.18632/oncotarget.2388

[140] Yang Y, Shi J, Tolomelli G, Xu H, Xia J, Wang H, et al. Raralpha2 expression confers myeloma stem cell features. Blood. 2013;**122**:1437-1447. DOI: 10.1182/blood-2013-02-482919

[141] Yang Y, Shi J, Gu Z, Salama ME, Das S, Wendlandt E, et al. Bruton tyrosine kinase is a therapeutic target in stem-like cells from multiple myeloma. Cancer Research. 2015;**75**: 594-604. DOI: 10.1158/0008-5472.CAN-14-2362

[142] Nishikawa SI, Osawa M. Niche for normal and cancer stem cells. Ernst Schering Foundation Symposium Proceedings. 2006;**5**:1-12

[143] Wallington-Beddoe CT, Kuss BJ, Sobieraj-Teague M, Pitson SM. Resistance to proteasome inhibitors and other targeted therapies in myeloma. British Journal of Haematology. 2018. DOI: 10.1111/bjh.15210

Chapter 5

Angiogenesis and Antiangiogenesis in Multiple Myeloma

Roberto Ria, Antonio Solimando, Assunta Melaccio, Azzurra Sportelli and Angelo Vacca

Additional information is available at the end of the chapter

http://dx.doi.org/10.5772/intechopen.76931

Abstract

Multiple myeloma progression is characterized by a dense interaction between cancer cells and bone marrow microenvironment. The interactions of myeloma cells with various stromal cells and extracellular matrix components are the main regulator of the biological processes that underlie the progression of the disease and of the classic symptomatology correlated. The bone marrow of myeloma patients has recognized autocrine and paracrine loops that regulate multiple signaling pathways and the malignant phenotype of plasma cells. One of the pivotal biological processes which are responsible for myeloma progression is the formation of new vessels from existing ones, known as angiogenesis. It represents a constant hallmark of disease progression and a characteristic feature of the active phase of the disease. Near angiogenesis, other two ancestral processes were active in the bone marrow: vasculogenesis and vasculogenic mimicry. These processes are mediated by the angiogenic cytokines, interleukins, and inflammatory cytokines directly secreted by plasma cells and stromal cells. Neovascularization is also mediated by direct interaction between plasma cells and the various components of bone marrow microenvironment. The observation of the increased bone marrow angiogenesis in multiple myeloma and its correlation with disease activity and overall survival led to consider angiogenesis as a new target in the treatment of multiple myeloma.

Keywords: angiogenesis, antiangiogenesis, bone marrow microenvironment, multiple myeloma, tumor progression, vasculogenesis, vasculogenic mimicry

1. Introduction

In the past decades, myeloma research has been focalized on the malignant cell leading to the identification of various genes (i.e., oncogenes and tumor suppressor genes) and of signaling pathways by which the identified genes themselves control survival and proliferation of cancer cells [1–4]. More recently, newly developed technologies have enabled us to investigate cancer cells at the genomic level. Such gene profiling studies are providing insight into the pathogenesis and risk stratification of plasma cell diseases, and help to predict both prognosis and treatment response [3, 4].

Cancer cells interact with all cells composing the microenvironment and with components of extracellular matrix (ECM) [5, 6]. These interactions play the most important role in the epigenetic control of the malignant phenotype, as in primary sites as in the metastatic ones [6, 7]. Moreover, interactions between host cells in the niche microenvironment and ECM represent an intense area of research [5–9]. The aim of these studies is the better understanding of the pathophysiological events in the tumor process, including malignant cells, surrounding cells, and ECM components [5–9].

Multiple myeloma (MM) is a malignancy of plasma cells that home to and expand in the bone marrow (BM) [9]. MM is characterized by a high genomic heterogeneity but, generally, it shows the same histological features, [8–10]. The interactions between MM plasma cells and BM microenvironment (stromal cells, hematopoietic cells, ahnd ECM) represent near genetic modifications an important factor for disease progression [11–14]. Pathophysiological interactions of myeloma cells with the components of BM microenvironment are pivotal during the progression-associated bone disease and neovascularization [13]. These interactions are mediated by autocrine and paracrine loops that regulate multiple signaling pathways and influence many fundamental biological aspects of the malignant phenotype (i.e., apoptosis, survival, proliferation, invasion, bone damage, and angiogenesis) [12–14].

Neovascularization is the formation of new vessels from existing ones (angiogenesis) or from endothelial precursors (vasculogenesis) and represents one of the principal biological process controlled by the interactions between plasma cells and BM microenvironment. It is a constant hallmark of disease progression [11–15]. Angiogenesis is controlled by several angiogenic cytokines [14, 15]. The major of these are vascular endothelial growth factor (VEGF), fibroblast growth factor-2 (FGF-2), and hepatocyte growth factor (HGF) directly secreted not only by the tumor plasma cells but also by stromal cells [14, 15].

The observation of an increased BM angiogenesis in MM, an overexpression of angiogenic cytokines, and their correlation with disease activity, overall survival and the development of new antiangiogenic compounds, led to consider angiogenesis as a new target in the treatment of MM [11–15].

2. Neovessels formation in multiple myeloma

Neovessels in the BM of patients with active MM appear thin, tortuous, and arborized and are highly permeable showing fenestrae, vesicles, transcellular holes, widened intercellular junctions, and a discontinuous basement membrane [16]. These alterations are consequent to the rapid neovascularization induced by tumor plasma cells by mean of three different processes: (i) angiogenesis, (ii) vasculogenesis, and (iii) vasculogenic mimicry [17].

2.1. Angiogenesis

In 1994, Vacca and colleagues [16] demonstrated for the first time that BM microvascular density was significantly increased in MM compared to monoclonal gammopathy of undetermined significance (MGUS) and moreover in active (diagnosis, relapse, and leukemic phase) versus non-active (complete/objective response and plateau) MM. The authors first hypothesized that progression from MGUS to MM is accompanied by an increase in BM microvascular density. Subsequent studies by other groups confirmed the observation of increased angiogenesis in active MM compared to healthy individuals or MGUS patients [17–20].

Angiogenesis is the sprouting of new blood vessels from pre-existing ones and is finely regulated [17, 18]. Angiogenesis is essential for tumor growth, invasion, and metastasis starting from the balanced early avascular phase of cancer up to being uncontrolled and unlimited in time during the vascular phase [6, 17, 20]. The angiogenic switch from the avascular to the vascular phase is controlled by the many oncogenes, among which c-myc, c-fos, c-jun, and ets-1 have been recognized [20, 21]. They are activated in tumor plasma cells as a consequence of immunoglobulin translocations and genetic instability [20, 21], and induce the angiogenic phenotype in MM plasma cells [21]. MM plasma cells become CD45-negative and begin to produce VEGF [22]. The same angiogenic switch represents a crucial event for the progression from asymptomatic to symptomatic MM [23]. So, angiogenesis represents an important process in MM progression as well as an important prognostic factor [17, 19, 20].

2.2. Vasculogenesis

Vasculogenesis is responsible for the primary development of the vascular system during embryogenesis and is fundamental for the formation of the yolk sac vasculature, of the heart, and of the dorsal aortae [24]. It derives from the differentiation of endothelial progenitors, namely angioblasts, deriving from mesoderm and aggregate into a primitive capillary plexus [24]. Important evidence suggests that vasculogenesis contributes to neovascularization in the bone marrow of MM patients [25–27]. In fact, putative endothelial progenitor cells have been isolated from peripheral blood and several studies have suggested that angioblasts contribute to the formation of tumor neovessels [25, 26]. It has been demonstrated that when CD34+ VEGFR-2+ cells isolated from peripheral blood of MM patients were cultured on fibronectin-coated plates and exposed to angiogenic cytokines, they acquire a typical spindle-shaped morphology and express endothelial cell markers (CD34, CD31, Flk-1, Tie-2, and E-selectins) [26]. Moreover, in the BM of MM patients, but not of MGUS patients, some endothelial cells of neovessel wall express on their surface the typical endothelial cell markers: factor VIII-related antigen (FVIII-RA), vascular endothelial-cadherin (VE-cadherin), VEGFR-2, and TIE/Tek, as well as the CD133 staminal antigen whose expression was found in the microvascular wall together with FVIII-RA or VE-cadherin in some active MM patients [26].

2.3. Vasculogenic mimicry

The phenomenon called "vasculogenesis mimicry" represent a model of neovascularization in aggressive solid and hematologic tumors, owing to the specific capacity of malignant cells and other non-endothelial cells to form vessel-like networks [27–33]. This phenomenon can be an escape mechanism for antiangiogenic drugs that are now incorporated into standard clinical practice [29]. Also, inflammatory cells (i.e. macrophages and mast cells) participate in this process [30–33] because they can generate endothelial progenitor and can produce functional capillary-like structures in vitro when stimulated by VEGF and/or FGF-2 [30–36].

Scavelli et al. demonstrated that when exposed to VEGF and FGF-2, macrophages isolated from BM of myeloma patients develop phenotypic and biologic properties similar to those of endothelial cells, and exhibit numerous cytoplasmic extroversions arranged in tube-like structures [35]. Finally, in BM biopsies of MM, the participation of inflammatory cells in the formation of the capillary network has been directly demonstrated [35, 36].

3. The BM microenvironment

The BM microenvironment plays a pivotal role during MM disease progression by mean neovascularization, bone disease, and activity of inflammatory cells. All the BM microenvironment components surround and support MM plasma cells proliferation, migration, and survival, and are implicated in drug resistance [34, 37].

3.1. Endothelial cells

BM endothelial cells of patients with MM are altered in shape and characterized by different phenotype (in term of expression of cell adhesion molecules, receptors for cytokines and growth factors together with FVIII-RA, and VE-cadherin) from those of normal resting endothelial cells and shows the capacity to proliferate rapidly and spontaneously enhanced angiogenesis [36–39]. In fact, Vacca et al. [38] demonstrated that the phenotype of MM endothelial cells is characterized by expression of surface receptors such as VEGFR-2 and Tie2/Tek (indicators of active angiogenesis), increased expression of the β3-integrin (that plays a pivotal role in the prevention of apoptosis, adhesion to the ECM, proliferation, migration, and capillarogenesis), expression of endoglin (implicated in the expression of the ligand of the plasma cell CD38 (CD31) enhancing plasma cells interaction with the new-formed blood vessels, favoring plasma cells entry into circulation, and disseminate). The expression of a water transporter, namely aquaporin 1, has been also demonstrated [39]. It enhances vascular permeability, facilitates plasma extravasation, increases interstitial pressure, induces hypoxia, and upregulates hypoxia-inducible factor-1 alpha (HIF-1α) and VEGF [39]. Some MM endothelial cells express the CD133 indicating their derivation from a subset of CD133+ progenitor cells which contribute to the formation of blood neovessels [26, 40, 41]. MM plasma cells recruit BM and circulating CD133+ progenitor cells into the tumor microenvironment by mean the release of a high quantity of VEGF, FGF-2, and IGF [26]. In the BM microenvironment, CD133+ progenitor cells differentiate into MM endothelial cells and complete the formation of the new vessel wall [26].

MM endothelial cells are functionally different from MGUS endothelial cells, are characterized by an overangiogenic phenotype, and resemble transformed cells because of they downregulate or upregulate some genes like tumor cells [41]. These changes are influenced by the MM microenvironmental and/or plasma cells factors (such as hypoxia, inflammation, expression of multiple cytokines, growth factors, etc.) that render endothelial cells unstable and heterogeneous, with progressive characteristics comparable with a cancer cell. In addition, those factors may have genetic causes and consequences (i.e., increased expression of oncogenes and loss of tumor suppressor genes) [41]. This reciprocal interrelationship and heterogeneity may translate into a site- and stage-specific changes in the regulation of BM-microvessel density and angiogenesis dependence, and ultimately to changes in the proliferation and antiapoptotic potential of MM tumor cells, even in the same patient [17]. Moreover, the overangiogenic activity of MM endothelial cells is linked to a well-defined protein expression [42]. This proteomic signature renders MM endothelial cells very similarly to transformed (such as tumor) cells than normal endothelial cells, confirming the results obtained in the studies at the genomic level [41].

3.2. Fibroblasts

The stromal microenvironment is characterized by a modified extracellular matrix, enhanced angiogenesis, and cells with an activated phenotype, including fibroblasts referred to as 'activated myofibroblasts' or 'cancer-associated fibroblasts' (CAFs) [6, 43–48]. In the poorly vascularized hypoxic or necrotic areas of tumors, they accumulate numerous tumor-associated fibroblasts [43, 44]. They respond to experimental hypoxia by producing high amounts of VEGF-2, FGF-2, tumor necrosis factor alpha (TNF-α), urokinase and matrix metalloproteinases and synthesizing inducible nitric oxide synthase, which increases blood flow and promotes angiogenesis [45]. In breast, prostate, and pancreatic carcinomas, the number of CAFs is associated with an increased malignancy grade, tumor progression, and poor prognosis [46]. CAFs are heterogeneous [45] and display phenotypes similar to those of myofibroblasts derived from quiescent fibroblasts that have undergone activation during tissue remodeling in wound healing, fibrosis [47]. CAFs can arise from resident fibroblasts, BM-derived progenitor cells and cells undergoing the endothelial-mesenchymal transition (EndMT) or mesenchymal transition (MT) [47] in the BM of MM patients, an important interplay between CAFs and plasma cells during MM initiation and progression has been demonstrated [48]. Plasma cells induce and maintain the CAF-activated phenotype, which, in turn, supports tumor progression by promoting extracellular matrix remodeling, cell proliferation, apoptosis resistance, and angiogenesis [48]. Moreover, CAFs play a key role in the bortezomib resistance of MM cells. The protective effect is not related to cell-to-cell interactions but to the ability of bortezomib to trigger bortezomib-resistant CAFs to release in the BM microenvironment several cytokine/growth factors with antiapoptotic effects, such as IGF-1, IL-6 IL-8, and exosomes [48].

3.3. Macrophages

There are several published data on the association between macrophage infiltration, vascularity, and prognosis in cancer [49–52].

In patients with active MM, macrophages contribute to building neovessels through vasculogenic mimicry [35]. Under a synergistic stimulation by VEGF/FGF-2, they undergo a phenotypic and functional adaptation but retain their own CD14 and CD68 lineage markers which can be evidenced in the neovessel wall [35]. They display oblong and spindle shape with thin cytoplasmic expansions, some of which are either arranged to form a microvessel-like lumen or anastomosed with each other and with those of nearby macrophages to form tubular-like structures [35]. In the BM of patients with active MM, plasma cells secrete VEGF and FGF-2 that bind to VEGFR-1 and FGFR-1, -2 and -3 expressed on monocytes/macrophages surface and induce monocyte migration and infiltration and macrophage to secrete their own VEGF and FGF-2 [17, 35, 49, 52]. These cytokine circuits further promote angiogenesis and vasculogenic mimicry [17].

3.4. Mast cells

Mast cells recruitment in the tumor bed has been associated with enhanced growth and invasion in solid and hematological malignancies [49, 53–56]. In MM, tumor plasma cells secrete stem cell factor (SCF), FGF-2, VEGF-2, and platelet-derived growth factor (PDGF) that recruit mast cells [14, 52]. The granules of mast cells contain several angiogenic factors: (i) tryptase and chymase that favor the formation of capillary structures via a direct action on endothelial cells and activate latent metalloproteinases and plasminogen activator [53]; (ii) heparin that induces endothelial cell proliferation and migration [54]; (iii) histamine, that has a direct angiogenic effect, induces VEGF production in the granulation tissue [54] and contributes to the hyperpermeability of newly formed microvessels, increasing leakage of plasma proteins and hence deposition of fibrin whose degradation products are angiogenic in vivo [55]; and (iv) TGF-β, TNF-α, IL-8, FGF-2, and VEGF, which are all angiogenic factors [52, 53]. Moreover, in the new vessels wall typical tryptase-positive mast cells connected by a junctional system with the endothelial cells can be evidenced. As macrophage, mast cells keep their lineage marker indicating their adaptation to contribute to vasculogenesis mimicry [33]. In patients with MM BM angiogenesis, evaluated as microvessel area, and mast cells counts are highly correlated [53, 56] and both parameters increase simultaneously in the active phase of disease [56].

3.5. Osteoclasts and osteoblasts

MM plasma cells that home and expand in the BM causes an unbalanced bone remodeling that induces osteolytic lesions and causes pain, the main symptom of MM [34]. In MM, plasma cell-dependent alterations of Runx2 and the Wnt pathways induce the differentiation of resident macrophages in osteoclasts and plasma cells themselves can transdifferentiate to functional osteoclasts [57, 58]. Bone disease results from the local production of osteoclast-activating factors (OAF), as well as IL-6, IL-1α or -1β, IL-11, TNF-α, TNF-β, and M-CSF [11]. In particular, the receptor activator of nuclear factor ligand (RANKL), the decoy receptor osteoprotegerin (OPG), its receptor (RANKR), and the chemokine macrophage inflammatory protein-1α (MIP-1α) trigger differentiation and activation signals in osteoclasts precursors, and thus promoting bone resorption [48]. Adhesion molecules, such as β1 integrins, mediate the binding of MM plasma cells to stromal cells and VCAM1 induces overexpression of RANKL in both cell types and suppresses OPG production by stromal cells. Furthermore, plasma cells interfere with the regulation of the bone resorption by the secretion of IL-7 and DKK1, a Wnt inhibitor [59].

It has demonstrated a close link between myeloma cells, osteoclasts, and vascular endothelial cells to form a vicious cycle between bone destruction, angiogenesis, and myeloma expansion in the MM bone marrow and that the inhibition of VEGF produced by plasma and stromal cells and osteopontin produced by osteoclasts, reduce angiogenesis and osteoclastogenic activity by vascular endothelial cells [11, 57].

Some issues demonstrated that CD38 is expressed by effectors and inhibitory cells, and by both osteoblasts and demonstrating the role of CD38 in bone remodeling, in mice and rabbit models [60] as in human [61]. Horenstein AL. et al. [62] recently shown that the ectoenzymatic network CD73/CD203a is active even in MM bone niche in the alternative production of ADO, which levels correlate with disease aggressiveness and ISS staging of MM patients [61]. Moreover, the role of CD38 in human OC differentiation and as well as the reduction of the area of osteoclast bone resorption in vitro by the anti-CD38 monoclonal antibody daratumumab have been also demonstrated [63]. Overall these findings suggest the possibility of a role of CD38 during osteoclast formation supporting the potential activity of daratumumab on MM bone disease and on the protection of MM plasma cells by stromal cells of the bone niche [60–63].

3.6. Hematopoietic stem cells

Hematopoietic stem cells (HSCs) reside in the BM in the endosteum niche and in the vascular niche, where they self-renew and differentiate into mature blood cells [64, 65]. This is a finely controlled-process by mean numerous signals from the bone marrow components [64, 65]. In MM, the BM niches (endosteum and vascular) components play a pivotal role in the regulation of vasculogenesis and angiogenesis [11, 14, 26, 64], and alterations of the signals in niche microenvironment modulate myeloma progression and spread [26, 64].

In the BM of patients with MM, the expression of the CD133 staminal antigen in some cells of the neovessel wall has been demonstrated [26, 38]. Moreover, a subset of CD34+/CD133+ cells mobilized in the peripheral blood for collection during transplant procedure express VEGFR-2 and are able to differentiate in mature endothelial cells in appropriate culture conditions [28].

3.7. Endothelial progenitor cells

Various studies have demonstrated that endothelial progenitor cells (EPCs) can be isolated from patients with MM [40, 66–69] and contribute to the formation of new blood vessels [40]. Moreover, circulating EPCs expressing CD146+, CD105+, and CD34+ are increased in MM patients compared to healthy controls [66, 67].

Rigolin et al. [69] have hypothesized a possible origin of EPCs and plasma cells from a common progenitor namely hemangioblast in MM patients. In their work, they demonstrated that EPCs, isolated from MM patients presents the 13q14 deletion and the great part of them are positive for the CD133 [69]. Finally, some evidence indicates a prognostic significance of the circulating EPCs also after treatment with new drugs [66, 68].

3.8. Mesenchymal stem cells

Mesenchymal stem cells (MSCs) are the major component of BM stroma [11, 57, 70–72]. These cells, of unclear origin in MM [71], are potentially able to differentiate into multiple histotypes (i.e. fibroblasts, adipocytes, chondrocytes, and osteoblasts) and in the BM form specialized niches namely "vascular niche" and "osteoblast niche" [57, 70, 71]. MSCs support tumor cell growth, metastasis, survival, bone marrow colonization, and evasion of the immune system [72]. MSCs can migrate toward primary tumors and metastatic sites, implying that these cells might modulate tumor growth and metastasis. In the BM of patients with MM, functional abnormalities of MSCs and complex interaction with MM plasma cells have been demonstrated indicating that they play a critical role in MM development and disease outcome [70, 71]. In fact, MSCs can induce bortezomib-resistance in MM plasma cell by increasing Bcl2 expression and enhance NF-κB activity via cell-cell contact [73, 74]. Moreover, MSCs are able to modulate engraftment of HSC, to suppress T- and B-lymphocyte activation and proliferation, and to affect dendritic cell maturation [71]. Finally, since MSCs represents the osteoblasts progenitors, in the BM of MM patients, MSCs play a critical role in the pathophysiology of myeloma bone disease [75]. They present reduced osteogenic potential and promoting osteoclasts formation and activity by increasing RANKL to OPG expression, augmenting secretion of activin A, uncoupling ephrinB2-EphB4 signaling, and augmenting Wnt5a production [75].

3.9. Adipocytes

The cancer-associated adipocytes (also namely peritumoral, intratumoral, or tumor-infiltrating adipocytes) influence tumor biology also by promoting angiogenesis [76–81]. A great number of signaling factors contributing to angiogenesis in both adipose tissue and tumors: VEGF, Ang-1 and -2, leptin, adiponectin, TNF-α, FGF, TGF-β, HGF, IL-6, and IL-8 [77–79, 81]. The VEGF/VEGFR system is the main mediator of angiogenic activity in adipose tissue [77]. In particular, adipocytes produce VEGF, Ang-2, and HGF [77, 81]. In MM, the hypoxic environment of BM favors the production of angiogenic factors by adipocytes, particularly VEGF, and decreases adipogenic differentiation increasing adipose-derived stem cell proliferation and migration [82, 83], supporting aberrant microvessel growth and neovascularization, and MM plasma cell proliferation [82, 83]. Paracrine and autocrine signaling of VEGFA between BM adipocytes and MM cells have been also demonstrating [77, 80, 81].

3.10. Soluble factors and transduction pathways

The progression from in situ to invasive and metastatic solid tumors are accompanied and enhanced by the switch from the perivascular to the vascular phase [84, 85]. The same process has been demonstrated in MM in which active disease represent the 'vascular phase' of plasma cell tumors, and non-active disease (remission or plateau phase), smoldering MM and MGUS their 'perivascular phase' [22, 26, 43].

VEGF is the main angiogenic cytokine secreted in the BM of patients with MM [86–88]. VEGF carries out its activity through the MEK-1/ERK pathway by the interaction with his receptors (VEGFR1–3) [86]. In the BM of patients with MM paracrine loops between endothelial cells and plasma cells [89] and autocrine loops on the same endothelial cells have been demonstrated [90]. Moreover, plasma cell-derived VEGF stimulates IL-6 and VEGF secretion in BM stromal cells, whereas stromal cells-derived IL-6 promotes proliferation, survival, and VEGF production in plasma cells, activating a loop between both growth factors [91].

Levels of FGF isoforms are significantly higher in the serum and plasma cell lysates of patients with active MM compared with non-active MM and MGUS patients [92–94]. Moreover, FGF-2 inhibition suppresses the angiogenic potential of plasma cells from patients with active MM in vitro and in vivo [92, 93]. Finally, FGF-2 triggers paracrine MM-stromal cell interactions in an IL-6/FGF-2 paracrine loop [92, 95] and syndecan-1 (CD138), a low-affinity receptor of FGF-2, is also expressed by MM cells [96]. The high expression/activation of the FGF2 signaling in active MM also overcomes the inhibitory effect of the Pentraxin 3 (PTX3) [97, 98], a soluble pattern recognition receptor that binds with high affinity and selectivity to FGF2 inhibiting its pro-angiogenic activity, autocrine loops usually activated to self-limit physiologic angiogenesis in a normal subject or MGUS patient [97].

HGF has been identified in human MM cell lines and in freshly isolated plasma cells from patients with MM [99, 100]. Serum levels of this factor are higher in newly diagnosed MM patients and decline after induction therapy in the responding patients. Ferrucci et al. demonstrated the co-expression of HGF and c-MET in MM endothelial cells, suggesting autocrine stimulation [99]. Moreover, BM stromal cells produce HGF, paracrine stimulation of MM cells within the BM microenvironment can also take place [99, 100]. The inhibition of this pathway causes reduction of spontaneous and plasma cell-induced angiogenesis in MM endothelial cells in vitro and in vivo [99–101].

The Ang-1/Ang-2 expression in MM patient serum and BM samples correlates with the BM microvascular density [102–106]. It has been demonstrated that Ang-1, as well as Ang-2 expression, is upregulated in MM cell lines and in plasma cells obtained from MM patients [103, 105] and that the angiopoietin receptor Tie-2 is upregulated in the BM endothelial cells in the presence of MM cells [104]. Moreover, anti-Tie-2 antibodies blocked the in vitro angiogenic activity of MM cells [104]. Higher levels of Ang-1 and Ang-2 have been detected in MM patients as compared to controls [102] and their ratio may represent an independent prognostic factor in these patients [106].

Osteopontin (OPN) contributes to angiogenesis in MM [107–109]. Its expression correlates with BM microvascular density, and OPN-immunodepleted conditioned media from myeloma cells fail to induce a pro-angiogenic effect [107, 108] and an anti-OPN antibody block myeloma-induced angiogenesis [107]. Moreover, OPN may represent a useful serum marker of bone disease and BM angiogenic extent in myeloma patients [109].

Matrix Metalloproteinase-2 and -9 (MMP-2 and MMP-9) secretion is increased in patients with active MM versus non-active MM or MGUS [92, 110, 111] and usually, the MMP-2 expression is stronger [92, 110]. MM cell lines and freshly isolated BM plasma cells of MM patients produce MMP-9 [112], and MMP secretion of MM cells is triggered by BM stromal or endothelial cells [92, 112].

PDGF-Receptor Beta (PDGF-Rbeta) is expressed in plasma cells of MM patients [111, 113], and PDGF-BB/PDGF-Rbeta kinase axis promotes MM tumor growth by activating ERK-1/2 and AKT [113, 114]. Dasatinib, an orally bioactive TK-inhibitor significantly delays MM tumor growth acting as an inhibitor of PDGF-Rbeta kinase activation [113].

Airoldi et al. [115] demonstrated that IL-12 receptor B2 (IL-12Rbeta2) is downregulated in MM plasma cells and IL-12 reduces their pro-angiogenic activity by downregulation of a wide panel of angiogenic factors, including FGF-2, VEGF, Ang-2, and IL-6 and upregulation of some inhibitors of angiogenesis, including CXCL-4, interferon alpha and gamma (IFN-α and IFN-γ), and tissue inhibitor of metalloproteinase-2 (TIMP-2).

IL-27 exert strong antitumor activities against MM cells from patients by binding with its specific IL-27 receptor [116, 117] inhibiting the angiogenic potential of MM plasma cells. In animals injected with the U266 MM cell line, the expression of the genes encoding the chemokines CCL-2, CXCL-3, CXCL-5, and CXCL-6 is significantly downregulated by IL-27 treatment [116, 117].

Another important paracrine loop between MM endothelial cells and plasma cells involves CXC-chemokines and their cognate receptors have been evidenced in the BM of MM patients [118, 119]. In fact, BM endothelial cells express and secrete high amounts of the CXC-chemokines CXCL8/IL-8, CXCL11/interferon-inducible T-cell alpha chemoattractant (I-TAC), CXCL12/stromal cell-derived factor (SDF)-1α, and CCL2/monocyte chemotactic protein (MPC)-1 [118] that mediate the interactions between plasma cells and stromal cells interacting with the respective chemokine receptors (CXCR and CCR) [118, 120].

HIF-1α has been demonstrated to be stabilized in MM plasma cells, in hypoxic as in normoxic conditions [82, 83, 119, 121–123]. The constitutive stabilization of HIF-1α in myeloma cells is associated with the oncogenic c-Myc activity, suggesting that a common signaling pathway is active in MM plasma cells [122]. Among target genes controlled by HIF-1α, the genes coding for the pro-angiogenic cytokines VEGF, IL-8, and OPN have been evidenced, and HIF-1α silencing significantly suppresses the pro-angiogenic properties of MM cells reducing their secretion [87]. Moreover, MM endothelial cells from relapsed/refractory MM patients, but not those of newly diagnosed or non-active MM patients, showed a stabilization and activation of the HIF-1α protein in normoxic conditions [124]. This stabilization is induced by ROS and correlated with the expression of HIF-1α pro-angiogenic targets [124]. The inhibition of HIF-1α in MM plasma cells [123] as well as in endothelial cells [124] impaired the MM plasma cells/stromal cells communication, the angiogenesis-related functions, and revert bortezomib- and lenalidomide-resistance [123, 124]. It may also have prognostic significance because patients with MM endothelial cells expressing the stabilized HIF-1α protein had shorter overall survival [124].

The mammalian target of rapamycin (mTOR) is an intracellular serine/threonine kinase that mediates intracellular metabolism, cell survival, and actin rearrangement. mTOR is made of two independent complexes, mTORC1, involved in protein synthesis and autophagy inhibition, and mTORC2, involved in progression promotion, survival, actin reorganization, and drug resistance [125–127]. In MM endothelial, a significantly higher activation of mTORC2 have been demonstrated. Its inhibition induces a reduction of the angiogenic abilities of MM endothelial cells, suggesting a major role of mTORC2 in the "angiogenic switch" and indicates that mTORC2 might be a new antiangiogenic target in MM [127].

In MM endothelial, cell-to-cell contact-dependent homotypic activation of Notch pathway has been shown [128, 129]. MM plasma cells cocultured with MM endothelial cells trigger Jagged1/2-mediated Notch activation enhancing endothelial angiogenic activity. Moreover, halting Notch axis reduces angiogenesis *in vitro* and *in vivo* suggesting Notch pathway as a novel therapeutic target in MM [129].

The ephrins (Efn) and their receptors (Eph), a large family of receptor tyrosine kinases, are involved in several biological processes including cancer growth, progression, and angiogenesis [130–133]. Caivano et al. [134] recently demonstrated that EphA3 is highly overexpressed in MM endothelial cells and its expression correlates with disease progression. They have also defined the biological role of EphA3 in MM angiogenesis and their preliminary data indicate that EphA3 could represent an angiogenic target in patients with MM [134].

Focal adhesion kinase (FAK) is a tyrosine kinase that localizes at focal adhesion sites of endothelial cell to the ECM [135–137]. It mediates signaling starting from integrin, is upregulated in many cancer types, controlling tumor aggressiveness, and metastasis [135], and is implicated in endothelial cell survival, proliferation, and migration [136, 137]. Integrin/FAK-mediated signaling cooperate with other growth factor receptor signaling (i.e. FGFR signaling) to promote angiogenesis in MM [138].

Various growth factor receptors induced an increase in DNA synthesis in MM endothelial cells by mean PI3K/Akt-MEK/ERK pathway inducing angiogenesis [17, 86, 138]. The role of this pathway in promoting angiogenesis is mainly related to the phosphorylation of eukaryotic translation initiation factor 4E-binding protein 1 (4E-BP1), S6-kinase (S6K), and MAP kinase interacting kinase mediated by ERK [139, 140]. This process leads to an increased rate of mRNA translation into HIF-1α protein in an oxygen-independent way [139, 140]. ERK is also able to activate the transcription of HIF-1α by the co-activator CBP/p300 that increases HIF-1α/p300 complex formation [139, 140].

MicroRNAs are small endogenous non-coding RNAs (21–25 nucleotides) involved in regulating normal physiological processes as well as cancer pathogenesis [141–143]. Particularly, some miRNA have been implicated in tumor angiogenesis individuate as potential therapeutic targets/therapy [143–145]. Evidence suggests that MM cells promote angiogenic activity via HIF-1α, a key transcription factor of hypoxia, leading to the overproduction of angiogenic cytokines [91, 104]. Moreover, communication between plasma cells, stromal cells, and endothelial cells is mediated also by mean the exosomes, small endosome-derived vesicles, containing a wide range of functional proteins, mRNA, and miRNA [146]. In BM of MM, miR-135b has been involved as the principal pro-angiogenic miRNA by targeting factor-inhibiting HIF-1 [147], whereas miR-199a-5p, which directly targets HIF1-α, miR-15a, and miR-16, and VEGF, have been demonstrated to be strong inhibitors of MM-induced angiogenesis [148, 149]. Overall, published data indicate that circulating microRNAs in exosomes and microvesicles can be useful biomarkers of angiogenesis, and synthetic miRNAs may be potential new antiangiogenic therapeutics tools in MM [150].

4. Antiangiogenesis in multiple myeloma

The combination of biological drugs in the actual therapeutic strategies of MM have improved the outcome of MM patients because of their activity on microenvironment [17, 151–153].

4.1. Proteasome inhibitors

Bortezomib, a potent, highly selective, and reversible proteasome inhibitor targeting the 26S proteasome complex [154, 155] act on key cellular processes, such as cell cycle progression, inflammation, immune surveillance, growth arrest, and apoptosis [154]. Bortezomib acts by mean the modulation of NF-κB transcription factor, which mediates the expression and secretion of cytokines, chemokines, cell adhesion molecules involved also in anti-apoptosis and cellular growth control [154–156]. After phosphorylation by IκB kinase, IκB is polyubiquitinated and degraded by the 26S proteasome, which allows p50/p65 NF-κB nuclear translocation and binding to consensus motifs in the promoter region of target genes [155, 156]. NF-κB regulated also the expression of adhesion molecules, such as ICAM-1 and VCAM-1, on both MM cells and BM stromal cells [156], so, its inhibition downregulates these adhesion molecules favoring the susceptibility of MM plasma cells to therapeutic agents [156]. Moreover, NF-κB activation controls the production of IL-6 by BM stromal cells that increase production and secretion of VEGF-2 and FGF-2 from MM plasma cells [91]. By blocking NF-kB, bortezomib inhibits MM cell adherence to the BM stromal cells reducing MM cell growth and VEGF-2 and FGF-2 secretion [17, 91, 154, 155].

Bortezomib is directly cytotoxic on MM plasma cells by blocking proteasome activity that causes the accumulation of misfolded polyubiquitinated proteins and causes ROS production [155, 156]. The accumulation of misfolded proteins in the endoplasmic reticulum triggers caspase-4 activation, and ROS accumulation causes disruption of membrane potential and the release of cytochrome c from mitochondria, and then the caspase-9 activation. These cytoplasmic alterations consequently, initiate the apoptotic cascades causing apoptosis of the cell [155, 156]. Finally, bortezomib downregulates VEGF, IL-6, IGF-I, Ang-1, and Ang-2 production and secretion by MM plasma cells and BM stromal cells, targeting aberrant blood vessel development through a potent inhibition of proliferation of activated endothelial cells [17, 154].

Ixazomib (MLN2238) is a second-generation proteasome inhibitor with a similar activity of bortezomib on the inhibition of NF-kB [157, 158]. It has been demonstrated that ixazomib affects BM stromal cells triggered MM cell growth and BM stromal cells-induced endothelial cell proliferation suggesting that ixazomib not only directly targets MM plasma cells but also overcomes the cytoprotective effects of the MM host BM microenvironment [158]. In fact, ixazomib is able to impact angiogenesis in vivo decreasing the expression of angiogenic markers in mice as well as in vitro reducing the capillary formation by HUVEC in the Matrigel™ system [159].

The antiangiogenic activity of another proteasome inhibitor, carfilzomib, has not been clearly demonstrated but it seems to have inhibitory activity on tumor-stromal interactions and angiogenesis [137, 160]. Moreover, VEGF pathway polymorphisms have been associated with clinical outcomes in MM patients [161], and have been reported that polymorphisms of VEGF pathway are associated with response to the combination of carfilzomib and lenalidomide [162].

4.2. Immunomodulators (IMIDs)

Thalidomide, a first generation immunomodulatory drug (IMiD), has a direct tumoricidal activity, an antiangiogenic effect and modulates TNF-α signaling through direct and/or indirect effects on the tumor microenvironment [15, 163–167], reduces FGF-2, VEGF, and IL-6 secretion in BM stromal cells and by MM cells [163]. It also interferes with NF-κB activity by blocking its ability to bind to DNA abrogating inflammatory/angiogenic cytokine production [165, 166], and disrupts the direct interactions between MM plasma cells and BM stromal cells by modulation of cell surface adhesion molecules [167].

Two new IMiDs, including lenalidomide and pomalidomide, demonstrating up to 50,000 times more potent inhibition of TNF-α than thalidomide, has been developed [168–170]. They inhibit VEGF and FGF-2 secretion from both myeloma and BM stromal cells and block endothelial cell migration and proliferation in vivo and in vitro [169]. Lenalidomide, a first derivative of thalidomide, is less toxic and more potent than the parent drug, and in patients with relapsed or refractory MM, lenalidomide can overcome resistance not only to conventional chemotherapy but also to thalidomide [169]. De Luisi et al. [170] demonstrated that lenalidomide inhibits angiogenesis and migration of MM endothelial cells and that lenalidomide-treated MM endothelial cells show changes in VEGF/VEGFR-2 signaling pathway, and in several proteins controlling EC motility, cytoskeleton remodeling, and energy metabolism pathways. Both thalidomide and lenalidomide downregulate VEGF. Pomalidomide is a third generation IMiD with increased activity in vitro compared with thalidomide and lenalidomide [171, 172], which exerts anti-MM effects through multiple mechanisms, including induction of apoptosis via caspase-8, reduction of proliferation, inhibition of NF-κ B activation, reduction of stromal cell stimulatory cytokine secretion, and angiogenesis inhibition [172].

4.3. Bisphosphonates

The bisphosphonates are other compounds that, although originally used to reduce bone loss in MM due to an anti-osteoclast activity, have also been shown to have antiangiogenic activity [173–175]. In fact, zoledronic acid has a direct cytotoxic activity on tumor cells and suppresses angiogenesis, inhibits FGF-2- and VEGF-dependent proliferation of endothelial cells and inhibits VEGFR-2 in an autocrine loop [173]. It has also been demonstrated that the addition of zoledronic acid to antimyeloma therapy, bortezomib-, lenalidomide-, or thalidomide-based, is associated with a benefit in term of skeletal-related event rate as well as in term of the progression-free survival rate of myeloma patients [174]. Neridronate exerts its antiangiogenic activity through both a direct effect on endothelial cell proliferative activity and inhibitory effect on the responsivity of the endothelial cells to the proliferative stimuli mediated by angiogenic cytokines [175].

4.4. Monoclonal antibodies and other drugs

The most successful therapeutic approach to target VEGF in cancer is the use of a humanized monoclonal antibody against VEGF, bevacizumab [176]. Several clinical trials in MM tested the effects of bevacizumab used in conjunction with other agents including lenalidomide, dexamethasone, or bortezomib with discouraging results [177].

In addition to bevacizumab, other VEGFRs targeting compounds (including aflibercept-VEGF-trap), tyrosine kinase inhibitors (cabozantinib, dasatinib, pazopanib, sorafenib, sunitinib, and semaxanib), PI3K/Akt-MEK/ERK pathway inhibitors, FAK inhibitors, interleukin inhibitors (atiprimod), farnesyltransferase inhibitors, other monoclonal antibodies (anti-CD40), and marine cartilage extract (neovastat) have shown antiangiogenic activity but no significant results or only preliminary preclinical data have been reported with the use of this drugs in MM [177–181].

5. Conclusions

Despite the good results obtained in the last decades, MM remains an incurable malignancy, indicating that our knowledge on the mechanisms responsible for disease progression and drug resistance is still not completely clear. The goal obtained with the introduction of the new target drugs for MM therapy is the improvement of the outcome of MM patients in term of progression-free and overall survival. The simultaneous block of plasma cell proliferation and survival, plasma cells/BM stromal cells interaction, and BM stromal cells activity by the novel agents help us to get these results. In fact, the BM microenvironment plays a crucial role in the pathophysiology of MM. An active crosstalk between MM plasma cells and stromal cells in the BM of myeloma patients is constantly working. It represents a hallmark of active MM favoring survival, proliferation, and migration of plasma cells, and modulates neovessel formation by mean angiogenesis favoring the disease progression. The crosstalk between MM plasma cells and BM microenvironment is not only responsible for drug resistance of plasma cells but also of endothelial cells and other cells composing the microenvironment. The better understanding of the biological mechanisms controlling the interactions between MM cells and BM stromal cells remain fundamental for our knowledge about disease progression and for developing novel drugs targeting these processes.

Conflict of interest

Authors have no conflict of interest to declare.

Author details

Roberto Ria*, Antonio Solimando, Assunta Melaccio, Azzurra Sportelli and Angelo Vacca

*Address all correspondence to: roberto.ria@uniba.it

Department of Biomedical Science and Human Oncology, University of Bari Medical School, Bari, Italy

References

[1] Kastrinakis NG, Gorgoulis VG, Foukas PG, et al. Molecular aspects of multiple myeloma. Annals of Oncology. 2000;**11**:1217-1228. DOI: 10.1023/A:1008331714186

[2] Bergsagel PL, Chesi MV. Molecular classification and risk stratification of myeloma. Hematological Oncology. 2013;**31**(Suppl 1):38-41. DOI: 10.1002/hon.2065

[3] Bhutani M, Landgren O, Usmani SZ. Multiple myeloma: Is it time for biomarker-driven therapy? American Society of Clinical Oncology Educational Book. 2015:e493-e503. DOI: 10.14694/EdBook_AM.2015.35.e493

[4] Patel U, Luthra R, Medeiros LJ, Patel KP. Diagnostic, prognostic, and predictive utility of recurrent somatic mutations in myeloid neoplasms. Clinical Lymphoma, Myeloma & Leukemia. 2017;**17S**:S62-S74. DOI: 10.1016/j.clml.2017.02.015

[5] Alzrigat M, Párraga AA, Jernberg-Wiklund H. Epigenetics in multiple myeloma: From mechanisms to therapy. Seminars in Cancer Biology. 2017. (in press) pii: S1044-579X(17)30104-9. DOI: 10.1016/j.semcancer.2017.09.007

[6] Hanahan D, Weinberg RA. Hallmarks of cancer: The next generation. Cell. 2011;**144**:646-674. DOI: 10.1016/j.cell.2011.02.013

[7] Langley RR, Fidler IJ. Tumor cell-organ microenvironment interactions in the pathogenesis of cancer metastasis. Endocrine Reviews. 2007;**28**:297-321. DOI: 10.1210/er.2006-0027

[8] Amodio N, D'Aquila P, Passarino G, et al. Epigenetic modifications in multiple myeloma: Recent advances on the role of DNA and histone methylation. Expert Opinion on Therapeutic Targets. 2017;**21**:91-101

[9] Glavey SV, Manier S, Sacco A, et al. Epigenetics in multiple myeloma. Cancer Treatment and Research. 2016;**169**:35-49

[10] Zhan F, Huang Y, Colla S, et al. The molecular classification of multiple myeloma. Blood. 2006;**108**:2020-2028. DOI: 10.1182/blood-2005-11-013458

[11] Ribatti D, Nico B, Vacca A. Multiple myeloma as a model for the role of bone marrow niches in the control of angiogenesis. International Review of Cell and Molecular Biology. 2015;**314**:259-282. DOI: 10.1016/bs.ircmb.2014.10.004

[12] Mondello P, Cuzzocrea S, Navarra M, Mian M. Bone marrow micro-environment is a crucial player for myelomagenesis and disease progression. Oncotarget. 2017;**8**:20394-20409. DOI: 10.18632/oncotarget.14610

[13] Ribatti D, Vacca A. The role of microenvironment in tumor angiogenesis. Genes & Nutrition. 2008;**3**:29-34. DOI: 10.1007/s12263-008-0076-3

[14] Ribatti D, Moschetta M, Vacca A. Microenvironment and multiple myeloma spread. Thrombosis Research. 2014;**133**(Suppl 2):102-106. DOI: 10.1016/S0049-3848(14)50017-5

[15] Moschetta M, Kawano Y, Podar K. Targeting the bone marrow microenvironment. Cancer Treatment and Research. 2016;**169**:63-102. DOI: 10.1007/978-3-319-40320-5_6

[16] Vacca A, Ribatti D, Roncali L, et al. Bone marrow angiogenesis and progression in multiple myeloma. British Journal of Haematology. 1994;**87**:503-508. DOI: 10.1111/j.1365-2141.1994.tb08304.x

[17] Ria R, Reale A, De Luisi A, et al. Bone marrow angiogenesis and progression in multiple myeloma. American Journal of Blood Research. 2011;**1**:76-89

[18] Stasi R, Amadori S. The role of angiogenesis in hematologic malignancies. Journal of Hematotherapy & Stem Cell Research. 2002;**11**:49-68. DOI: 10.1089/152581602753448531

[19] Vacca A, Ribatti D. Bone marrow angiogenesis in multiple myeloma. Leukemia. 2006;**20**:193-199. DOI: 10.1038/sj.leu.2404067

[20] Vacca A, Ria R, Reale A, Ribatti D. Angiogenesis in multiple myeloma. Chemical Immunology and Allergy. 2014;**99**:180-196. DOI: 10.1159/000353312

[21] Vacca A, Ribatti D, Roccaro AM, et al. Bone marrow angiogenesis in patients with active multiple myeloma. Seminars in Oncology. 2001;**28**:543-550

[22] Asosingh K, De Raeve H, Menu E, et al. Angiogenic switch during 5T2MM murine myeloma tumorigenesis: Role of CD45 heterogeneity. Blood. 2004;**103**:3131-3177. DOI: 10.1182/blood-2003-08-2946

[23] Calcinotto A, Ponzoni M, Ria R, et al. Modifications of the mouse bone marrow microenvironment favour angiogenesis and correlate with disease progression from asymptomatic to symptomatic multiple myeloma. Oncoimmunology. May 7, 2015;**4**(6):e1008850. eCollection Jun 2015. DOI: 10.1080/2162402X.2015.1008850

[24] Risau W, Flamme I. Vasculogenesis. Annual Review of Cell and Developmental Biology. 1995;**11**:73-91. DOI: 10.1146/annurev.cb.11.110195.000445

[25] Ribatti D. Postnatal vasculogenesis. Mechanisms of Development. 2001;**100**:157-163. DOI: 10.1016/S0925-4773(00)00522-0

[26] Reale A, Melaccio A, Lamanuzzi A, et al. Functional and biological role of endothelial precursor cells in tumour progression: A new potential therapeutic target in haematological malignancies. Stem Cells International. 2016;**2016**:7954580. DOI: 10.1155/2016/7954580

[27] Moschetta M, Mishima Y, Sahin I, et al. Role of endothelial progenitor cells in cancer progression. Biochimica et Biophysica Acta. 2014;**1846**:26-39. DOI: 10.1016/j.bbcan.2014.03.005

[28] Ria R, Piccoli C, Cirulli T, et al. Endothelial differentiation of hematopoietic stem and progenitor cells from patients with multiple myeloma. Clinical Cancer Research. 2008;**14**:1678-1685. DOI: 10.1158/1078-0432.CCR-07-4071

[29] Döme B, Hendrix MJ, Paku S, Tóvári J, Tímár J. Alternative vascularisation mechanisms in cancer: Pathology and therapeutic implications. The American Journal of Pathology. 2007;**170**:1-15. DOI: 10.2353/ajpath.2007.060302

[30] Yang Z, Yao H, Fei F, et al. Generation of erythroid cells from polyploid giant cancer cells: Re-thinking about tumor blood supply. Journal of Cancer Research and Clinical Oncology. 2018;**144**:617-627. DOI: 10.1007/s00432-018-2598-4

[31] Pinto MP, Sotomayor P, Carrasco-Avino G, et al. Escaping antiangiogenic therapy: Strategies employed by cancer cells. International Journal of Molecular Sciences. 2016;**17**:1489. pii: E1489. DOI: 10.3390/ijms17091489

[32] Vacca A, Ribatti D. Angiogenesis and vasculogenesis in multiple myeloma: Role of inflammatory cells. Recent Results in Cancer Research. 2011;**183**:187-195. DOI: 10.1007/978-3-540-85772-3_4

[33] Rehman J, Li J, Orschell CM, March KL. Peripheral blood "endothelial progenitor cells" are derived from monocyte/macrophages and secrete angiogenic growth factors. Circulation. 2003;**107**:1164-1169. DOI: 10.1161/01.CIR.0000058702.69484.A0

[34] Kumar SK, Rajkumar V, Kyle RA, et al. Multiple myeloma. Nature Reviews Disease Primers. 2017;**3**:17046. DOI: 10.1038/nrdp.2017.46

[35] Scavelli C, Nico B, Cirulli T, et al. Vasculogenic mimicry by bone marrow macrophages in patients with multiple myeloma. Oncogene. 2008;**27**:663-674. DOI: 10.1038/sj.onc.1210691

[36] Nico B, Mangieri D, Crivellato E, et al. Mast Cells contribute to vasculogenic mimicry in multiple myeloma. Stem Cells and Development. 2008;**17**:19-22. DOI: 10.1089/scd.2007.0132

[37] Manier S, Sacco A, Leleu X, et al. Bone marrow microenvironment in multiple myeloma progression. Journal of Biomedicine & Biotechnology. 2012;**2012**:157496. DOI: 10.1155/2012/157496

[38] Vacca A, Ria R, Semeraro F, et al. Endothelial cells in the bone marrow of patients with multiple myeloma. Blood. 2003;**102**:3340-3348. DOI: 10.1182/blood-2003-04-1338

[39] Vacca A, Frigeri A, Ribatti D, et al. Microvessel overexpression of aquaporin 1 parallels bone marrow angiogenesis in patients with active multiple myeloma. British Journal of Haematology. 2001;**113**:415-421. DOI: 10.1046/j.1365-2141.2001.02738.x

[40] Tenreiro MM, Correia ML, Brito MA. Endothelial progenitor cells in multiple myeloma neovascularization: A brick to the wall. Angiogenesis. 2017;**20**:443-462. DOI: 10.1007/s10456-017-9571-8

[41] Ria R, Todoerti K, Berardi S, et al. Gene expression profiling of bone marrow endothelial cells in patients with multiple myeloma. Clinical Cancer Research. 2009;**15**:5369-5378. DOI: 10.1158/1078-0432.CCR-09-0040

[42] Berardi S, Caivano A, Ria R, et al. Four proteins governing overangiogenic endothelial cell phenotype in patients with multiple myeloma are plausible therapeutic targets. Oncogene. 2012;**31**:2258-2269. DOI: 10.1038/onc.2011.412. Epub Oct 3, 2011

[43] Ribatti D, Vacca A. Role of endothelial cells and fibroblasts in multiple myeloma angiogenic switch. Cancer Treatment and Research. 2016;**169**:51-61. DOI: 10.1007/978-3-319-40320-5_5

[44] Franco OE, Shaw AK, Strand DW, Hayward SW. Cancer associated fibroblasts in cancer pathogenesis. Seminars in Cell & Developmental Biology. 2010;**21**:33-39. DOI: 10.1016/j.semcdb.2009.10.010

[45] Santi A, Kugeratski FG, Zanivan S. Cancer associated fibroblasts: The architects of stroma remodeling. Proteomics. 2018;**18**:e1700167. DOI: 10.1002/pmic.201700167

[46] Paulsson J, Micke P. Prognostic relevance of cancer-associated fibroblasts in human cancer. Seminars in Cancer Biology. 2014;**25**:61-68. DOI: 10.1016/j.semcancer.2014.02.006

[47] Hinz B, Phan SH, Thannickal VJ, et al. The myofibroblasts: One function, multiple origins. The American Journal of Pathology. 2007;**170**:1807-1816. DOI: 10.2353/ajpath.2007.070112

[48] Frassanito MA, Rao L, Moschetta M, et al. Bone marrow fibroblasts parallel multiple myeloma progression in patients and mice: In vitro and in vivo studies. Leukemia. 2014;**28**:904-916. DOI: 10.1038/leu.2013.254

[49] Ribatti D, Vacca A. The role of inflammatory cells in angiogenesis in multiple myeloma. Advances in Experimental Medicine and Biology. 2014;**816**:361-376. DOI: 10.1007/978-3-0348-0837-8_14

[50] Salmi M. Macrophages and cancer. Duodecim. 2017;**133**:829-837

[51] Kim J, Bae JS. Tumor-associated macrophages and neutrophils in tumor microenvironment. Mediators of Inflammation. 2016;**2016**:6058147. DOI: 10.1155/2016/6058147

[52] Barleon B, Sozzani S, Zhou D, et al. Migration of human monocytes in response to vescular endothelial growth factor (VEGF) is mediated via the VEGF receptor Flt-1. Blood. 1996;**87**:3336-3343

[53] Ribatti D, Crivellato E, Roccaro AM, Ria R, Vacca A. Mast cell contribution to angiogenesis related to tumour progression. Clinical and Experimental Allergy. 2004;**34**:1660-1664. DOI: 10.1111/j.1365-2222.2004.02104.x

[54] Sörbo J, Jakobsson A, Norrby K. Mast cell histamine is angiogenic through receptors for histamine 1 and histamine 2. International Journal of Experimental Pathology. 1994;**75**:43-50

[55] Thompson WD, Campbell R, Evans T. Fibrin degradation and angiogenesis: Quantitative analysis of the angiogenic response in the chick chorioallantoic membrane. The Journal of Pathology. 1995;**145**:27-37. DOI: 10.1002/path.1711450103

[56] Ribatti D, Vacca A, Nico B, et al. Bone marrow angiogenesis and mast cell density increase simultaneously with progression of human multiple myeloma. British Journal of Cancer. 1999;**79**:451-455. DOI: 10.1038/sj.bjc.6690070

[57] Jurczyszyn A, Czepiel J, Gdula-Argasińska J, et al. The analysis of the relationship between multiple myeloma cells and their microenvironment. Journal of Cancer. 2015;**6**:160-168. DOI: 10.7150/jca.10873

[58] Giuliani N, Colla S, Morandi F, et al. Myeloma cells block RUNX2/CBFA1 activity in human bone marrow osteoblast progenitors and inhibit osteoblast formation and differentiation. Blood. 2005;**106**:2472-2483. DOI: 10.1182/blood-2004-12-4986

[59] Tian E, Zhan F, Walker R, et al. The role of the Wnt-signaling antagonist DKK1 in the development of osteolytic lesions in multiple myeloma. The New England Journal of Medicine. 2003;**349**:2483-2494. DOI: 10.1056/NEJMoa030847

[60] Sun L, Iqbal J, Dolgilevich S, et al. Disordered osteoclast formation and function in a CD38 (ADP-ribosyl cyclase)-deficient mouse establishes an essential role for CD38 in bone resorption. The FASEB Journal. 2003;**17**:369-375. DOI: 10.1096/fj.02-0205com

[61] An G, Acharya C, Feng X, et al. Osteoclasts promote immune suppressive microenvironment in multiple myeloma: Therapeutic implication. Blood. 2016;**128**:1590-1603. DOI: 10.1182/blood-2016-03-707547

[62] Horenstein AL, Quarona V, Toscani D, et al. Adenosine generated in the bone marrow niche through a CD38-mediated pathway correlates with progression of human myeloma. Molecular Medicine. 2016;**22**:694-704. DOI: 10.2119/molmed.2016.00198

[63] Costa F, Toscani D, Chillemi A, et al. Expression of CD38 in myeloma bone niche: A rational basis for the use of anti-CD38 immunotherapy to inhibit osteoclast formation. Oncotarget. 2017;**8**:56598-56611. DOI: 10.18632/oncotarget.17896

[64] Tamma R, Ribatti D. Bone niches, hematopoietic stem cells, and vessel formation. International Journal of Molecular Sciences. 2017;**18**:1-13. pii: E151. DOI: 10.3390/ijms18010151

[65] Birbrair A, Frenette PS. Niche heterogeneity in the bone marrow. Annals of the New York Academy of Sciences. 2016;**1370**:82-96. DOI: 10.1111/nyas.13016

[66] Bhaskar A, Gupta R, Kumar L, et al. Circulating endothelial progenitor cells as potential prognostic biomarker in multiple myeloma. Leukemia & Lymphoma. 2012;**53**:635-640. DOI: 10.3109/10428194.2011.628880

[67] Zhang H, Vakil V, Braunstein M, et al. Circulating endothelial progenitor cells in multiple myeloma: Implications and significance. Blood. 2005;**105**:3286-3294. DOI: 10.1182/blood-2004-06-2101

[68] Wang L, Du F, Zhang HM, et al. Changes in circulating endothelial progenitor cells predict responses of multiple myeloma patients to treatment with bortezomib and dexamethasone. Brazilian Journal of Medical and Biological Research. 2015;**48**:736-742. DOI: 10.1590/1414-431X20154558

[69] Rigolin GM, Fraulini C, Ciccone M, et al. Neoplastic circulating endothelial cells in multiple myeloma 13q14 deletion. Blood. 2006;**107**:2531-2535

[70] Xu S, De Veirman K, De Becker A, et al. Mesenchymal stem cells in multiple myeloma: A therapeutical tool or target? Leukemia. 2018. (in press) DOI: 10.1038/s41375-018-0061-9

[71] Reagan MR, Ghobrial IM. Multiple myeloma mesenchymal stem cells: Characterization, origin, and tumor-promoting effects. Clinical Cancer Research. 2012;**18**:342-349. DOI: 10.1158/1078-0432.CCR-11-2212

[72] Herrero C, Pérez-Simón JA. Immunomodulatory effect of mesenchymal stem cells. Brazilian Journal of Medical and Biological Research. 2010;**43**:425-430

[73] Markovina S, Callander NS, O'Connor SL, et al. Bone marrow stromal cells from multiple myeloma patients uniquely induce bortezomib resistant NF-kappaB activity in myeloma cells. Molecular Cancer. 2010;**9**:176. DOI: 10.1186/1476-4598-9-176

[74] Hao M, Zhang L, An G, et al. Bone marrow stromal cells protect myeloma cells from bortezomib induced apoptosis by suppressing microRNA-15a expression. Leukemia & Lymphoma. 2011;**52**:1787-1794. DOI: 10.3109/10428194.2011.576791

[75] Garcia-Gomez A, Sanchez-Guijo F, Del Cañizo MC, et al. Multiple myeloma mesenchymal stromal cells: Contribution to myeloma bone disease and therapeutics. World Journal of Stem Cells. 2014;**6**:322-343. DOI: 10.4252/wjsc.v6.i3.322

[76] Soukas A, Socci ND, Saatkamp BD, et al. Distinct transcriptional profiles of adipogenesis in vivo and in vitro. The Journal of Biological Chemistry. 2001;**276**:34167-34174. DOI: 10.1074/jbc.M104421200

[77] Baek JH, Jang JE, Kang CM, et al. Hypoxia-induced VEGF enhances tumor survivability via suppression of serum deprivation-induced apoptosis. Oncogene. 2000;**19**:4621-4631. DOI: 10.1038/sj.onc.1203814

[78] Cozzo AJ, Fuller AM, Makowski L. Contribution of adipose tissue to development of cancer. Comprehensive Physiology. 2017;**8**:237-282. DOI: 10.1002/cphy.c170008

[79] Wagner M, Dudley AC. A three-party alliance in solid tumors: Adipocytes, macrophages and vascular endothelial cells. Adipocytes. 2013;**2**:67-73. DOI: 10.4161/adip.23016

[80] Nieman KM, Romero IL, Van Houten B, Lengyel E. Adipose tissue and adipocytes support tumorigenesis and metastasis. Biochimica et Biophysica Acta. 2013;**1831**:1533-1541. DOI: 10.1016/j.bbalip.2013.02.010

[81] Falank C, Fairfield H, Reagan MR. Signaling interplay between bone marrow adipose tissue and multiple myeloma cells. Frontiers in Endocrinology (Lausanne). 2016;**7**:67. DOI: 10.3389/fendo.2016.00067

[82] Spencer JA, Ferraro F, Roussakis E, et al. Direct measurement of local oxygen concentration in the bone marrow of live animals. Nature. 2014;**508**:269-273. DOI: 10.1038/nature13034

[83] Kakudo N, Morimoto N, Ogawa T, et al. Hypoxia enhances proliferation of human adipose-derived stem cells via HIF-1α activation. PLoS One. 2015;**10**:e0139890. DOI: 10.1371/journal.pone.0139890

[84] Baeriswyl V, Christofori G. The angiogenic switch in carcinogenesis. Seminars in Cancer Biology. Oct 2009;**19**(5):329-337. DOI: 10.1016/j.semcancer.2009.05.003

[85] Kazerounian S, Lawler J. Integration of pro- and anti-angiogenic signals by endothelial cells. Journal of Cell Communication and Signaling. 2018;**12**:171-179. DOI: 10.1007/s12079-017-0433-3

[86] Ria R, Roccaro AM, Merchionne F, et al. Vascular endothelial growth factor and its receptors in multiple myeloma. Leukemia. 2003;**17**:1961-1966. DOI: 10.1038/sj.leu.2403076

[87] Ramakrishnan V, D'Souza A. Signaling pathways and emerging therapies in multiple myeloma. Current Hematologic Malignancy Reports. Apr 2016;**11**(2):156-164. DOI: 10.1007/s11899-016-0315-4

[88] Medinger M, Passweg J. Role of tumour angiogenesis in haematological malignancies. Swiss Medical Weekly. Nov 6, 2014;**144**:w14050. DOI: 10.4414/smw.2014.14050

[89] Vacca A, Ria R, Ribatti D, et al. A paracrine loop in the vascular endothelial growth factor pathway triggers tumor angiogenesis and growth in multiple myeloma. Haematologica. 2003;**88**:176-185

[90] Ria R, Vacca A, Russo F, et al. A VEGF-dependent autocrine loop mediates proliferation and capillarogenesis in bone marrow endothelial cells of patients with multiple myeloma. Thrombosis and Haemostasis. 2004;**93**:1438-1445. DOI: 10.1160/TH04-06-0334

[91] Dankbar B, Padro T, Leo R, et al. Vascular endothelial growth factor and interleukin-6 in paracrine tumor-stromal cell interactions in multiple myeloma. Blood. 2000;**95**:2630-2636

[92] Vacca A, Ribatti D, Presta M, et al. Bone marrow neovascularization, plasma cell angiogenic potential, and matrix metalloproteinase-2 secretion parallel progression of human multiple myeloma. Blood. 1999;**93**:3064-3073

[93] Suvannasankha A, Tompkins DR, Edwards DF, et al. FGF23 is elevated in multiple myeloma and increases heparanase expression by tumor cells. Oncotarget. 2015;**6**:19647-19660. DOI: 10.18632/oncotarget.3794

[94] Sucak GT, Aki SZ, Yüzbaşioğlu B, et al. Prognostic value of bone marrow microvessel density and angiogenic cytokines in patients with multiple myeloma undergoing autologous stem cell transplant. Leukemia & Lymphoma. 2011;**52**:1281-1289. DOI: 10.3109/10428194.2011.569695

[95] Bisping G, Leo R, Wenning D, et al. Paracrine interactions of basic fibroblast growth factor and interleukin-6 in multiple myeloma. Blood. 2003;**101**:2775-2783. DOI: 10.1182/blood-2002-09-2907

[96] Witzig T, Kimlinger T, Stenson M, Thereneau T. Syndecan-1 expression on malignant cells from the blood and marrow of patients with plasma cell proliferative disorders and B-cell chronic lymphocytic leukemia. Leukemia & Lymphoma. 1998;**31**:167-175. DOI: 10.3109/10428199809057596

[97] Basile A, Moschetta M, Ditonno P, et al. Pentraxin 3 (PTX3) inhibits plasma cell/stromal cell cross-talk in the bone marrow of multiple myeloma patients. The Journal of Pathology. 2013;**229**:87-98. DOI: 10.1002/path.4081

[98] Yamamoto S, Hagihara T, Horiuchi Y, et al. Mediator cyclin-dependent kinases upregulate transcription of inflammatory genes in cooperation with NF-κB and C/EBPβ on stimulation of toll-like receptor 9. Genes to Cells. 2017;**22**:265-276. DOI: 10.1111/gtc.12475

[99] Ferrucci A, Moschetta M, Frassanito MA, et al. A HGF/cMET autocrine loop is operative in multiple myeloma bone marrow endothelial cells and may represent a novel therapeutic target. Clinical Cancer Research. 2014;**20**:5796-5807. DOI: 10.1158/1078-0432.CCR-14-0847

[100] Gambella M, Palumbo A, Rocci A. MET/HGF pathway in multiple myeloma: From diagnosis to targeted therapy? Expert Review of Molecular Diagnostics. 2015;**15**:881-893. DOI: 10.1586/14737159.2015.1046436

[101] Jurczyszyn A, Zebzda A, Gdula-Argasińska J, et al. Blocking MET receptor signaling in multiple myeloma cells in vitro and in vivo. Advances in Clinical and Experimental Medicine. 2018;**27**:153-158. DOI: 10.17219/acem/68271

[102] Ting KR, Henry M, Meiller J, et al. Novel panel of protein biomarkers to predict response to bortezomib-containing induction regimens in multiple myeloma patients. BBA Clinical. 2017;**8**:28-34. DOI: 10.1016/j.bbacli.2017.05.003

[103] Belloni D, Marcatti M, Ponzoni M, et al. Angiopoietin-2 in bone marrow milieu promotes multiple myeloma-associated angiogenesis. Experimental Cell Research. 2015;**330**:1-12. DOI: 10.1016/j.yexcr.2014.10.017

[104] Giuliani N, Colla S, Lazzaretti M, et al. Proangiogenic properties of human myeloma cells: Production of angiopoietin-1 and its potential relationship to myeloma-induced angiogenesis. Blood. 2003;**102**:638-645. DOI: 10.1182/blood-2002-10-3257

[105] Pappa CA, Tsirakis G, Samiotakis P, et al. Serum levels of angiopoietin-2 are associated with the growth of multiple myeloma. Cancer Investigation. 2013;**31**:385-389. DOI: 10.3109/07357907.2013.800093

[106] Terpos E, Anargyrou K, Katodritou E, et al. Greek myeloma study group, Greece. Circulating angiopoietin-1 to angiopoietin-2 ratio is an independent prognostic factor for survival in newly diagnosed patients with multiple myeloma who received therapy with novel antimyeloma agents. International Journal of Cancer. 2012;**130**:735-742. DOI: 10.1002/ijc.26062

[107] Cheriyath V, Husein MA. Osteopontin, angiogenesis and multiple myeloma. Leukemia. 2005;**19**:2203-2205. DOI: 10.1038/sj.leu.2403978

[108] Babarović E, Valković T, Budisavljević I, et al. The expression of osteopontin and vascular endothelial growth factor in correlation with angiogenesis in monoclonal gammopathy of undetermined significance and multiple myeloma. Pathology, Research and Practice. 2016;**212**:509-516. DOI: 10.1016/j.prp.2015.11.021

[109] Sfiridaki A, Miyakis S, Pappa C, et al. Circulating osteopontin: A dual marker of bone destruction and angiogenesis in patients with multiple myeloma. Journal of Hematology & Oncology. 2011;**4**:22. DOI: 10.1186/1756-8722-4-22

[110] Bolkun L, Lemancewicz D, Sobolewski K, et al. The evaluation of angiogenesis and matrix metalloproteinase-2 secretion in bone marrow of multiple myeloma patients before and after the treatment. Advances in Medical Sciences. 2013;**58**:118-125. DOI: 10.2478/v10039-012-0048-0

[111] Bilalis A, Pouliou E, Roussou M, et al. Increased expression of platelet derived growth factor receptor β on trephine biopsies correlates with advanced myeloma. Journal of Balkan Union of Oncology. 2017;**22**:1032-1037

[112] Barillé S, Akhoundi C, Collette M, et al. Metalloproteinases in multiple myeloma: Production of matrix metalloproteinase-9 (MMP-9), activation of pro MMP-2, and induction of MMP-1 by myeloma cells. Blood. 1997;**90**:1649-1655

[113] Coluccia AML, Cirulli T, Neri P, et al. Validation of PDGFRβ and c-Src tyrosine kinases as tumor/vessel targets in patients with multiple myeloma: Preclinical efficacy of the novel, orally available inhibitor dasatinib. Blood. 2008;**12**:1346-1356. DOI: 10.1182/blood-2007-10-116590

[114] Tsirakis G, Pappa CA, Kanellou P, et al. Role of platelet-derived growth factor-AB in tumour growth and angiogenesis in relation with other angiogenic cytokines in multiple myeloma. Hematological Oncology. 2012;**30**:131-136. DOI: 10.1002/hon.1014

[115] Airoldi I, Cocco C, Giuliani N, et al. Constitutive expression of IL-12Rb2 on human multiple myeloma cells delineates a novel therapeutic target. Blood. 2008;**112**:750-759. DOI: 10.1182/blood-2008-02-139378

[116] Cocco C, Giuliani N, Di Carlo E, et al. Interleukin-27 acts as multifunctional antitumor agent in multiple myeloma. Clinical Cancer Research. 2010;**16**:4188-4197. DOI: 10.1158/1078-0432.CCR-10-0173

[117] Dondero A, Casu B, Bellora F, et al. NK cells and multiple myeloma-associated endothelial cells: Molecular interactions and influence of IL-27. Oncotarget. 2017;**8**:35088-35102. DOI: 10.18632/oncotarget.17070

[118] Pellegrino A, Ria R, Di Pietro G, et al. Bone marrow endothelial cells in multiple myeloma secrete CXC-chemokines that mediate interactions with plasma cells. British Journal of Haematology. 2005;**129**:248-256. DOI: 10.1111/j.1365-2141.2005.05443.x

[119] Colla S, Storti P, Donofrio G, et al. Low bone marrow oxygen tension and hypoxia-inducible factor-1α overexpression characterize patients with multiple myeloma: Role on the transcriptional and proangiogenic profiles of CD138(+) cells. Leukemia. 2010;**24**:1967-1970. DOI: 10.1038/leu.2010.193

[120] Pappa CA, Tsirakis G, Kanellou P, et al. Monitoring serum levels ELR+ CXC chemokines and the relationship between microvessel density and angiogenic growth factors in multiple myeloma. Cytokine. 2011;**56**:616-620. DOI: 10.1016/j.cyto.2011.08.034

[121] Bhaskar A, Tiwary BN. Hypoxia inducible factor-1 alpha and multiple myeloma. International Journal of Advanced Research (Indore). 2016;**4**:706-715

[122] Zhang J, Sattler M, Tonon G, et al. Targeting angiogenesis via a c-Myc/hypoxia-inducible factor-1alpha-dependent pathway in multiple myeloma. Cancer Research. 2009;**69**:5082-5090. DOI: 10.1158/0008-5472.CAN-08-4603

[123] Borsi E, Perrone G, Terragna C, et al. HIF-1α inhibition blocks the cross talk between multiple myeloma plasma cells and tumor microenvironment. Experimental Cell Research. 2014;**328**:444-455. DOI: 10.1016/j.yexcr.2014.09.018

[124] Ria R, Catacchio I, Berardi S, et al. HIF-1α of bone marrow endothelial cells implies relapse and drug resistance in patients with multiple myeloma and may act as a therapeutic target. Clinical Cancer Research. 2014;**20**:847-858. DOI: 10.1158/1078-0432.CCR-13-1950

[125] Conciatori F, Ciuffreda L, Bazzichetto C, et al. mTOR cross-talk in cancer and potential for combination therapy. Cancers (Basel). 2018;**10**:1-30. pii: E23. DOI: 10.3390/cancers10010023

[126] Janku F, Yap TA, Meric-Bernstam F. Targeting the PI3K pathway in cancer: Are we making headway? Nature Reviews. Clinical Oncology. 2018;**15**:273-291. DOI: 10.1038/nrclinonc.2018.28

[127] Lamanuzzi A, Saltarella I, Desantis V, et al. Inhibition of mTOR Complex 2 Restrains Tumor Angiogenesis in Multiple Myeloma Oncotarget. 2018 (in press)

[128] LaFoya B, Munroe JA, Mia MM, et al. Notch: A multi-functional integrating system of microenvironmental signals. Developmental Biology. 2016;**418**:227-241. DOI: 10.1016/j.ydbio.2016.08.023

[129] Colombo M, Mirandola L, Platonova N, et al. Notch-directed microenvironment reprogramming in myeloma: A single path to multiple outcomes. Leukemia. 2013;**27**:1009-1018. DOI: 10.1038/leu.2013.6

[130] Pasquale EB. Eph receptors and ephrins in cancer: Bidirectional signalling and beyond. Nature Reviews. Cancer. 2010;**10**:165-180. DOI: 10.1038/nrc2806

[131] Feldheim DA, O'Leary DD. Visual map development: Bidirectional signaling, bifunctional guidance molecules, and competition. Cold Spring Harbor Perspectives in Biology. 2010;**2**:a001768-a001768. DOI: 10.1101/cshperspect.a001768

[132] Janes PW, Slape CI, Farnsworth RH, et al. EphA3 biology and cancer. Growth Factors. 2014;**32**:176-189. DOI: 10.3109/08977194.2014.982276

[133] Brantley DM, Cheng N, Thompson EJ, et al. Soluble Eph A receptors inhibit tumor angiogenesis and progression in vivo. Oncogene. 2002;**21**:7011-7026. DOI: 10.1038/sj.onc.1205679

[134] Caivano A, La Rocca F, Laurenzana I, et al. Epha3 acts as proangiogenic factor in multiple myeloma. Oncotarget. 2017;**8**:34298-34309. DOI: 10.18632/oncotarget.16100

[135] Lechertier T, Hodivala-Dilke K. Focal adhesion kinase and tumour angiogenesis. The Journal of Pathology. 2012;**226**:404-412. DOI: 10.1002/path.3018

[136] Coelho NM, Llopis-Hernández V, Salmerón-Sánchez M, Altankov G. Dynamic reorganization and enzymatic remodeling of type IV collagen at cell-biomaterial Interface. Advances in Protein Chemistry and Structural Biology. 2016;**105**:81-104. DOI: 10.1016/bs.apcsb.2016.06.001

[137] Infusino GA, Jacobson JR. Endothelial FAK as a therapeutic target in disease. Microvascular Research. 2012;**83**:89-96. DOI: 10.1016/j.mvr.2011.09.011

[138] Tanghetti E, Ria R, Dell'Era P, et al. Biological activity of substrate-bound basic fibroblast growth factor (FGF2): Recruitment of FGF receptor-1 in endothelial cell adhesion contacts. Oncogene. 2002;**21**:3889-3897. DOI: 10.1038/sj.onc.1205407

[139] Masoud GN, Li W. HIF-1α pathway: Role, regulation and intervention for cancer therapy. Acta Pharmaceutica Sinica B. 2015;**5**:378-389. DOI: 10.1016/j.apsb.2015.05.007

[140] Sang N, Stiehl DP, Bohensky J, et al. MAPK signaling up-regulates the activity of hypoxia-inducible factors by its effects on p300. The Journal of Biological Chemistry. 2003;**278**:14013-14019. DOI: 10.1074/jbc.M209702200

[141] Bartel DP. MicroRNAs: Genomics, biogenesis, mechanism, and function. Cell. 2004;**116**:281-297

[142] Winter J, Diederichs S. MicroRNA biogenesis and cancer. Methods in Molecular Biology. 2011;**676**:3-22. DOI: 10.1007/978-1-60761-863-8_1

[143] Wang Y, Wang L, Chen C, Chu X. New insights into the regulatory role of microRNA in tumor angiogenesis and clinical implications. Molecular Cancer. 2018;**17**:22. DOI: 10.1186/s12943-018-0766-4

[144] Wang W, Zhang E, Lin C. MicroRNAs in tumor angiogenesis. Life Sciences. 2015;**136**:28-35. DOI: 10.1016/j.lfs.2015.06.025

[145] Yin R, Guo L, Zhang W, Zheng J. The pleiotropic effects of miRNAs on tumor angiogenesis. Journal of Cellular Biochemistry. 2015;**116**:1807-1815. DOI: 10.1002/jcb.24679

[146] Ohyashiki JH, Umezu T, Ohyashiki K. Exosomes promote bone marrow angiogenesis in hematologic neoplasia: The role of hypoxia. Current Opinion in Hematology. 2016;**23**:268-273. DOI: 10.1097/MOH.0000000000000235

[147] Umezu T, Tadokoro H, Azuma K, et al. Exosomal miR-135b shed from hypoxic multiple myeloma cells enhances angiogenesis by targeting factor-inhibiting HIF-1. Blood. 2014;**124**:3748-3757. DOI: 10.1182/blood-2014-05-576116

[148] Raimondi L, Amodio N, Di Martino MT, et al. Targeting of multiple myeloma-related angiogenesis by miR-199a-5p mimics: In vitro and in vivo anti-tumor activity. Oncotarget. 2014;**5**:3039-3054. DOI: 10.18632/oncotarget.1747

[149] Sun CY, She XM, Qin Y, et al. miR-15a and miR-16 affect the angiogenesis of multiple myeloma by targeting VEGF. Carcinogenesis. 2013;**34**:426-435. DOI: 10.1093/carcin/bgs333

[150] Katoh M. Therapeutics targeting angiogenesis: Genetics and epigenetics, extracellular miRNAs and signaling networks (review). International Journal of Molecular Medicine. 2013;**32**:763-767. DOI: 10.3892/ijmm.2013.1444

[151] Ria R, Reale A, Vacca A. Novel agents and new therapeutic approaches for treatment of multiple myeloma. World Journal of Methodology. 2014;**4**:73-90. DOI: 10.5662/wjm.v4.i2.73

[152] Barchnicka A, Olejniczak-Nowakowska M, Krupa-Kotara K, Grosicki S. The importance of antiangiogenic effect in multiple myeloma treatment. Advances in Clinical and Experimental Medicine. 2018;**27**:291-297. DOI: 10.17219/acem/68826

[153] Kumar S. Emerging options in multiple myeloma: Targeted, immune, and epigenetic therapies. Hematology. American Society of Hematology. Education Program. 2017;**2017**:518-524. DOI: 10.1182/asheducation-2017.1.518

[154] Roccaro AM, Hideshima T, Raje N, et al. Bortezomib mediates antiangiogenesis in multiple myeloma via direct and indirect effects on endothelial cells. Cancer Research. 2006;**66**:184-191. DOI: 10.1158/0008-5472.CAN-05-1195

[155] Roccaro AM, Hideshima T, Richardson PG, et al. Bortezomib as an antitumor agent. Current Pharmaceutical Biotechnology. 2006;**7**:441-448

[156] Hideshima T, Chauhan D, Richardson P, et al. NF-kappa B as a therapeutic target in multiple myeloma. The Journal of Biological Chemistry. 2002;**277**:16639-16647. DOI: 10.1074/jbc.M200360200

[157] Gandolfi S, Laubach JP, Hideshima T, et al. The proteasome and proteasome inhibitors in multiple myeloma. Cancer Metastasis Reviews. 2017;**36**:561-584. DOI: 10.1007/s10555-017-9707-8

[158] Moreau P, Touzeau C. Multiple myeloma: From front-line to relapsed therapies. American Society of Clinical Oncology Educational Book. 2015:e504-e511. DOI: 10.14694/EdBook_AM.2015.35.e504

[159] Chauhan D, Tian Z, Zhou B, et al. In vitro and in vivo selective antitumor activity of a novel orally bioavailable proteasome inhibitor MLN9708 against multiple myeloma cells. Clinical Cancer Research. 2011;**17**:5311-5321. DOI: 10.1158/1078-0432.CCR-11-0476

[160] McConkey DJ, Zhu K. Mechanisms of proteasome inhibitor action and resistance in cancer. Drug Resistance Updates. 2008;**11**:164-179. DOI: 10.1016/j.drup.2008.08.002

[161] Brito AB, Lourenço GJ, Oliveira GB, et al. Associations of VEGF and VEGFR2 polymorphisms with increased risk and aggressiveness of multiple myeloma. Annals of Hematology. 2014;**93**:1363-1369. DOI: 10.1007/s00277-014-2062-8

[162] Sissung TM, Peer CJ, Korde N, et al. Carfilzomib and lenalidomide response related to VEGF and VEGFR2 germline polymorphisms. Cancer Chemotherapy and Pharmacology. 2017;**80**:217-221. DOI: 10.1007/s00280-017-3323-8

[163] D'Amato RJ, Loughnan MS, Flynn E, Folkman J. Thalidomide is an inhibitor of angiogemesis. Proceedings of the National Academy of Sciences of the United States of America. 1994;**91**:4082-4085

[164] Mercurio A, Adriani G, Catalano A, et al. A mini-review on thalidomide: Chemistry, mechanisms of action, therapeutic potential and anti-angiogenic properties in multiple myeloma. Current Medicinal Chemistry. 2017;**24**:2736-2744. DOI: 10.2174/0929867324666170601074646

[165] Gao Y, Ma G, Liu S, et al. Thalidomide and multiple myeloma serum synergistically induce a hemostatic imbalance in endothelial cells in vitro. Thrombosis Research. 2015;**135**:1154-1159. DOI: 10.1016/j.thromres.2015.03.019

[166] Ribatti D, Vacca A. Novel therapeutic approches targeting vascular endothelial growth factor and its receptors in haematological malignancies. Current Cancer Drug Targets. 2005;**5**:573-578. DOI: 10.2174/156800905774932806

[167] Gupta D, Treon SP, Shima Y, et al. Adherence of multiple myeloma cells to bone marrow stromal cells upregulates vascular endothelial growth factoor secretion: Therapeutic application. Leukemia. 2001;**15**:1950-1961

[168] Dredge K, Marriott JB, Macdonald CD, et al. Novel thalidomide analogues display anti-angiogenic activity independently of immunomodulatory effects. British Journal of Cancer. 2002;**87**:1166-1172. DOI: 10.1038/sj.bjc.6600607

[169] Bartlett JB, Dredge K, Dalgleish AG. The evolution of thalidomide and its IMiD derivatives as anticancer agents. Nature Reviews. Cancer. 2004;**4**:314-322. DOI: 10.1038/nrc1323

[170] De Luisi A, Ferrucci A, Coluccia AM, et al. Lenalidomide restrains motility and overangiogenic potential of bone marrow endothelial cells in patients with active multiple myeloma. Clinical Cancer Research. 2011;**17**:1935-1946. DOI: 10.1158/1078-0432.CCR-10-2381

[171] Saini N, Mahindra A. Novel immunomodulatory compounds in multiple myeloma. Expert Opinion on Investigational Drugs. 2013;**22**:207-215. DOI: 10.1517/13543784.2013.749235

[172] Mark TM, Coleman M, Niesvizky R. Preclinical and clinical results with pomalidomide in the treatment of relapsed/refractory multiple myeloma. Leukemia Research. 2014 May;**38**(5):517-524. DOI: 10.1016/j.leukres.2014.02.008

[173] Scavelli C, Di Pietro G, Cirulli T, et al. Zoledronic acid affects ocer-angiogenic phenotype of endothelial cells in patients with multiple myeloma. Molecular Cancer Therapeutics. 2007;**6**(12 Pt 1):3256-3262. DOI: 10.1158/1535-7163.MCT-07-0311

[174] Ria R, Reale A, Moschetta M, et al. A retrospective study of skeletal and disease-free survival benefits of zoledronic acid therapy in patients with multiple myeloma treated with novel agents. International Journal of Clinical and Experimental Medicine. 2013;**6**:30-38

[175] Ribatti D, Nico B, Mangieri D, et al. Neridronate inhibits angiogenesis in vitro and in vivo. Clinical Rheumatology. 2007;**26**:1094-1098. DOI: 10.1007/s10067-006-0455-3

[176] Ferrara N, Hillan KJ, Gerber HP, Novotny W. Discovery and development of bevacizumab, an anti-VEGF antibody for treating cancer. Nature Reviews. Drug Discovery. 2004;**3**:391-400. DOI: 10.1038/nrd1381

[177] Podar K, Anderson KC. The pathophysiologic role of VEGF in hematologic malignancies: Therapeutic implications. Blood. 2005;**105**:1383-1395. DOI: 10.1182/blood-2004-07-2909

[178] Zagouri F, Terpos E, Kastritis E, Dimopoulos MA. Emerging antibodies for the treatment of multiple myeloma. Expert Opinion on Emerging Drugs. 2016;**21**:225-237. DOI: 10.1080/14728214.2016.1186644

[179] Cook KM, Figg WD. Angiogenesis inhibitors: Current strategies and future prospects. CA: A Cancer Journal for Clinicians. 2010;**60**:222-243. DOI: 10.3322/caac.20075

[180] Mo HN, Liu P. Targeting MET in cancer therapy. Chronic Diseases and Translational Medicine. 2017;**3**:148-153. DOI: 10.1016/j.cdtm.2017.06.002

[181] Lopuch S, Kawalec P, Wiśniewska N. Effectiveness of targeted therapy as monotherapy or combined therapy in patients with relapsed or refractory multiple myeloma: A systematic review and meta-analysis. Hematology. 2015;**20**:1-10. DOI: 10.1179/1607845414Y.0000000159

Section 3

Clinical Aspects of Multiple Myeloma

Chapter 6

Hematopoietic Stem Cell Transplantation in Multiple Myeloma in the Era of Novel Therapies

Khalid Ahmed Al-Anazi

Additional information is available at the end of the chapter

http://dx.doi.org/10.5772/intechopen.79999

Abstract

Multiple myeloma is the second commonest hematologic malignancy. It is characterized by neoplastic proliferation of a single clone of plasma cells in the bone marrow producing a monoclonal immunoglobulin and ultimately causing various complications and organ dysfunction. Over the last 10 years, management of multiple myeloma has dramatically changed due to the introduction of several novel therapies that have improved the disease outcome and prognosis, as well as the quality of life of patients with myeloma due to their safety, tolerability and efficacy. Additionally, the widespread utilization of autologous hematopoietic stem cell transplantation, which is still the standard of care for transplant-eligible patients, and the implementation of new therapeutic strategies such as drug combinations in addition to consolidation and maintenance therapies have resulted in further improvements in response rates and survival in patients with multiple myeloma. This book chapter will be an update on the novel therapies and the recent treatment strategies in myeloma. The role of stem cell treatments in the era of novel therapies will be discussed thoroughly.

Keywords: multiple myeloma, hematopoietic stem cell transplantation, novel therapies, monoclonal antibodies

1. Introduction

Multiple myeloma (MM) is an incurable, debilitating and heterogeneous malignancy that has highly variable clinical course [1–6]. It is a plasma cell neoplasm characterized by neoplastic proliferation of a single clone of plasma cells in the bone marrow (BM) producing a monoclonal immunoglobulin and causing anemia, renal failure, bone destruction and infectious complications [7–9]. It is the second most commonly diagnosed hematologic malignancy (HM) and it accounts for approximately 10% of all HMs [8]. The median age of MM at diagnosis is 70 years in the United States of America (USA) and 72 years in Europe [9].

2. Diagnosis, staging, genetics and risk stratification

The diagnostic criteria for MM are: (1) clonal BM plasma cells ≥10% or biopsy-proven bony or extramedullary plasmacytoma and (2) at least one of the following: (a) evidence of end-organ damage such as anemia, lytic bone lesions, hypercalcemia and renal insufficiency, (b) clonal BM plasma cells ≥60%, (c) involved:uninvolved serum free light chain ratio ≥100 and (d) at least two focal lesions on magnetic resonance imaging [8, 10–15].

MM is usually classified into three stages: (1) stage I; all the following: serum albumin ≥3.5 g/dL, serum beta 2 microglobulin (B2M) < 3.5 mg/L, normal serum lactic dehydrogenase (LDH) and no high-risk (HR) cytogenetics; (2) stage II: not fitting stages I and III with serum B2M: 3.5–5.5 mg/L, and (3) stage III; all the following: serum B2M > 3.5 mg/L and HR cytogenetics or elevated serum LDH level [8, 13].

The following cytogenetic abnormalities have been reported in patients with MM: trisomies; monosomies; 17 p deletion; amp (1q20); t(14,16); t(14,20); t(4,14); t(6,14) and t(11,14) [8, 13, 16]. Also, the following molecular mutations have been reported in MM patients: NRAS, KRAS, TP53, BRAF, CCND1, FAM46C, MYC, XBP1, EZH2 and CHST15 [17–21]. Recently, the following laboratory techniques have been utilized in the diagnosis and follow-up of patients with MM: (1) next-generation sequencing (NGS), (2) genomic and epigenetic studies, (3) microRNA and (4) minimal residual disease (MRD) evaluation by flow cytometry, polymerase chain reaction, and NGS [17–22]. Mass accumulation rate will be used in the near future for susceptibility of human MM cell lines to standard-of-care therapies [23].

The HR features in MM include: (1) cytogenetic and molecular abnormalities that include: hypodiploid, 17 p deletion, t(4,14), t(14,16), t(14,20) and EZH2; (2) international scoring system stage II or III; (3) presence of comorbid medical conditions that limit therapy; (4) extramedullary disease (EMD) and (5) renal failure, high serum LDH level and plasma cell leukemia [13, 16, 21, 24, 25]. MM patients are stratified into three risk groups based on their cytogenetic profiles as follows: (1) HR that includes 17 p deletion, t(14,16) or t(14,20); (2) intermediate risk that includes: t(4,14) and amp (1q20)/gain (1q) and (3) standard risk that includes: trisomies, t(11,14) and t(6,14) [8, 13, 16]. Additional poor prognostic features include: age ≥60 years and refractory and/or relapsed MM (R/R-MM) [26].

3. New insights into the pathogenesis of MM

Despite the recent progress in understanding MM, the pathogenesis of the disease is incompletely understood and is apparently multifactorial in nature [27]. The 10 hallmarks of cancer are: (1) self-sufficiency in growth signaling, (2) evasion of apoptosis, (3) insensitivity to anti-growth mechanisms, (4) tissue invasion and metastases, (5) limitless replicative potential, (6) sustained angiogenesis, (7) avoidance of immune destruction, (8) reprogramming of energy metabolism, (9) tumor-promoting inflammation and (10) genome instability and mutation.

All the 10 hallmarks of cancer are present and active in MM and they contribute to tumor initiation, drug resistance, disease progression and relapse [28–30].

BM adipose tissue is a newly recognized contributor to MM oncogenesis and disease progression, particularly affecting MM cell metabolism, immune action and inflammation in addition to influencing angiogenesis [28]. BM adipose tissue may support MM through: (1) bioactive lipids such as fuel source, signaling molecule and substrate for lipid peroxidation and (2) MM supportive adipokines such as interleukin (IL)-6, tumor necrosis factor-α, MCP-1, PAI-1, resistin and leptin. The interaction between hypoxia, BM adipose tissue and angiogenesis is complicated [28].

The BM niche in patients with MM appears to play an important role in differentiation, migration, survival and drug resistance of malignant plasma cells [31, 32]. The BM niche is composed of (1) cellular compartment that contains the following constituents: hematopoietic and nonhematopoietic cells, stromal cells, osteoblasts, osteoclasts, endothelial cells and immune cells and (2) noncellular compartment, which has the following constituents: extracellular matrix (ECM) and liquid milieu that has cytokines, chemokines and growth factors [31–34]. MM cells home to the BM, adhere to the ECM and BM stromal cells. Trafficking or homing ingress allows progression or metastasis of disease to new BM sites [31].

Bone destruction is the hallmark of MM and is mediated by osteoblasts [35]. Osteoblasts are the most important components of the MM microenvironment. They largely affect disease progression either directly or indirectly. Also, they may slow MM growth [36]. Normally, there is a balance between osteoblastic and osteoclastic activity and imbalance leads to development of disease lesions. Hence, increased osteoclastic activity is associated with MM [37]. Osteoclasts are the primary mediators of bone resorption in both healthy and pathological bone turnover. Bone anabolic agents hold potential for antimyeloma and antiosteolysis therapies [36].

MM pathophysiology is the result of the interaction between clonal plasma cells and the surrounding BM microenvironment [31, 32, 38–40]. BM angiogenesis represents a constant hallmark of MM progression partly driven by the release of proangiogenic cytokines from the tumor plasma cells, BM stromal cells and osteoclasts such as vascular endothelial growth factor (VEGF), basic fibroblast growth factor (bFGF) and metalloproteinases [31]. Also, BM stromal cells from MM patients express several proangiogenic molecules such as VEGF, bFGF, angiopoietin-1, transforming growth factor-β, hepatocyte growth factor, platelet-derived growth factor and IL-1 [31]. The signaling pathways that are active in MM microenvironment include Ras GAP, FAK, phosphoinositide 3-kinase (PI-3K)-akt, MEK-ERK and STAT [38]. Other signaling pathways that may also become new therapeutic targets in MM include RANKL, DKK1, sclerostin and activing-A [31, 39].

MicroRNAs play a crucial role in cancer progression [40]. They are the novel crossroads between MM cells and MM microenvironment [41]. Several microRNAs are dysregulated in MM [40]. Dysregulation of microRNAs in MM cells and MM microenvironment has important impacts on initiation of MM, disease progression and drug resistance [42, 43]. Approximately 95 microRNAs are expressed at high levels in MM, particularly miR-125b, miR-133a, miR-1 and miR-124a [40]. Deregulated microRNAs target genes regulating cell cycle, apoptosis, survival and cell growth [40]. Interactions between various constituents of BM microenvironment, particularly MM mesenchymal stem cells and MM cancer stem cells, may be involved in disease initiation such as bone involvement, disease progression, relapse and drug resistance, so microRNAs may become very useful in designing targeted therapies in the field of precision medicine [27, 44–52]. Additionally, circulating microRNAs may serve as diagnostic and prognostic markers due to their impact on gene expression, biological function and survival, and microRNA-based assays may help in improving risk stratification in MM [27, 53–58].

4. Management of MM

Over the past two decades, management of MM has dramatically changed and this has translated into significant improvements in disease outcomes and prognosis. This unprecedented progress can be attributed to (1) the application of high-dose (HD) chemotherapy followed by autologous hematopoietic stem cell transplantation (HSCT), (2) improvement in supportive care strategies and (3) the introduction of several novel agents particularly immunomodulatory agents and proteasome inhibitors in the treatment of patients with MM [10, 13, 16, 59–61].

Cytotoxic agents that have been used in the treatment of MM include (1) corticosteroids such as dexamethasone and prednisolone, (2) conventional chemotherapies including melphalan, cyclophosphamide, liposomal doxorubicin, bendamustine, carmustine (BCNU), D-PACE (dexamethasone, cisplatin, doxorubicin, cyclophosphamide, etoposide) and DCEP (dexamethasone, cyclophosphamide, etoposide, cisplatin) [62]. However, remarkable improvements in survival of patients with MM have been achieved following the introduction of thalidomide, bortezomib and lenalidomide, as well as the recent introduction and approval of the following novel therapeutic agents: (1) newer proteasome inhibitors such as carfilzomib and ixazomib; (2) histone deacetylase inhibitors such as panobinostat and vorinostat; (3) new immunomodulatory drugs such as pomalidomide; (4) monoclonal antibodies such as daratumumab and elotuzumab; (5) Bruton tyrosine kinase inhibitors such as ibrutinib; (6) IL-6 inhibitors such as siltuximab; (7) PI-3 K inhibitors and (8) various immunotherapeutic strategies including chimeric antigen receptor (CAR) T cells [10, 13, 15, 62–64].

5. Frontline and induction therapies in MM

Several studies have shown that VRD (bortezomib, lenalidomide, dexamethasone) regimen is well tolerated and highly effective in the treatment of newly diagnosed MM patients [65–70]. Once used as first-line therapy for MM, VRD has been shown to be superior to the doublet regimen of lenalidomide plus dexamethasone, as well as the triplet regimens VCD (bortezomib, cyclophosphamide, dexamethasone) and VTD (bortezomib, thalidomide, dexamethasone) [68]. Carfilzomib, lenalidomide, dexamethasone (KRD) is an alternative promising regimen but has only been evaluated in small phase II studies in the frontline setting [68].

Response criteria in patients with MM subjected to various therapeutic regimens include MRD evaluation by multicolor flow cytometry or sequencing on bone marrow samples and imaging for EMD [59, 71]. MRD has recently been incorporated into the International

Myeloma Working Group response criteria and new studies have demonstrated that achievement of MRD negativity is a stronger predictor of survival than is traditional complete response (CR) [72].

6. HSCT in patients with MM

6.1. Autologous HSCT

Autologous HSCT, performed at the time of initial diagnosis or at relapse, is considered the standard of care for patients with newly diagnosed MM who are younger than 70 years [8, 73, 74]. Even in the era of novel therapies, timing of performance of autologous HSCT, whether upfront or at relapse, is still controversial although there is global consensus strongly in favor of early autologous HSCT [75].

Autologous HSCT is not curative for MM [8, 73]. Allogeneic HSCT is the only curative therapy for MM but at the expense of increased treatment-related mortality (TRM), so candidates for allografts should be carefully selected from the pool of young patients with R/R-MM [76]. Several randomized clinical trials have shown that, compared with conventional chemotherapy alone, HD chemotherapy followed by stem cell rescue is associated with prolonged event-free survival (EFS) and overall survival (OS) [8, 73, 74]. The recent widespread implementation of autologous HSCT in conjunction with novel therapies has revolutionized the management of MM and has markedly altered the natural history of the disease by improving disease responses and response duration ultimately leading to significant improvement in OS [73].

Eligibility for autologous HSCT is determined by age, performance status, presence and severity of comorbid medical conditions, and frailty score as frailty has been shown to be a predictor of short survival and is considered an exclusion criterion for autologous HSCT [8].

6.2. Cryopreservation versus noncryopreservation of stem cells

For most types of transplants, cryopreservation of HSCs is necessary and is an essential component of the clinical protocol [77]. Dimethyl sulfoxide (DMSO) is widely used as a cryopreservant for various types of stem cells and other body tissues. It has the following adverse effects: skin irritation, garlic breath or body odor; abdominal pain, nausea, vomiting and diarrhea; bronchospasm, chest tightness and dyspnea; altered heart rate and blood pressure, arrhythmias, heart block and myocardial ischemia; various degrees of organ dysfunction and death [77, 78]. Additionally, DMSO has in vitro toxicity in the form of induction of red blood cell hemolysis and reduction in platelet aggregation and activity [78].

Several studies and one meta-analysis have shown that noncryopreserved autologous HSCT for MM is simple, safe and cost-effective and gives results that are at least equivalent to autologous HSCT with cryopreservation [79–84]. TRM at day 100 post-HSCT has ranged between 0.0 and 3.4% [80, 82–84]. Noncryopreserved stem cells can be infused till day 5 postapheresis without viability loss provided they are stored at +4°C in conventional blood bank refrigerator [79, 81, 82, 84]. In a systematic review that included 16 studies having 560 patients with various HMs including MM, hematopoietic engraftment was universal and only one graft failure was reported [79, 81]. The median times for engraftment following noncryopreserved autografts were 9–14 days for neutrophils and 14–25 days for platelets [79, 81]. Other recent studies on noncryopreserved autologous HSCT in patients with MM have shown the following results: neutrophil engraftment between 10 and 14 days and platelet engraftment between 13 and 25 days postautologous HSCT [85–92].

Melphalan is the standard chemotherapeutic agent that is used in the conditioning therapy prior to autologous HSCT in MM. The dose ranges between 140 and 200 mg/m^2, given intravenously (IV) [79, 81, 82, 93]. It is cleared from plasma and urine in 1 and 6 hours, respectively. Stem cells can be safely infused as early as 8–24 hours following melphalan administration [79, 81].

Recently, other drugs have been used in the conditioning therapy prior to autologous HSCT in MM either alone or in combination with HD melphalan [94–97]. Compared to HD melphalan, the use of ixazomib, BCNU, bortezomib and IV busulfan either alone or in various combinations with HD melphalan in the conditioning therapies has increased the overall response rates and the median OS without additional toxicity [93–97].

HSCT without cryopreservation has several advantages including (1) simplicity of implementation, (2) allowing autologous HSCT to be performed entirely as outpatient, (3) reduction of transplantation costs, (4) reducing the time between the last induction therapy and HD chemotherapy, (5) prevention of DMSO toxicity, (6) no significant loss of viability of the collected HSCs provided stem cell infusion is made within 5 days of apheresis, (7) expansion of the number of medical institutions performing stem cell therapies and (8) potent engraftment syndrome and autologous graft versus host disease (GVHD) [79–84, 98, 99]. HSCT without cryopreservation has the following disadvantages: (1) plenty of coordination is needed between various teams regarding timing of stem cell mobilization, apheresis, administration of conditioning therapy and infusion of stem cells; (2) limitation of the use of standard HD chemotherapy schedules such as BEAM (BCNU, etoposide, cytarabine and melphalan) employed in the autologous HSCT for lymphoma and (3) inability to store part of the collection and reserving it for a second autologous HSCT in case a rich product is obtained [79–84].

6.3. Outpatient HSCT

MM is the leading indication for autologous HSCT worldwide. Patients with MM are ideal candidates for outpatient autologous HSCT because of the following reasons: the ease of administering HD melphalan, the relatively low extra-hematological toxicity and the short period of neutropenia [85].

Outpatient autologous HSCT for MM is not yet established as a routine procedure, due to reluctance of certain centers and due to the absence of guidelines. However, reduction of costs and period of hospitalization are the driving forces behind the adoption of outpatient HSCT. The mixed inpatient/outpatient model has been shown to be highly feasible with very low rates of rehospitalization and TRM [100, 101].

Several studies have shown safety, feasibility and cost-effectiveness of outpatient autologous HSCT for MM [86–90]. Selection criteria for outpatient autologous HSCT include expected compliance, proximity to the HSCT center for daily visits, 24-hour caregiver support, favorable performance status and favorable comorbidity profile [91]. Lack of caregiver is a limiting factor for outpatient autologous HSCT [92].

6.4. Tandem and second AHSCT

Even before the era of novel therapies, tandem autologous HSCT had been performed in patients with MM and the results of tandem transplants showed superior outcomes compared to single autologous HSCTs [102, 103]. Later on, two single-center retrospective analyses showed higher rates of progression-free survival (PFS) and OS in patients subjected to tandem autologous HSCT compared to recipients of single autologous HSCT [104, 105]. A meta-analysis that included six studies comparing tandem to single autologous HSCT in patients with MM showed: (1) no difference between the two forms of autologous HSCT with respect to OS and EFS and (2) tandem autologous HSCT was associated with improved response rates but at the expense of increased TRM [106]. However, this meta-analysis was criticized as it included a study with significant statistical errors [107].

Several studies have shown that a second autologous HSCT used as part of salvage therapy in patients with MM relapsing after the first autologous HSCT has been found to be safe and feasible particularly in carefully selected patients [108–112]. Factors associated with the success of second autologous HSCT include younger age, B2M < 2.5 mg/L at diagnosis, remission duration >9 months from first autologous HSCT, > partial response achieved in response to the first autologous HSCT and performance of second autologous HSCT before relapse and within 6–12 months from the first autologous HSCT [113, 114].

6.5. Allogeneic HSCT in MM

Although allogeneic HSCT represents the only potentially curative therapeutic modality in patients with MM, it is associated with relatively high TRM [76, 115, 116]. The advent of reduced intensity conditioning (RIC) and the application of autologous-allogeneic tandem HSCT approaches have broadened the use of allogeneic HSCT in patients with MM. Autologous-allogeneic tandem HSCT may overcome the negative impact of 17 p deletion and/or t(4,14) and the achievement of molecular remission in patients having HR cytogenetics has resulted in long-term freedom from disease [117].

In patients with HR disease or those relapsing after autologous HSCT, particularly younger patients who are fit for allografts, salvage therapy with novel agents followed by RIC allogeneic HSCT has been shown to provide significant PFS benefit [76, 118–121]. In patients lacking human leukocyte antigen (HLA)-matching sibling donors, alternate donors such as matched unrelated donors, cord blood transplantation and haploidentical forms of allogeneic HSCT have been employed and they have shown feasibility and effectiveness [115, 122–124].

7. Consolidation and maintenance therapies in MM

Almost all patients with MM relapse after autologous HSCT. Hence, treatment given in the postautologous HSCT period is aimed at suppression of residual disease in order to prolong duration of response, OS and PFS while minimizing toxicity [125, 126].

The use of novel therapies in the consolidation phase following single or tandem autologous HSCT has been shown to enhance the rate as well as the quality of response thus contributing to improvements in clinical outcomes including prolongation of PFS [126]. Bortezomib-based regimens used as consolidation therapy after autologous HSCT in patients with MM have been shown to be effective in the improving PFS and decreasing relapse rate [127].

Maintenance therapy represents an important therapeutic strategy to delay disease progression and relapse [125, 126]. The following drugs have been used in postautologous HSCT maintenance: interferon, thalidomide, bortezomib and carfilzomib [125, 126, 128–130]. Bortezomib is safe, well tolerated and efficacious and it can be used with no risk of second malignancy till disease progression, but its disadvantages include cost and effects on quality of life (QoL) [126, 130].

In February 2017, the Food and Drug Administration in the USA approved the use of lenalidomide as maintenance therapy after autologous HSCT for patients with MM, after showing efficacy and safety in several studies [131]. Lenalidomide has tumoricidal and immunomodulatory activities against MM [132]. Several studies have shown the efficacy of lenalidomide maintenance after autologous HSCT as this therapy has been shown to be associated with significant improvements in OS, PFS and longer time to disease progression [133–136]. A multicenter, randomized double-blind study that included 306 patients with newly diagnosed MM ≥65 years of age and ineligible for autologous HSCT treated initially with melphalan, prednisolone and lenalidomide induction followed by lenalidomide versus placebo maintenance showed the following results: (1) significant prolongation of PFS, (2) maximum benefit was achieved in patients 65–75 years of age and (3) 3-year second primary tumor of 7% in the lenalidomide arm versus 3% in the placebo arm [132]. Other studies on lenalidomide maintenance have shown more toxicity and low rate of development of second tumors [133, 134]. Lenalidomide maintenance can be initiated as early as day 100 postautologous HSCT [133]. Duration of lenalidomide maintenance longer than 3 years has been associated with further improvement in survival [134]. Several studies performed in patients with newly diagnosed MM subjected to autologous HSCT have shown continuous therapy to be more effective in prolongation of OS and PFS that limited the duration of treatment [137–141].

8. Novel therapies in MM

The novel therapies that have recently been introduced into the treatment of MM include (1) proteasome inhibitors such as bortezomib, carfilzomib and ixazomib; (2) immunomodulatory agents such as thalidomide, lenalidomide and pomalidomide; (3) monoclonal antibodies such as daratumumab and elotuzumab and (4) histone deacetylase inhibitors such as panobinostat, in addition to other classes of medications that can also be used in the treatment of MM such as glucocorticoids, DNA alkylating agents, as well as doxorubicin, cisplatinum and etoposide [10, 13, 15, 62–64]. Novel agents and targeted therapies that are either currently used or under development for the treatment of MM are shown in **Table 1** [61, 62, 142–150].

Several cell cycle regulatory proteins have been proposed as therapeutic targets in patients with MM. Other targets that have already been identified in MM include microtubules,

1. **Monoclonal antibodies:** Anti-CD 38 (daratumumab, elotuzumab, isatuximab, MOR202), anti-CD138 (indatuximab ravtansine), anti-interleukin-6 (siltuximab), anti-RANKL (denosumab), anti-KIR2DL1/2/4 (IPH2101)
2. **Immunomodulatory agents:** thalidomide, lenalidomide, pomalidomide
3. **Proteasome inhibitors:** bortezomib, carfilzomib, ixazomib
4. **Histone deacetylase inhibitors:** panobinostat, vorinostat, romidepsin, ricolinostat
5. **mTOR inhibitors:** everolimus, temsirolimus
6. **Checkpoint (programmed cell death protein 1) inhibitors:** nivolumab, pembrolizumab
7. **Bruton's tyrosine kinase inhibitors:** ibrutinib
8. **BCL2 antagonists (BH3 mimetics):** venetoclax, obatoclax, navitoclax
9. **Cyclin-dependent kinase inhibitors:** dinaciclib
10. **MEK inhibitors:** selumetinib
11. **Kinesin spindle protein 1 inhibitors**: filanesib, array 520
12. **Selective inhibitors of nuclear transport**: selinexor
13. **Phosphoinositide 3-kinase-Akt inhibitors:** perifosine, afuresertib
14. **PIM kinase inhibitors:** LGH 447
15. **Vaccines:** PVH-410
16. **Chimeric antigen receptor T cells (CAR T cells):** directed against:
    - **a.** CD-19
    - **b.** CD-38
    - **c.** B-cell maturation antigen
    - **d.** Cell surface glycoprotein

Table 1. Novel agents and targeted therapies that are either currently used or under development for the treatment of multiple myeloma.

kinesin motor proteins, aurora kinases, polo-like kinases and the anaphase-promoting complex/cyclosome [151]. The novel therapies that are used in the treatment of MM differ in their modes of action. Nevertheless, each drug has its own side effects that should be considered particularly once treating patients with comorbid medical conditions and once these novel agents are used in combination with other drugs [152].

8.1. Daratumumab

Daratumumab is a human IgG_k monoclonal antibody that targets CD38, which is a cell surface protein that is overexpressed in MM cells. It is given IV at a dose of 16 mg/kg weekly [153–156]. It induces death of MM cells by several mechanisms including (1) complement-dependent cytotoxicity, (2) antibody-dependent cell-mediated cytotoxicity, (3) antibody-dependent cellular phagocytosis and (4) apoptosis [153–156].

Daratumumab has shown substantial efficacy as monotherapy in heavily pretreated patients with MM as well as in combination with bortezomib in patients with newly diagnosed MM [154]. Two phase III randomized clinical trials in R/R MM using daratumumab in combination with either bortezomib and dexamethasone or lenalidomide and dexamethasone showed significantly longer PFS with manageable toxicity [154, 156]. In a phase III randomized clinical trial performed in patients with newly diagnosed MM, not eligible for autologous HSCT, the addition of daratumumab to bortezomib, melphalan and prednisolone decreased the risk of death and disease progression but was also associated with higher rates of infections [155]. The adverse effects of daratumumab include infusion-related reactions, hematologic toxicity in the form of neutropenia and thrombocytopenia and various infectious complications [153–156].

8.2. Elotuzumab

Elotuzumab is an immunostimulatory monoclonal antibody targeting signaling lymphocyte activation molecule F7 (SLAMF7) [157]. While no responses to elotuzumab as a single agent were obtained, the addition of elotuzumab to lenalidomide and dexamethasone in RR-MM patients resulted in overall response rate (ORR) of 79% compared to 66% ORR obtained with lenalidomide and dexamethasone alone [142, 158]. Also, in a phase III randomized clinical trial in patients with R/R-MM, the combination of elotuzumab, lenalidomide and dexamethasone decreased the risks of death and disease progression by 30% [157].

8.3. Pomalidomide

Pomalidomide is a third-generation immunomodulatory agent that has been approved for patients with progressive MM or those who have received at least two lines of therapy [159]. It has been shown to be effective in combination with dexamethasone ± carfilzomib or other agents in patients with R/R-MM or in those with HR cytogenetics [159–162]. The use of pomalidomide combined with low-dose dexamethasone in heavily pretreated patients with R/R-MM has been shown to be cost-effective as the combination has produced clinical outcomes comparable to those obtained by daratumumab alone or carfilzomib alone [5].

8.4. Carfilzomib

Carfilzomib is a second-generation proteasome inhibitor [163]. It is well tolerated and causes minimal neurotoxicity. It has demonstrated promising activity in patients with MM who are refractory to bortezomib or immunomodulatory agents [163–165]. It can be combined with dexamethasone or other novel agents [164–166].

It is able to sensitize 24% of bortezomib-refractory MM patients. When combined with dexamethasone in R/R-MM, it resulted in superior outcome in terms of ORR and PFS compared to bortezomib and dexamethasone combination [158]. Also, it is under evaluation for patients with newly diagnosed MM [166].

8.5. Panobinostat

Histone deacetylase inhibitors such as panobinostat and vorinostat have demonstrated some activity against MM and they have multiple proposed mechanisms of actions once used in the treatment of MM [167]. Panobinostat is a potent oral pan-deacetylase inhibitor. It affects growth and survival of MM cells through alteration of (1) gene expression through epigenetic modification and (2) protein metabolism by inhibiting protein degradation [168–171]. The approval of panobinostat for the treatment of MM was based on the results of phase III randomized double-blind clinical trial (PANORAMA 1), which demonstrated improvement in median PFS of 7.8 months for panobinostat, bortezomib and dexamethasone in comparison with placebo, bortezomib and dexamethasone [168–171]. Panobinostat, in combination with bortezomib and dexamethasone, was recently approved in the USA, Europe and Japan for the treatment of patients with MM who had failed at least two prior regimens including bortezomib and an immunomodulatory agent [168–171]. A meta-analysis that included 11 clinical trials and 700 patients with R/R-MM treated with panobinostat demonstrated not only efficacy but also safety of panobinostat in combination with other agents [172]. The main toxic effects of panobinostat are thrombocytopenia and diarrhea. However, several studies showed other adverse effects including lymphopenia, neutropenia and anemia, nausea, vomiting, constipation and abdominal pain, asthenia, fatigue, peripheral edema and peripheral neuropathy [167–172]. Ongoing clinical trials are evaluating the role of panobinostat in combination with drugs other than bortezomib in R/R-MM, in combination with various drugs in newly diagnosed disease and in maintenance therapy of myeloma [169].

8.6. CAR T cells

CAR is a hybrid antigen receptor that is composed of an extracellular antigen-binding domain and an intracellular signaling domain. T cells genetically targeted with a CAR to B-cell malignancies have demonstrated tremendous clinical outcome [173]. Immunotherapy using CAR-mediated T cells has demonstrated high response rates in patients with B-cell malignancies. CAR T-cell therapy is a cellular therapy that redirects a patient's T cells to specifically target and destroy tumor cells [174]. CARs are genetically engineered fusion proteins composed of antigen recognition domain derived from a monoclonal antibody as well as an intracellular T-cell signaling domain and a costimulatory domain [174].

There are multiple steps in the production of CAR T cells and these include (1) leukapheresis to separate leukocytes; (2) enrichment of leukapheresis product with T cells; (3) separation of T-cell subsets at the level of CD4/CD8 composition using specific antibody-based conjugates or markers; (4) T-cell selection or activation, gene transfer or genetic modification and viral transduction; (5) volume expansion of T cells, isolation, washing and culture followed by cryopreservation and (6) infusion of CAR T cells [174, 175].

Adverse effects of CAR T-cell therapy include cytokine release syndrome (CRS), neurotoxicity, on target/off tumor recognition and anaphylaxis. Additionally, theoretical toxicities of CAR T cells include clonal expansion secondary to insertional oncogenesis, GVHD and off-target antigen recognition [176]. Management of CAR T-cell toxicity includes supportive measures, immunosuppression with tocilizumab (IL-6) receptor blockade for CRS and suicide or elimination genes to allow for selective depletion of CAR T cells [176].

CAR expressing T cells have demonstrated success in the treatment of B-cell lymphoid malignancies particularly CD19+ acute lymphoblastic leukemia and chronic lymphocytic leukemia [177]. Cell surface glycoprotein (CS1) is highly expressed on MM cells and is an ideal target for the treatment of MM, that is, CS1 can be targeted by CAR natural killer cells to treat MM [177]. A patient with advanced and refractory MM received myeloablative treatment with melphalan 140 mg/m^2, followed by autologous HSCT, and then infusion of CTL019 CAR resulted in CR with no disease progression for 12 months after CAR T-cell infusion [178]. CAR T cells can target the following antigens in patients with MM: B-cell maturation antigen (BCMA), CD138, CD19 and kappa-light chain [179]. A bispecific T-cell engager (BiTE) targeting BCMA and $CD3_E$ (BI 836909) has been developed and it has been shown to be highly potent and efficacious to selectively deplete BCMA-positive MM cells; thus, it represents a novel immunotherapeutic approach in the treatment of MM [180]. CARs are proteins that incorporate antigen domain, costimulatory domains and T-cell activation domains [181]. Only a limited number of patients with MM received CAR T-cell therapy, but preliminary results are encouraging [179].

BCMA is only expressed on some B cells, normal plasma cells and malignant plasma cells. The first clinical trial using CAR T cells targeting BCMA that is expressed in most cases of MM included 12 patients [181]. After dose escalation in the infusion of CAR-BCMA cells was used, the trial showed remarkable success and impressive activity against MM cells as BM plasma cells became undetectable by flow cytometry and patients entered stringent CR lasting for 17 weeks before relapse [181]. Another clinical trial using CAR-BCMA that included 21 patients showed increase in response rate from 89 to 100% after dose escalation [182].

9. Refractory and/or relapsed MM (R/R-MM)

The course of MM progression is highly variable as almost all patients with MM who respond to initial therapy will eventually relapse and require further treatment [6]. The introduction of novel agents over the last 15 years, the implementation of new therapeutic strategies and the adoption of drug combinations that include highly effective and tolerable drugs have improved (1) the clinical outcome dramatically as response rates have increased from approximately 30% with single agents to about 90% with combination therapies and (2) the QoL even in heavily pretreated patients. However, determining the optimal sequence and combination as well as timing of each agent is necessary [6]. In a retrospective analysis of 628 patients with newly diagnosed MM who developed relapse after initial therapy, it was found that prolonged duration of treatment was associated with improved survival [141]. Unfortunately, secondary plasma cell leukemia and EMD still present difficult therapeutic challenges [16].

There is no standard of care for MM relapse after autologous HSCT [183, 184]. Regimens that are composed of combination therapy with (1) drugs having synergistic effect and no cross-resistance and (2) one or two novel therapies are generally preferred as they lead to deeper and longer responses that are translated into improved survival [16, 183–185]. However, treatment should be individualized based on toxicity as well as patient and disease characteristics [184]. A meta-analysis of phase III randomized controlled trials showed that, compared to doublet regimens, triplets resulted in improved OS, PFS, very good partial response and CR although the risk of having grade III/IV drug adverse effects was higher with triplet regimens [185].

Mechanisms of drug resistance in MM include (1) multidrug-resistant gene polymorphism, (2) P-glycoprotein overexpression in MM cells, (3) microenvironmental changes, (4) clonal evolution including, (5) cancer stem cells, (6) upregulation and downregulation of various micro-RNAs and (7) selected CD34+, CD 138+, B7-, H1+, CD19- plasma cell accumulation after treatment [40].

Therapeutic options for patients with R/R-MM include (1) salvage therapy; combination of old and new therapies such as (a) bortezomib, thalidomide, cisplatin, cyclophosphamide, etoposide and doxorubicin (VTD-PACE); (b) KRD/carfilzomib, pomalidomide and dexamethasone

http://dx.doi.org/10.5772/intechopen.79999

(KPD) ± PACE or (c) daratumumab-based therapy; (2) second autologous HSCT; (3) allogeneic HSCT in carefully selected patients and (4) enrollment in clinical trials [8, 11, 13, 16]. Specific agents that are used in the treatment of R/R-MM include (1) immunomodulatory agents such as thalidomide, lenalidomide and pomalidomide; (2) proteasome inhibitors such as bortezomib, carfilzomib and ixazomib; (3) monoclonal antibodies such as daratumumab and elotuzumab; (4) histone deacetylase inhibitors such as panobinostat and (5) pembrolizumab [6, 142, 157, 158, 164, 186]. The use of pembrolizumab (antiprogrammed cell death 1) in combination with lenalidomide and dexamethasone in patients with R/R-MM resulted in 76% ORR [142, 158].

10. Management of MM patients having renal failure

Renal impairment (RI) is one of the most common complications of MM as 20–50% of patients with newly diagnosed MM present with RI, while 40–50% of patients develop RI during the course of the disease and about 5% of myeloma patients have dialysis-dependent renal failure (RF) at presentation [187–191]. In patients with MM, the causes of RI include myeloma cast nephropathy, excess of monoclonal free light chains causing proximal renal tubular damage, dehydration, infectious complications, hypercalcemia, hyperuricemia, use of nephrotoxic drugs and contrast media, hyperviscosity, myeloma cell infiltration and amyloid deposition [187–189, 192].

Bortezomib, thalidomide, lenalidomide and dexamethasone in various combinations can be used in the treatment of MM patients having RF and their use has been associated with high response rates and recovery of even partial or complete recovery of renal function [187–189, 191, 192]. In early chemotherapy trials, RF was considered a predictor of poor prognosis, patients with hemodialysis were reported to have a poorer prognosis and RF was considered an exclusion criterion from autologous HSCT because of the concerns about higher rates of treatment-related toxicity and nonrelapse mortality (NRM) due to mucositis, infectious complications and encephalopathy [187, 190]. However, recent studies have shown that autologous HSCT in patients with MM and RF has been associated with partial or complete recovery of renal function even in dialysis-dependent patients [190]. Therefore, autologous HSCT can be offered to patients with MM and RF with acceptable toxicity and NRM and a significant improvement in renal function that may be encountered in approximately one third of patients [187, 190]. In patients with MM and RF, a melphalan dose of 200 mg/m^2 can be administered in the conditioning therapy of auto-HSCT without an increase in toxicity and NRM [190].

Kidney transplantation is the treatment of choice for most patients with end-stage renal failure (ESRD) as it is associated with improved survival and QoL compared to hemodialysis [193]. Even in patients with MM having RF, kidney transplantation is a valid therapeutic option in well-selected patients who achieve control of their disease and maintain a durable remission preferably for 3–5 years and have stable light chain levels but this option should be considered early in the course of the disease [194–197]. Combined HSCT, predominantly autologous HSCT, and renal transplantation have been performed for patients having various hematological disorders such as plasma cell dyscrasias [198–202]. Patients with MM having ESRD, either on regular hemodialysis or not, can be offered not only HSCT but also combined HSCT and renal transplantation either simultaneously or sequentially [198, 199, 203–206].

11. Conclusions and future directions

The introduction of several novel agents and targeted therapies over the last 10 years has revolutionized the management of MM and has produced unprecedented outcomes in terms of disease control and OS. Currently, novel agents and targeted therapies are used in the following settings: (1) prior to HSCT to reduce tumor burden and to optimally control MM, (2) following HSCT as consolidation and maintenance therapy to allow long-term disease control and (3) as salvage therapy in case of relapse of MM after HSCT.

However, novel agents and targeted therapies should not be considered as a form of replacement to HSCT, but instead these two valuable therapeutic interventions should be considered complementary to each other. The smart combination of novel agents and targeted therapies with various forms of HSCT in the new treatment paradigm of MM will ultimately lead to higher cure rates and longer disease controls.

Author details

Khalid Ahmed Al-Anazi

Address all correspondence to: kaa_alanazi@yahoo.com

Department of Adult Hematology and Hematopoietic Stem Cell Transplantation,
Oncology Center, King Fahad Specialist Hospital, Dammam, Saudi Arabia

References

[1] Dimopoulos MA, Kaufman JL, White D, Cook G, Rizzo M, Xu Y, et al. A comparison of the efficacy of immunomodulatory-containing regimens in relapsed/refractory multiple myeloma: a network meta-analysis. Clinical Lymphoma, Myeloma & Leukemia. 2018;**18**(3):163-173.e6. DOI: 10.1016/j.clml.2017.12.011. [Epub Jan 5, 2018]

[2] Maiese EM, Ainsworth C, Le Moine JG, Ahdesmäki O, Bell J, Hawe E. Comparative efficacy of treatments for previously treated multiple myeloma: A systematic literature review and network meta-analysis. Clinical Therapeutics. 2018;**40**(3):480-494.e23. DOI: 10.1016/j.clinthera.2018.01.014. [Epub Feb 28, 2018]

[3] Walters DK, Arendt BK, Tschumper RC, Wu X, Jelinek DF. Characterization and use of the novel human multiple myeloma cell line MC-B11/14 to study biological consequences of CRISPR-mediated loss of immunoglobulin A heavy chain. Experimental Hematology. 2018;**57**:42-49.e1. DOI: 10.1016/j.exphem.2017.09.010 [Epub Oct 13, 2017]

[4] Jakab S, Lázár E, Benedek I, Köpeczi J, Pakucs A, Benedek I. New treatment methods in multiple myeloma. Journal of Interdisciplinary Medicine. 2017;**2**(2):144-149. DOI: 10.1515/jim-2017-0055

[5] Pelligra CG, Parikh K, Guo S, Chandler C, Mouro J, Abouzaid S, et al. Cost-effectiveness of pomalidomide, carfilzomib, and daratumumab for the treatment of patients with

heavily pretreated relapsed-refractory multiple myeloma in the United States. Clinical Therapeutics. 2017;**39**(10):1986-2005.e5. DOI: 10.1016/j.clinthera.2017.08.010 [Epub Sep 28, 2017]

[6] Sonneveld P, De Wit E, Moreau P. How have evolutions in strategies for the treatment of relapsed/refractory multiple myeloma translated into improved outcomes for patients? Critical Reviews in Oncology/Hematology. 2017;**112**:153-170. DOI: 10.1016/j.critrevonc.2017.02.007 [Epub Feb 14, 2017]

[7] Fonseca R, Abouzaid S, Bonafede M, Cai Q, Parikh K, Cosler L, et al. Trends in overall survival and costs of multiple myeloma, 2000-2014. Leukemia. 2017;**31**(9):1915-1921. DOI: 10.1038/leu.2016.380 [Epub Dec 23, 2016]

[8] Rajkumar SV. Clinical features, laboratory manifestations, and diagnosis of multiple myeloma. Up to date 2018. Edited by Kyle RA, Connor RF

[9] Ludwig H, Bolejack V, Crowley J, Bladé J, Miguel JS, Kyle RA, et al. Survival and years of life lost in different age cohorts of patients with multiple myeloma. Journal of Clinical Oncology. 2010;**28**(9):1599-1605. DOI: 10.1200/JCO.2009.25.2114 [Epub Feb 22, 2010]

[10] Rajkumar SV, Kumar S. Multiple myeloma: Diagnosis and treatment. Mayo Clinic Proceedings. 2016;**91**(1):101-119. DOI: 10.1016/j.mayocp.2015.11.007

[11] Sonneveld P, Avet-Loiseau H, Lonial S, Usmani S, Siegel D, et al. Treatment of multiple myeloma with high-risk cytogenetics:A consensus of the International Myeloma Working Group. Blood. 2016;**127**(24):2955-2962. DOI: 10.1182/blood-2016-01-631200 [Epub Mar 21, 2016]

[12] Johnson SK, Heuck CJ, Albino AP, Qu P, Zhang Q, Barlogie B, et al. The use of molecular-based risk stratification and pharmacogenomics for outcome prediction and personalized therapeutic management of multiple myeloma. International Journal of Hematology. 2011;**94**(4):321-333. DOI: 10.1007/s12185-011-0948-y [Epub Oct 15, 2011]

[13] Rajkumar SV. Multiple myeloma: 2016 update on diagnosis, risk-stratification, and management. American Journal of Hematology. 2016;**91**(7):719-734. DOI: 10.1002/ajh.24402

[14] Fonseca R, Monge J, Dimopoulos MA. Staging and prognostication of multiple myeloma. Expert Review of Hematology. 2014;**7**(1):21-31. DOI: 10.1586/17474086.2014. 882224

[15] Raza S, Safyan RA, Rosenbaum E, Bowman AS, Lentzsch S. Optimizing current and emerging therapies in multiple myeloma: A guide for the hematologist. Therapeutic Advances in Hematology. 2017;**8**(2):55-70. DOI: 10.1177/2040620716680548 [Epub Dec 9, 2016]

[16] Dingli D, Ailawadhi S, Bergsagel PL, Buadi FK, Dispenzieri A, Fonseca R, et al. Therapy for relapsed multiple myeloma: Guidelines from the Mayo stratification for myeloma and risk-adapted therapy. Mayo Clinic Proceedings. 2017;**92**(4):578-598. DOI: 10.1016/j.mayocp.2017.01.003 [Epub Mar 11, 2017]

[17] Rossi A, Voigtlaender M, Janjetovic S, Thiele B, Alawi M, März M, et al. Mutational landscape reflects the biological continuum of plasma cell dyscrasias. Blood Cancer Journal. 2017;**7**(2):e537. DOI: 10.1038/bcj.2017.19

[18] Bolli N, Avet-Loiseau H, Wedge DC, Van Loo P, Alexandrov LB, Martincorena I, et al. Heterogeneity of genomic evolution and mutational profiles in multiple myeloma. Nature Communications. 2014;**5**:2997. DOI: 10.1038/ncomms3997

[19] Talley PJ, Chantry AD, Buckle CH. Genetics in myeloma: Genetic technologies and their application to screening approaches in myeloma. British Medical Bulletin. 2015;**113**(1):15-30. DOI: 10.1093/bmb/ldu041

[20] Rustad EH, Coward E, Skytøen ER, Misund K, Holien T, Standal T, et al. Monitoring multiple myeloma by quantification of recurrent mutations in serum. Haematologica. 2017;**102**(7):1266-1272. DOI: 10.3324/haematol.2016.160564 [Epub Apr 6, 2017]

[21] Pawlyn C, Bright MD, Buros AF, Stein CK, Walters Z, Aronson LI, et al. Overexpression of EZH2 in multiple myeloma is associated with poor prognosis and dysregulation of cell cycle control. Blood Cancer Journal. 2017;**7**(3):e549. DOI: 10.1038/bcj.2017.27

[22] Lionetti M, Neri A. Utilizing next-generation sequencing in the management of multiple myeloma. Expert Review of Molecular Diagnostics. 2017;**17**(7):653-663. DOI: 10.1080/14737159.2017.1332996 [Epub May 26, 2017]

[23] Cetin AE, Stevens MM, Calistri NL, Fulciniti M, Olcum S, Kimmerling RJ, et al. Determining therapeutic susceptibility in multiple myeloma by single-cell mass accumulation. Nature Communications. 2017;**8**(1):1613. DOI: 10.1038/s41467-017-01593-2

[24] Celotto K, Lee K, Holstein SA. End-stage myeloma with extramedullary plasmacytomas in the era of novel therapies. American Journal of Hematology Oncology. 2017;**13**(2):21-23

[25] Lancman G, Tremblay D, Barley K, Barlogie B, Cho HJ, Jagannath S, et al. The effect of novel therapies in high-molecular-risk multiple myeloma. Clinical Advances in Hematology & Oncology. 2017;**15**(11):870-879

[26] Thoennissen GB, Görlich D, Bacher U, Aufenberg T, Hüsken AC, Hansmeier AA, et al. Autologous stem cell transplantation in multiple myeloma in the era of novel drug induction: A retrospective single-center analysis. Acta Haematologica. 2017;**137**(3):163-172. DOI: 10.1159/000463534 [Epub Apr 12, 2017]

[27] Yamamoto T, Kosaka N, Hattori Y, Ochiya T. A challenge to aging society by microRNA in extracellular vesicles: MicroRNA in extracellular vesicles as promising biomarkers and novel therapeutic targets in multiple myeloma. Journal of Clinical Medicine. 2018; **7**(3). DOI: 10.3390/jcm7030055

[28] Falank C, Fairfield H, Reagan MR. Signaling interplay between bone marrow adipose tissue and multiple Myeloma cells. Frontiers in Endocrinology (Lausanne). 2016;**7**:67. DOI: 10.3389/fendo.216.00067 [eCollection 2016]

[29] Hanahan D, Weinberg RA. The hallmarks of cancer. Cell. 2000;**100**(1):57-70

[30] Hanahan D, Weinberg RA. Hallmarks of cancer: The next generation. Cell. 2011;**144**(5):646-674. DOI: 10.1016/j.cell. 2011.02.013

[31] Manier S, Sacco A, Leleu X, Ghobrial IM, Roccaro AM. Bone marrow microenvironment in multiple myeloma progression. Journal of Biomedicine & Biotechnology. 2012;**2012**:157496. DOI: 10.1155/2012/157496 [Epub Oct 3, 2012]

[32] Jurczyszyn A, Czepiel J, Gdula-Argasińska J, Perucki W, Skotnicki AB, Majka M. The analysis of the relationship between multiple myeloma cells and their microenvironment. Journal of Cancer. 2015;**6**(2):160-168. DOI: 10.7150/jca.10873 [eCollection 2015]

[33] Kawano Y, Moschetta M, Manier S, Glavey S, Görgün GT, Roccaro AM, et al. Targeting the bone marrow microenvironment in multiple myeloma. Immunological Reviews. 2015;**263**(1):160-172. DOI: 10.1111/imr.12233

[34] Podar K, Chauhan D, Anderson KC. Bone marrow microenvironment and the identification of new targets for myeloma therapy. Leukemia. 2009;**23**(1):10-24. DOI: 10.1038/leu.2008.259 [Epub Oct 9, 2008]

[35] Shay G, Hazlehurst L, Lynch CC. Dissecting the multiple myeloma-bone microenvironment reveals new therapeutic opportunities. Journal of Molecular Medicine (Berl). 2016;**94**(1):21-35. DOI: 10.1007/s00109-015-1345-4 [Epub Oct 1, 2015]

[36] Reagan MR, Liaw L, Rosen CJ, Ghobrial IM. Dynamic interplay between bone and multiple myeloma: Emerging roles of the osteoblast. Bone. 2015;**75**:161-169. DOI: 10.1016/j.bone. 2015.02.021 [Epub Feb 26, 2015]

[37] Qiao M, Wu D, Carey M, Zhou X, Zhang L. Multi-scale agent-based multiple myeloma cancer modeling and the related study of the balance between osteoclasts and osteoblasts. PLoS One. 2015;**10**(12):e0143206. DOI: 10.1371/journal.pone. 0143206 [eCollection 2015]

[38] Fairfield H, Falank C, Avery L, Reagan MR. Multiple myeloma in the marrow: Pathogenesis and treatments. Annals of the New York Academy of Sciences. 2016;**1364**:32-51. DOI: 10.1111/nyas.13038

[39] Flodr P, Latalova P, Pusciznova P, Pika T, Bacovsky J, Scudla V, et al. Multiple myeloma and bone marrow microenvironment immunohistochemical study of the expression of 15 proteins related to myeloma bone disease. Blood. 2015;**126**:5318

[40] Yang WC, Lin SF. Mechanisms of drug resistance in relapse and refractory multiple myeloma. BioMed Research International. 2015;**2015**:341430. DOI: 10.1155/2015/341430 [Epub Nov 16, 2015]

[41] Raimondi L, De Luca A, Morelli E, Giavaresi G, Tagliaferri P, Tassone P, et al. MicroRNAs: Novel crossroads between myeloma cells and the bone marrow microenvironment. BioMed Research International. 2016;**2016**:6504593. DOI: 10.1155/2016/6504593 [Epub Jan 4, 2016]

[42] Zhang J, Xiao X, Liu J. The role of circulating miRNAs in multiple myeloma. Science China. Life Sciences. 2015;**58**(12):1262-1269. DOI: 10.1007/s11427-015-4969-2 [Epub Nov 25, 2015]

[43] Abdi J, Jian H, Chang H. Role of micro-RNAs in drug resistance of multiple myeloma. Oncotarget. 2016;**7**(37):60723-60735. DOI: 10.18632/oncotarget.11032 [Epub Aug 2, 2016]

[44] Brennan SK, Matsui W. Cancer stem cells: Controversies in multiple myeloma. Journal of Molecular Medicine (Berl). 2009;**87**(11):1079-1085. DOI: 10.1007/s00109-009-0531-7 [Epub Sep 17, 2009]

[45] Gao M, Kong Y, Yang G, Gao L, Shi J. Multiple myeloma cancer stem cells. Oncotarget. 2016;**7**(23):35466-35477. DOI: 10.18632/oncotarget.8154

[46] Huff CA, Matsui W. Multiple myeloma cancer stem cells. Journal of Clinical Oncology. 2008;**26**(17):2895-2900. DOI: 10.1200/JCO.2007. 15.8428

[47] Kellner J, Liu B, Kang Y, Li Z. Fact or fiction—Identifying the elusive multiple myeloma stem cell. Journal of Hematology & Oncology. 2013;**6**:91. DOI: 10.1186/1756-8722-6-91

[48] Johnsen HE, Bøgsted M, Schmitz A, Bødker JS, El-Galaly TC, Johansen P, et al. The myeloma stem cell concept, revisited: From phenomenology to operational terms. Haematologica. 2016;**101**(12):1451-1459. DOI: 10.3324/haematol.2015.138826 [Epub Nov 10, 2016]

[49] Franqui-Machin R, Wendlandt EB, Janz S, Zhan F, Tricot G. Cancer stem cells are the cause of drug resistance in multiple myeloma: fact or fiction? Oncotarget. 2015;**6**(38):40496-40506. DOI: 10.18632/oncotarget.5800

[50] Basak GW, Carrier E. The search for multiple myeloma stem cells: The long and winding road. Biology of Blood and Marrow Transplantation. 2010;**16**(5):587-594. DOI: 10.1016/j.bbmt.2009. 10.024 [Epub Nov 4, 2009]

[51] Matsui W, Wang Q, Barber JP, Brennan S, Smith BD, Borrello I, et al. Clonogenic multiple myeloma progenitors, stem cell properties, and drug resistance. Cancer Research. 2008;**68**(1):190-197. DOI: 10.1158/0008-5472.CAN-07-3096

[52] Bleker de Oliveira M, Eugenio AI, Fook Alves VL, Zanatta D, Yamamoto M, Strauss BE, et al. Heat shock protein 70 inhibitor, alone or in combination with bortezomib, prevented plasmacytoma development in immunodeficient mice transplanted with myeloma cell lines. Blood. 2016;**128**:5658

[53] Xu YN, Xiao CR, Huang YD, Lu QY. Circulating serum microRNA as diagnostic biomarkers for multiple myeloma. Zhongguo Shi Yan Xue Ye Xue Za Zhi. 2017;**25**(2):471-475. DOI: 10.7534/j.issn.1009-2137.2017.02.029

[54] Seckinger A, Meißner T, Moreaux J, Benes V, Hillengass J, Castoldi M, et al. MiRNAs in multiple myeloma—A survival relevant complex regulator of gene expression. Oncotarget. 2015;**6**(36):39165-39183. DOI: 10.18632/oncotarget.5381

[55] Kubiczkova L, Kryukov F, Slaby O, Dementyeva E, Jarkovsky J, Nekvindova J, et al. Circulating serum microRNAs as novel diagnostic and prognostic biomarkers for multiple myeloma and monoclonal gammopathy of undetermined significance. Haematologica. 2014;**99**(3):511-518. DOI: 10.3324/haematol.2013.093500 [Epub Nov 15, 2013]

[56] Jones CI, Zabolotskaya MV, King AJ, Stewart HJS, Horne GA, Chevassut TJ, et al. Identification of circulating microRNAs as diagnostic biomarkers for use in multiple

myeloma. British Journal of Cancer. 2012;**107**(12):1987-1996. DOI: 10.1038/bjc.2012.525 [Epub Nov 20, 2012]

[57] Manier S, Liu CJ, Avet-Loiseau H, Park J, Shi J, Campigotto F, et al. Prognostic role of circulating exosomal miRNAs in multiple myeloma. Blood. 2017;**129**(17):2429-2436. DOI: 10.1182/blood-2016-09-742296 [Epub Feb 17, 2017]

[58] Wu P, Agnelli L, Walker BA, Todoerti K, Lionetti M, Johnson DC, et al. Improved risk stratification in myeloma using a microRNA-based classifier. British Journal of Haematology. 2013;**162**(3):348-359. DOI: 10.1111/bjh.12394 [Epub May 30, 2013]

[59] Anderson KC. Progress and paradigms in multiple myeloma. Clinical Cancer Research. 2016;**22**(22):5419-5427. DOI: 10.1158/1078-0432.CCR-16-0625

[60] Cavo MS, Rajkumar V, Palumbo A, Moreau P, Orlowski R, Bladé J, et al., on behalf of the International Myeloma Working Group. International Myeloma Working Group consensus approach to the treatment of multiple myeloma patients who are candidates for autologous stem cell transplantation. Blood. 2011;**117**(23):6063-6073. DOI: 10.1182/blood-2011-02-297325 [Epub Mar 29, 2011]

[61] Nijhof IS, van de Donk NWCJ, Zweegman S, Lokhorst HM. Current and new therapeutic strategies for relapsed and refractory multiple myeloma: An update. Drugs. 2018;**78**(1):19-37. DOI: 10.1007/s40265-017-0841-y

[62] Tremblay D, Chari A. Novel targets in multiple myeloma. American Journal of Hematology Oncology. 2016;**12**(10):18-25

[63] Naymagon L, Abdul-Hay M. Novel agents in the treatment of multiple myeloma: A review about the future. Journal of Hematology & Oncology. 2016;**9**(1):52. DOI: 10.1186/s13045-016-0282-1

[64] Mikkilineni L, Kochenderfer JN. Chimeric antigen receptor T-cell therapies for multiple myeloma. Blood. 2017;**130**(24):2594-2602. DOI: 10.1182/blood-2017-06-793869 [Epub Sep 19, 2017]

[65] Roussel M, Lauwers-Cances V, Robillard N, Hulin C, Leleu X, Benboubker L, et al. Front-line transplantation program with lenalidomide, bortezomib, and dexamethasone combination as induction and consolidation followed by lenalidomide maintenance in patients with multiple myeloma: A phase II study by the Intergroupe Francophone du Myélome. Journal of Clinical Oncology. 2014;**32**(25):2712-2717. DOI: 10.1200/JCO.2013.54.8164

[66] Richardson PG, Weller E, Lonial S, Jakubowiak AJ, Jagannath S, Raje NS, et al. Lenalidomide, bortezomib, and dexamethasone combination therapy in patients with newly diagnosed multiple myeloma. Blood. 2010;**116**(5):679-686. DOI: 10.1182/blood-2010-02-268862 [Epub Apr 12, 2010]

[67] Attal M, Lauwers-Cances V, Hulin C, Leleu X, Caillot D, Escoffre M, et al., IFM 2009 Study. Lenalidomide, bortezomib, and dexamethasone with transplantation for myeloma. New England Journal of Medicine 2017;**376**(14):1311-1320. DOI: 10.1056/NEJMoa1611750

[68] Rajan AM, Rajkumar V. Treatment of newly diagnosed myeloma: Bortezomib-based triplet. Seminars in Oncology. 2016;**43**(6):700-702. DOI: 10.1053/j.seminoncol.2016.11.003

[69] Chakraborty R, Muchtar E, Kumar S, Buadi FK, Dingli D, Dispenzieri A, et al. The impact of induction regimen on transplant outcome in newly diagnosed multiple myeloma in the era of novel agents. Bone Marrow Transplantation. 2017;**52**(1):34-40. DOI: 10.1038/bmt.2016.214 [Epub Aug 22, 2016]

[70] Durie BG, Hoering A, Abidi MH, Rajkumar SV, Epstein J, Kahanic SP, et al. Bortezomib with lenalidomide and dexamethasone versus lenalidomide and dexamethasone alone in patients with newly diagnosed myeloma without intent for immediate autologous stem-cell transplant (SWOG S0777): A randomised, open-label, phase 3 trial. Lancet. 2017;**389**(10068):519-527. DOI: 10.1016/S0140-6736(16)31594-X [Epub Dec 23, 2016]

[71] Jelinek T, Bezdekova R, Zatopkova M, Burgos L, Simicek M, Sevcikova T, et al. Current applications of multiparameter flow cytometry in plasma cell disorders. Blood Cancer Journal. 2017;**7**(10):e617. DOI: 10.1038/bcj.2017.90

[72] Holstein SA, Avet-Loiseau H, Hahn T, Ho CM, Lohr JG, Munshi NC, et al. BMT CTN myeloma intergroup workshop on minimal residual disease and immune profiling: Summary and recommendations from the organizing committee. Biology of Blood and Marrow Transplantation. 2018;**24**(4):641-648. DOI: 10.1016/j.bbmt.2017.12.774 [Epub Dec 11, 2017]

[73] Bhatnagar B, Badros AZ. Controversies in autologous stem cell transplantation for the treatment of multiple myeloma. In: Demirer T, editor. Innovations in Stem Cell Transplantation. Intech Open; 2013. DOI: 10.5772/54115

[74] Mohty M, Harousseau JL. Treatment of autologous stem cell transplant-eligible multiple myeloma patients: Ten questions and answers. Haematologica. 2014;**99**(3):408-416. DOI: 10.3324/haematol.2013.096149

[75] Brioli A. First line vs delayed transplantation in myeloma: Certainties and controversies. World Journal of Transplantation. 2016;**6**(2):321-330. DOI: 10.5500/wjt.v6.i2.321

[76] Patriarca F, Einsele H, Spina F, Bruno B, Isola M, Nozzoli C, et al. Allogeneic stem cell transplantation in multiple myeloma relapsed after autograft: A multicenter retrospective study based on donor availability. Biology of Blood and Marrow Transplantation. 2012;**18**(4):617-626. DOI: 10.1016/j.bbmt.2011. 07.026 [Epub Aug 3, 2011]

[77] Shu Z, Heimfeld S, Gao D. Hematopoietic stem cell transplantation with cryopreserved grafts: adverse reactions after transplantation and cryoprotectant removal prior to infusion. Bone Marrow Transplantation. 2014;**49**(4):469-476. DOI: 10.1038/bmt.2013.152. [Epub Sep 30, 2013]

[78] Yi X, Liu M, Luo Q, Zhuo H, Cao H, Wang J, et al. Toxic effects of dimethyl sulfoxide on red blood cells, platelets, and vascular endothelial cells in vitro. FEBS Open Bio. 2017;**7**:485-494

[79] Wannesson L, Panzarella T, Mikhael J, Keating A. Feasibility and safety of autotransplants with noncryopreserved marrow or peripheral blood stem cells: A systematic review. Annals of Oncology. 2007;**18**(4):623-632

[80] Jasuja SK, Kukar (jasuja) N, Jain R, Bhateja A, Jasuja A, Rohit Jain, et al. A simplified method at lowest cost for autologous, non-cryopreserved, unmanipulated, peripheral hematopoietic stem cell transplant in multiple myeloma and non-Hodgkin's lymphoma: Asian scenario. Journal of Clinical Oncology. 2010;**28**(15):ė18545

[81] Al-Anazi KA. Autologous hematopoietic stem cell transplantation for multiple myeloma without cryopreservation. Bone Marrow Research. 2012;**2012**:917361

[82] Ramzi M, Zakerinia M, Nourani H, Dehghani M, Vojdani R, Haghighinejad H. Non-cryopreserved hematopoietic stem cell transplantation in multiple myeloma, a single center experience. Clinical Transplantation. 2012;**26**(1):117-122

[83] Kayal S, Sharma A, Iqbal S, Tejomurtula T, Cyriac SL, Raina V, et al. High-dose chemotherapy and autologous stem cell transplantation in multiple myeloma: A single institution experience at All India Institute of Medical Sciences, New Delhi, using non-cryopreserved peripheral blood stem cells. Clinical Lymphoma, Myeloma & Leukemia. 2014;**14**(2):140-147. DOI: 10.1016/j.clml.2013.09.001 Epub 2013 Sep 28

[84] Bekadja MA, Brahimi M, Osmani S, Arabi A, Bouhass R, Yafour N, et al. A simplified method for autologous stem cell transplantation in multiple myeloma. Hematology Oncology and Stem Cell Therapy. 2012;**5**(1):49-53. DOI: 10.5144/1658-3876.2012.49

[85] Martino M, Lemoli RM, Girmenia C, Castagna L, Bruno B, Cavallo F, et al. Italian consensus conference for the outpatient autologous stem cell transplantation management in multiple myeloma. Bone Marrow Transplantation. 2016;**51**(8):1032-1040. DOI: 10.1038/bmt.2016.79 [Epub Apr 4, 2016]

[86] Jagannath S, Vesole DH, Zhang M, Desikan KR, Copeland N, Jagannath M, et al. Feasibility and cost-effectiveness of outpatient autotransplants in multiple myeloma. Bone Marrow Transplantation. 1997;**20**(6):445-450. DOI: 10.1038/sj.bmt.1700900

[87] Ferrara F, Palmieri S, Viola A, Copia C, Schiavone EM, De Simone M, et al. Outpatient-based peripheral blood stem cell transplantation for patients with multiple myeloma. The Hematology Journal. 2004;**5**(3):222-226. DOI: 10.1038/sj.thj.6200349

[88] Holbro A, Ahmad I, Cohen S, Roy J, Lachance S, Chagnon M, et al. Safety and cost-effectiveness of outpatient autologous stem cell transplantation in patients with multiple myeloma. Biology of Blood and Marrow Transplantation. 2013;**19**(4):547-551. DOI: 10.1016/j.bbmt.2012.12.006 [Epub Dec 16, 2012]

[89] Graff TM, Singavi AK, Schmidt W, Eastwood D, Drobyski WR, Horowitz M, et al. Safety of outpatient autologous hematopoietic cell transplantation for multiple myeloma and lymphoma. Bone Marrow Transplantation. 2015;**50**(7):947-953. DOI: 10.1038/bmt.2015.46 [Epub Apr 13, 2015]

[90] Lisenko K, Sauer S, Bruckner T, Egerer G, Goldschmidt H, Hillengass J, et al. High-dose chemotherapy and autologous stem cell transplantation of patients with multiple myeloma in an outpatient setting. BMC Cancer. 2017;**17**(1):151. DOI: 10.1186/s12885-017-3137-4

[91] Kroll TM, Singavi A, Schmidt W, Eastwood D, Drobski W, Horowitz MM, et al. Safety of outpatient autologous hematopoietic cell transplantation (AuHCT) for multiple myeloma and lymphoma. Biology of Blood and Marrow Transplantation. 2014;**20**(Suppl 2):S114. DOI: 10.1016/j.bbmt.2013.12.166

[92] Frey P, Stinson T, Siston A, Knight SJ, Ferdman E, Traynor A, et al. Lack of caregivers limits use of outpatient hematopoietic stem cell transplant program. Bone Marrow Transplantation. 2002;**30**(11):741-748. DOI: 10.1038/sj.bmt. 1703676

[93] Sivaraj D, Bacon W, Long GD, Rizzieri DA, Horwitz ME, Sullivan KM, et al. High-dose BCNU/melphalan conditioning regimen before autologous stem cell transplantation in newly diagnosed multiple myeloma. Bone Marrow Transplantation. 2018;**53**(1):34-38. DOI: 10.1038/bmt.2017.208 [Epub Oct 30, 2017]

[94] Striha A, Ashcroft AJ, Hockaday A, Cairns DA, Boardman K, Jacques G, Williams C, et al. The role of ixazomib as an augmented conditioning therapy in salvage autologous stem cell transplant (ASCT) and as a post-ASCT consolidation and maintenance strategy in patients with relapsed multiple myeloma (ACCoRd [UK-MRA myeloma XII] trial): Study protocol for a phase III randomised controlled trial. Trials. 2018;**19**(1):169. DOI: 10.1186/s13063-018-2524-8

[95] Jimenez-Zepeda VH, Duggan P, Neri P, Chaudhry A, Murray K, Culham M, et al. Bortezomib and melphalan conditioning increases the rate of complete response and MRD negativity for patients with multiple myeloma undergoing single autologous stem cell transplant. Leukemia & Lymphoma. 2016;**57**(4):973-976. DOI: 10.3109/10428194. 2015.1085534 [Epub Oct 8, 2015]

[96] Blanes M, Lahuerta JJ, González JD, Ribas P, Solano C, Alegre A, et al. Intravenous busulfan and melphalan as a conditioning regimen for autologous stem cell transplantation in patients with newly diagnosed multiple myeloma: A matched comparison to a melphalan-only approach. Biology of Blood and Marrow Transplantation. 2013;**19**(1):69-74. DOI: 10.1016/j.bbmt.2012.08. 009 [Epub Aug 13, 2012]

[97] Barta SK, Jain R, Mazumder A, Carter J, Almanzar L, Browne R, et al. Pharmacokinetics-directed intravenous busulfan combined with high-dose melphalan and bortezomib as a conditioning regimen for atients with multiple myeloma. Clinical Lymphoma, Myeloma & Leukemia. 2017;**17**(10):650-657. DOI: 10.1016/j.clml.2017.06.005 [Epub Jun 17, 2017]

[98] Mutahar E, Al-Anazi KA. Engraftment syndrome: An updated review. Journal of Stem Cell and Transplantation. 2017;**1**(3):16. DOI: 10.21767/2575-7725.100016

[99] Kanfar S, Al-Anazi KA. Autologous graft versus host disease: An updated review. Annals of Stem Cells and Regenerative Medicine. 2018;**1**(1):1002

[100] Morabito F, Martino M, Stelitano C, Oliva E, Kropp M, Irrera G, et al. Feasibility of a mixed inpatient-outpatient model of peripheral blood stem cell transplantation for multiple myeloma. Haematologica. 2002;**87**(11):1192-1199

[101] Clemens AB, Anderegg S. Mixed outpatient-inpatient autologous stem cell transplant for multiple myeloma: A cost-saving initiative in a resource constrained environment. Journal of Oncology Pharmacy Practice. 2017;**23**(5):384-388. DOI: 10.1177/1078155216639753 [Epub Mar 21, 2016]

[102] Barlogie B, Jagannath S, Vesole DH, Naucke S, Cheson B, Mattox S, et al. Superiority of tandem autologous transplantation over standard therapy for previously untreated multiple myeloma. Blood. 1997;**89**(3):789-793

[103] Attal M, Harousseau JL, Facon T, Guilhot F, Doyen C, Fuzibet JG, et al., InterGroupe Francophone du Myélome. Single versus double autologous stem-cell transplantation for multiple myeloma. New England Journal of Medicine. 2003;**349**(26):2495-2502. DOI: 10.1056/NEJMoa032290

[104] Bergantim R, Trigo F, Guimarães JE. Impact of tandem autologous stem cell transplantation and response to transplant in the outcome of multiple myeloma. Experimental Hematology & Oncology. 2012;**1**(1):35. DOI: 10.1186/2162-3619-1-35

[105] Elice F, Raimondi R, Tosetto A, D'Emilio A, Di Bona E, Piccin A, et al. Prolonged overall survival with second on-demand autologous transplant in multiple myeloma. American Journal of Hematology. 2006;**81**(6):426-431. DOI: 10.1002/ajh.20641

[106] Kumar A, Kharfan-Dabaja MA, Glasmacher A, Djulbegovic B. Tandem versus single autologous hematopoietic cell transplantation for the treatment of multiple myeloma: A systematic review and meta-analysis. Journal of the National Cancer Institute. 2009;**101**(2):100-106. DOI: 10.1093/jnci/djn439 [Epub Jan 13, 2009]

[107] Mehta J. Re: Tandem vs single autologous hematopoietic cell transplantation for the treatment of multiple myeloma: A systematic review and meta-analysis. Journal of the National Cancer Institute. 2009;**101**(20):1430-1431

[108] Singh Abbi KK, Zheng J, Devlin SM, Giralt S, Landau H. Second autologous stem cell transplant: An effective therapy for relapsed multiple myeloma. Biology of Blood and Marrow Transplantation. 2015;**21**(3):468-472. DOI: 10.1016/j.bbmt. 2014. 11.677 [Epub Dec 18, 2014]

[109] Olin RL, Vogl DT, Porter DL, Luger SM, Schuster SJ, Tsai DE, et al. Second auto-SCT is safe and effective salvage therapy for relapsed multiple myeloma. Bone Marrow Transplantation. 2009;**43**(5):417-422. DOI: 10.1038/bmt.2008.334 [Epub Oct 13, 2008]

[110] Jimenez-Zepeda VH, Mikhael J, Winter A, Franke N, Masih-Khan E, Trudel S, et al. Second autologous stem cell transplantation as salvage therapy for multiple myeloma: Impact on progression-free and overall survival. Biology of Blood and Marrow Transplantation. 2012;**18**(5):773-779. DOI: 10.1016/j.bbmt. 2011.10. 044 [Epub Nov 4, 2011]

[111] Gonsalves WI, Gertz MA, Lacy MQ, Dispenzieri A, Hayman SR, Buadi FK, et al. Second auto-SCT for treatment of relapsed multiple myeloma. Bone Marrow Transplantation. 2013;**48**(4):568-573. DOI: 10.1038/bmt.2012.183. [Epub Sep 24, 2012]

[112] Atanackovic D, Schilling G. Second autologous transplant as salvage therapy in multiple myeloma. British Journal of Haematology. 2013;**163**(5):565-572. DOI: 10.1111/bjh.12579 [Epub Sep 24, 2013]

[113] Cook G, Liakopoulou E, Pearce R, Cavet J, Morgan GJ, Kirkland K, et al., British Society of Blood & Marrow Transplantation Clinical Trials Committee. Factors influencing the outcome of a second autologous stem cell transplant (ASCT) in relapsed multiple myeloma: A study from the British Society of Blood and Marrow Transplantation Registry. Biology of Blood and Marrow Transplantation 2011;**17**(11):1638-1645. DOI: 10.1016/j.bbmt. 2011.04.005. [Epub Apr 23, 2011]

[114] Morris C, Iacobelli S, Brand R, Bjorkstrand B, Drake M, Niederwieser D, et al., Chronic Leukaemia Working Party Myeloma Subcommittee, European Group for Blood and Marrow Transplantation. Benefit and timing of second transplantations in multiple myeloma: Clinical findings and methodological limitations in a European Group for Blood and Marrow Transplantation registry study. Journal of Clinical Oncology. 2004;**22**(9):1674-1681. DOI: 10.1200/JCO.2004.06.144 [Epub Mar 22, 2004]

[115] Castagna L, Mussetti A, Devillier R, Dominietto A, Marcatti M, Milone G, et al. Haploidentical allogeneic hematopoietic cell transplantation for multiple myeloma using post-transplantation cyclophosphamide graft-versus-host disease prophylaxis. Biology of Blood and Marrow Transplantation. 2017;**23**(9):1549-1554. DOI: 10.1016/j.bbmt.2017.05.006 [Epub May 10, 2017]

[116] Mir MA, Kapoor P, Kumar S, Pandey S, Dispenzieri A, Lacy MQ, et al. Trends and outcomes in allogeneic hematopoietic stem cell transplant for multiple myeloma at Mayo Clinic. Clinical Lymphoma, Myeloma & Leukemia. 2015;**15**(6):349-357.e2. DOI: 10.1016/j.clml.2015.03.016 [Epub Apr 2, 2015]

[117] Kröger N, Badbaran A, Zabelina T, Ayuk F, Wolschke C, Alchalby H, et al. Impact of high-risk cytogenetics and achievement of molecular remission on long-term freedom from disease after autologous-allogeneic tandem transplantation in patients with multiple myeloma. Biology of Blood and Marrow Transplantation. 2013;**19**(3):398-404. DOI: 10.1016/j.bbmt.2012.10.008 [Epub Oct 16, 2012]

[118] Giaccone L, Evangelista A, Patriarca F, Sorasio R, Pini M, Carnevale-Schianca F, et al. Impact of new drugs on the long-term follow-up of upfront tandem autograft-allograft in multiple myeloma. Biology of Blood and Marrow Transplantation. 2018;**24**(1):189-193. DOI: 10.1016/j.bbmt.2017.09.017 [Epub Oct 4, 2017]

[119] Gay F, Engelhardt M, Terpos E, Wäsch R, Giaccone L, Auner HW, et al. From transplant to novel cellular therapies in multiple myeloma: European Myeloma Network guidelines and future perspectives. Haematologica. 2018;**103**(2):197-211. DOI: 10.3324/haematol.2017.174573 [Epub Dec 7, 2017]

[120] Pawarode A, Mineishi S, Reddy P, Braun TM, Khaled YA, Choi SW, et al. Reducing treatment-related mortality did not improve outcomes of allogeneic myeloablative hematopoietic cell transplantation for high-risk multiple myeloma: A university of Michigan prospective series. Biology of Blood and Marrow Transplantation. 2016;**22**(1):54-60. DOI: 10.1016/j.bbmt.2015.07.021 [Epub Jul 26, 2015]

[121] Rasche L, Röllig C, Stuhler G, Danhof S, Mielke S, Grigoleit GU, et al. Allogeneic hematopoietic cell transplantation in multiple myeloma: Focus on longitudinal assessment of donor chimerism, extramedullary disease, and high-risk cytogenetic features. Biology of Blood and Marrow Transplantation. 2016;**22**(11):1988-1996. DOI: 10.1016/j.bbmt.2016.08.024 [Epub Aug 31, 2016]

[122] Kawamura K, Takamatsu H, Ikeda T, Komatsu T, Aotsuka N, Amano I, et al. Cord blood transplantation for multiple myeloma: A study from the multiple myeloma working group of the Japan society for hematopoietic cell transplantation. Biology of Blood and Marrow Transplantation. 2015;**21**(7):1291-1298. DOI: 10.1016/j.bbmt.2015.02.015 [Epub Feb 21, 2015]

[123] Ghosh N, Ye X, Tsai HL, Bolaños-Meade J, Fuchs EJ, Luznik L, et al. Allogeneic blood or marrow transplantation with post-transplantation cyclophosphamide as graft-versus-host disease prophylaxis in multiple myeloma. Biology of Blood and Marrow Transplantation. 2017;**23**(11):1903-1909. DOI: 10.1016/j.bbmt.2017.07.003 [Epub Jul 12, 2017]

[124] Passera R, Pollichieni S, Brunello L, Patriarca F, Bonifazi F, Montefusco V, et al. Allogeneic hematopoietic cell transplantation from unrelated donors in multiple myeloma: Study from the Italian bone marrow donor registry. Biology of Blood and Marrow Transplantation. 2013;**19**(6):940-948. DOI: 10.1016/j.bbmt.2013.03.012 [Epub Mar 26, 2013]

[125] Cornell RF, D'Souza A, Kassim AA, Costa LJ, Innis-Shelton RD, Zhang MJ, et al. Maintenance versus induction therapy choice on outcomes after autologous transplantation for multiple myeloma. Biology of Blood and Marrow Transplantation. 2017;**23**(2):269-277. DOI: 10.1016/j.bbmt.2016.11.011 [Epub Nov 15, 2016]

[126] Lee HS, Min CK. Optimal maintenance and consolidation therapy for multiple myeloma in actual clinical practice. The Korean Journal of Internal Medicine. 2016;**31**(5):809-819. DOI: 10.3904/kjim.2016.110 [Epub Sep 1, 2016]

[127] Talhi S, Osmani S, Brahimi M, Amani K, Ouldjeriouat H, Bouchama S, et al. Bortezomib-based regimens as consolidation therapy after autologous hematopoietic stem cell transplantation in multiple myeloma: A single center experience from Oran (Algeria). Blood. 2016;**128**:5121

[128] Alexanian R, Weber D, Giralt S, Delasalle K. Consolidation therapy of multiple myeloma with thalidomide-dexamethasone after intensive chemotherapy. Annals of Oncology. 2002;**13**(7):1116-1119

[129] Mohty M, Richardson PG, McCarthy PL, Attal M. Consolidation and maintenance therapy for multiple myeloma after autologous transplantation: Where do we stand? Bone Marrow Transplantation. 2015;**50**(8):1024-1029. DOI: 10.1038/bmt.2015.83 [Epub Apr 20, 2015]

[130] Sivaraj D, Green MM, Li Z, Sung AD, Sarantopoulos S, Kang Y, et al. Outcomes of maintenance therapy with bortezomib after autologous stem cell transplantation for patients with multiple myeloma. Biology of Blood and Marrow Transplantation. 2017;**23**(2):262-268. DOI: 10.1016/j.bbmt.2016.11.010 [Epub Nov 14, 2016]

[131] Pulte ED, Dmytrijuk A, Nie L, Goldberg KB, McKee AE, Farrell AT, et al. FDA approval summary: Lenalidomide as maintenance therapy after autologous stem cell transplant in newly diagnosed multiple myeloma. Oncologist. 2018;**23**(6):734-739. DOI: 10.1634/theoncologist.2017-0440

[132] Palumbo A, Hajek R, Delforge M, Kropff M, Petrucci MT, Catalano J, et al., MM-015 Investigators. Continuous lenalidomide treatment for newly diagnosed multiple myeloma. The New England Journal of Medicine. 2012;**366**(19):1759-1769. DOI: 10.1056/NEJMoa1112704

[133] McCarthy PL, Owzar K, Hofmeister CC, Hurd DD, Hassoun H, Richardson PG, et al. Lenalidomide after stem-cell transplantation for multiple myeloma. The New England Journal of Medicine. 2012;**366**(19):1770-1781. DOI: 10.1056/NEJMoa1114083

[134] Mian M, Tinelli M, De March E, Turri G, Meneghini V, Pescosta N, et al. Bortezomib, thalidomide and lenalidomide: Have they really changed the outcome of multiple myeloma? Anticancer Research. 2016;**36**(3):1059-1065

[135] McCarthy PL, Holstein SA, Petrucci MT, Richardson PG, Hulin C, Tosi P, et al. Lenalidomide maintenance after autologous stem-cell transplantation in newly diagnosed multiple myeloma: A meta-analysis. Journal of Clinical Oncology. 2017;**35**(29):3279-3289. DOI: 10.1200/JCO.2017.72.6679 [Epub Jul 25, 2017]

[136] Attal M, Lauwers-Cances V, Marit G, Caillot D, Moreau P, Facon T, et al., IFM Investigators. Lenalidomide maintenance after stem-cell transplantation for multiple myeloma. The New England Journal of Medicine. 2012;**366**(19):1782-1791. DOI: 10.1056/NEJMoa1114138

[137] Ludwig H, Zojer N. Fixed duration vs continuous therapy in multiple myeloma. Hematology. American Society of Hematology. Education Program. 2017;**2017**(1):212-222. DOI: 10.1182/asheducation-2017.1.212

[138] Palumbo A, Gay F, Cavallo F, Di Raimondo F, Larocca A, Hardan I, et al. Continuous therapy versus fixed duration of therapy in patients with newly diagnosed multiple myeloma. Journal of Clinical Oncology. 2015;**33**(30):3459-3466. DOI: 10.1200/JCO.2014.60.2466 [Epub Aug 17, 2015]

[139] Guglielmelli T, Palumbo A. Multiple myeloma: Is a shift toward continuous therapy needed to move forward? Expert Review of Hematology. 2015;**8**(3):253-256. DOI: 10.1586/17474086.2015.1001360 [Epub Jan 12, 2015]

[140] Bahlis NJ, Corso A, Mugge LO, Shen ZX, Desjardins P, Stoppa AM, et al. Benefit of continuous treatment for responders with newly diagnosed multiple myeloma in the randomized FIRST trial. Leukemia. 2017;**31**(11):2435-2442. DOI: 10.1038/leu.2017.111 [Epub Apr 4, 2017]

[141] Hari P, Romanus D, Palumbo A, Luptakova K, Rifkin RM, Tran LM, et al. Prolonged duration of therapy is associated with improved survival in patients treated for relapsed/refractory multiple myeloma in routine clinical care in the United States. Clinical Lymphoma, Myeloma & Leukemia. 2018;**18**(2):152-160. DOI: 10.1016/j.clml.2017.12.012 [Epub Jan 5, 2018]

[142] Zhang T, Wang S, Lin T, Xie J, Zhao L, Liang Z, et al. Systematic review and meta-analysis of the efficacy and safety of novel monoclonal antibodies for treatment of relapsed/refractory multiple myeloma. Oncotarget. 2017;**8**(20):34001-34017. DOI: 10.18632/oncotarget.16987

[143] Kumar SK, LaPlant B, Chng WJ, Zonder J, Callander N, Fonseca R, et al., Mayo Phase 2 Consortium. Dinaciclib, a novel CDK inhibitor, demonstrates encouraging single-agent activity in patients with relapsed multiple myeloma. Blood. 2015;**125**(3):443-448. DOI: 10.1182/blood-2014-05-573741. [Epub Nov 13, 2014]

[144] Richardson PG, Bensinger WI, Huff CA, Costello CL, Lendvai N, Berdeja JG, et al. Ibrutinib alone or with dexamethasone for relapsed or relapsed and refractory multiple myeloma: Phase 2 trial results. British Journal of Haematology. 2018;**180**(6):821-830. DOI: 10.1111/bjh.15058 [Epub Feb 13, 2018]

[145] Ashjian E, Redic K. Multiple myeloma: Updates for pharmacists in the treatment of relapsed and refractory disease. Journal of Oncology Pharmacy Practice. 2016;**22**(2):289-302. DOI: 10.1177/1078155215572036 [Epub Feb 17, 2015]

[146] El-Amm J, Tabbara IA. Emerging therapies in multiple myeloma. American Journal of Clinical Oncology. 2015;**38**(3):315-321. DOI: 10.1097/COC.0b013e3182a4676b

[147] Rosean TR, Tompkins VS, Tricot G, Holman CJ, Olivier AK, Zhan F, et al. Preclinical validation of interleukin 6 as a therapeutic target in multiple myeloma. Immunologic Research. 2014;**59**(1-3):188-202. DOI: 10.1007/s12026-014-8528-x

[148] Redic KA, Hough SM, Price EM. Clinical developments in the treatment of relapsed or relapsed and refractory multiple myeloma: Impact of panobinostat, the first-in-class histone deacetylase inhibitor. OncoTargets and Therapy. 2016;**9**:2783-2793. DOI: 10.2147/OTT.S87962 [eCollection 2016]

[149] de la Puente P, Muz B, Azab F, Luderer M, Azab AK. Molecularly targeted therapies in multiple myeloma. Leukemia Research and Treatment. 2014;**2014**:976567. DOI: 10.1155/2014/976567. [Epub Apr 16, 2014]

[150] Gonsalves WI, Milani P, Derudas D, Buadi FK. The next generation of novel therapies for the management of relapsed multiple myeloma. Future Oncology. 2017;**13**(1):63-75. DOI: 10.2217/fon-2016-0200 [Epub Aug 11, 2016]

[151] Maes A, Menu E, Veirman K, Maes K, Vand Erkerken K, De Bruyne E. The therapeutic potential of cell cycle targeting in multiple myeloma. Oncotarget. 2017;**8**(52):90501-90520. DOI: 10.18632/oncotarget.18765 [eCollection Oct 27, 2107]

[152] Ludwig H, Delforge M, Facon T, Einsele H, Gay F, Moreau P, et al. Prevention and management of adverse events of Novel agents in multiple myeloma: A consensus of the european myeloma network. Leukemia. 2018. DOI: 10.1038/s41375-018-0040-1 [Epub ahead of print]

[153] Sanchez L, Wang Y, Siegel DS, Wang ML. Daratumumab: A first-in-class CD38 monoclonal antibody for the treatment of multiple myeloma. Journal of Hematology & Oncology. 2016;**9**(1):51. DOI: 10.1186/s13045-016-0283-0

[154] Palumbo A, Chanan-Khan A, Weisel K, Nooka AK, Masszi T, Beksac M, et al., CASTOR Investigators. Daratumumab, bortezomib, and dexamethasone for multiple myeloma. The New England Journal of Medicine. 2016;**375**(8):754-766. DOI: 10.1056/NEJMoa1606038

[155] Mateos MV, Dimopoulos MA, Cavo M, Suzuki K, Jakubowiak A, Knop S, et al., ALCYONE Trial Investigators. Daratumumab plus bortezomib, melphalan, and prednisone for untreated myeloma. The New England Journal of Medicine. 2018;**378**(6):518-528. DOI: 10.1056/NEJMoa1714678. [Epub Dec 12, 2017]

[156] Dimopoulos MA, Oriol A, Nahi H, San-Miguel J, Bahlis NJ, Usmani SZ, et al., POLLUX Investigators. Daratumumab, lenalidomide, and dexamethasone for multiple myeloma. The New England Journal of Medicine. 2016;**375**(14):1319-1331. DOI: 10.1056/NEJMoa1607751

[157] Lonial S, Dimopoulos M, Palumbo A, White D, Grosicki S, Spicka I, et al., ELOQUENT-2 Investigators. Elotuzumab therapy for relapsed or refractory multiple myeloma. The New England Journal of Medicine. 2015;**373**(7):621-631. DOI: 10.1056/NEJMoa1505654 [Epub Jun 2, 2015]

[158] Wallington-Beddoe CT, Pitson SM. Novel therapies for multiple myeloma. Aging (Albany NY). 2017;**9**(8):1857-1858. DOI: 10.18632/aging.101284 [Epub Aug 28, 2017]

[159] Ríos-Tamayo R, Martín-García A, Alarcón-Payer C, Sánchez-Rodríguez D, de la Guardia AMDVD, García Collado CG, et al. Pomalidomide in the treatment of multiple myeloma: Design, development and place in therapy. Drug Design, Development and Therapy. 2017;**11**:2399-2408. DOI: 10.2147/DDDT.S115456 [eCollection 2017]

[160] Richardson PG, Baz R, Wang M, Jakubowiak AJ, Laubach JP, Harvey RD, et al. Phase 1 study of twice-weekly ixazomib, an oral proteasome inhibitor, in relapsed/refractory multiple myeloma patients. Blood. 2014;**124**(7):1038-1406. DOI: 10.1182/blood-2014-01-548826 [Epub Jun 11, 2014]

[161] Uccello G, Petrungaro A, Mazzone C, Recchia AG, Greco R, Mendicino F, et al. Pomalidomide in multiple myeloma. Expert Opinion on Pharmacotherapy. 2017;**18**(2): 133-137. DOI: 10.1080/14656566.2016.1274973 [Epub Dec 26, 2016]

[162] Sriskandarajah P, Jolly H, Pawlyn C, Mohammed K, Dearden C, Potter M, et al. Retrospective cohort analysis examining the efficacy and safety of (V) DTPACE in newly diagnosed and relapsed/refractory myeloma patients-the UK experience. Clinical Lymphoma, Myeloma & Leukemia. 2016;**16**(Suppl 2):S80. DOI: 10.1016/j.clml.2016.07.112

[163] Jain S, Diefenbach CM, Zain JM, O'Connor OA. Emerging role of carfilzomib in treatment of relapsed and refractory lymphoid neoplasms and multiple myeloma. Core Evidence. 2011;**6**:43-57. DOI: 10.2147/CE.S13838 [Epub Apr 4, 2011]

[164] Dimopoulos MA, Kimball AS. Carfilzomib for relapsed or refractory multiple myeloma -Authors' reply. The Lancet Oncology. 2018;**19**(1):e2. DOI: 10.1016/S1470-2045(17)30920-8

[165] Tanimoto T, Tsuda K, Oshima K, Mori J, Shimmura H. Carfilzomib for relapsed or refractory multiple myeloma. The Lancet Oncology. 2018;**19**(1):e1. DOI: 10.1016/S1470-2045(17)30859-8

[166] Muchtar E, Gertz MA, Magen H. A practical review on carfilzomib in multiple myeloma. European Journal of Haematology. 2016;**96**(6):564-577. DOI: 10.1111/ejh.12749 [Epub Mar 9, 2016]

[167] Afifi S, Michael A, Azimi M, Rodriguez M, Lendvai N, Landgren O. Role of histone deacetylase inhibitors in relapsed refractory multiple myeloma: A focus on vorinostat and panobinostat. Pharmacotherapy. 2015;**35**(12):1173-1188. DOI: 10.1002/phar.1671

[168] Richardson PG, Hungria VT, Yoon SS, Beksac M, Dimopoulos MA, Elghandour A, et al. Panobinostat plus bortezomib and dexamethasone in previously treated multiple myeloma: Outcomes by prior treatment. Blood. 2016;**127**(6):713-721. DOI: 10.1182/blood-2015-09-665018 [Epub Dec 2, 2015]

[169] Laubach JP, Moreau P, San-Miguel JF, Richardson PG. Panobinostat for the treatment of multiple myeloma. Clinical Cancer Research. 2015;**21**(21):4767-4773. DOI: 10.1158/1078-0432.CCR-15-0530 [Epub Sep 11, 2015]

[170] Mu S, Kuroda Y, Shibayama H, Hino M, Tajima T, Corrado C, et al. Panobinostat PK/PD profile in combination with bortezomib and dexamethasone in patients with relapsed and relapsed/refractory multiple myeloma. European Journal of Clinical Pharmacology. 2016;**72**(2):153-161. DOI: 10.1007/s00228-015-1967-z [Epub Oct 22, 2015]

[171] San-Miguel JF, Einsele H, Moreau P. The role of panobinostat plus bortezomib and dexamethasone in treating relapsed or relapsed and refractory multiple myeloma: A European perspective. Advances in Therapy. 2016;**33**(11):1896-1920. DOI: 10.1007/s12325-016-0413-7 [Epub Sep 27, 2016]

[172] Liu JD, Sun CY, Tang L, Wu YY, Wang QY, Hu B, et al. Efficacy and safety of panobinostat in relapsed or/and refractory multiple myeloma: Meta analyses of clinical trials and systematic review. Scientific Reports. 2016;**6**:27361. DOI: 10.1038/srep27361

[173] Abate-Daga D, Davila ML. CAR models: Next-generation CAR modifications for enhanced T-cell function. Molecular Therapy—Oncolytics. 2016;**3**:16014. DOI: 10.1038/mto.2016.14 [eCollection 2016]

[174] Levine BL, Miskin J, Wonnacott K, Keir C. Global manufacturing of CAR T cell therapy. Molecular Therapy—Methods and Clinical Development. 2016;**4**:92-101. DOI: 10.1016/j.omtm.2016.12.006 [eCollection Mar 17, 2017]

[175] Wang X, Xiao Q, Wang Z, Feng WL. CAR-T therapy for leukemia: Progress and challenges. Translational Research. 2017;**182**:135-144. DOI: 10.1016/j.trsl.2016.10.008 [Epub Oct 27, 2016]

[176] Bonifant CL, Jackson HJ, Brentjens RJ, Curran KJ. Toxicity and management in CAR T-cell therapy. Molecular Therapy—Oncolytics. 2016;**3**:16011. DOI: 10.1038/mto.2016.11 [eCollection 2016]

[177] Chu J, Deng Y, Benson DM, He S, Hughes T, Zhang J, et al. CS1-specific chimeric antigen receptor (CAR)-engineered natural killer cells enhance in vitro and in vivo antitumor activity against human multiple myeloma. Leukemia. 2014;**28**(4):917-927. DOI: 10.1038/leu.2013.279 [Epub Sep 26, 2013]

[178] Garfall AL, Maus MV, Hwang WT, Lacey SF, Mahnke YD, Melenhorst JJ, et al. Chimeric antigen receptor T cells against CD19 for multiple myeloma. The New England Journal of Medicine. 2015;**373**(11):1040-1047. DOI: 10.1056/NEJMoa1504542

[179] Ormhøj M, Bedoya F, Frigault MJ, Maus MV. CARs in the lead against multiple myeloma. Current Hematologic Malignancy Reports. 2017;**12**(2):119-125. DOI: 10.1007/s11899-017-0373-2

[180] Hipp S, Tai YT, Blanset D, Deegen P, Wahl J, Thomas O, et al. A novel BCMA/CD3 bispecific T-cell engager for the treatment of multiple myeloma induces selective lysis in vitro and in vivo. Leukemia. 2017;**31**(8):1743-1751. DOI: 10.1038/leu.2016.388 [Epub Dec 27, 2016]

[181] Ali SA, Shi V, Maric I, Wang M, Stroncek DF, Rose JJ, et al. T cells expressing an anti-B-cell maturation antigen chimeric antigen receptor cause remissions of multiple myeloma. Blood. 2016;**128**(13):1688-1700. DOI: 10.1182/blood-2016-04-711903 [Epub Jul 13, 2016]

[182] Yee AJ, Raje N. Best of 2017 in multiple myeloma. American Society of Hematology. The Hematologist, ASH News and Reports. January-February 2018:**15**(1)

[183] Chim CS, Kumar SK, Orlowski RZ, Cook G, Richardson PG, Gertz MA, et al. Management of relapsed and refractory multiple myeloma: Novel agents, antibodies, immunotherapies and beyond. Leukemia. 2018;**32**(2):252-262. DOI: 10.1038/leu.2017.329 [Epub Nov 16, 2017]

[184] Malard F, Harousseau JL, Mohty M. Multiple myeloma treatment at relapse after autologous stem cell transplantation: A practical analysis. Cancer Treatment Reviews. 2017;**52**:41-47. DOI: 10.1016/j.ctrv.2016.11.005 [Epub Nov 15, 2016]

[185] Sun Z, Zheng F, Wu S, Liu Y, Guo H, Liu Y. Triplet versus doublet combination regimens for the treatment of relapsed or refractory multiple myeloma: A meta-analysis of phase III randomized controlled trials. Critical Reviews in Oncology/Hematology. 2017;**113**:249-255. DOI: 10.1016/j.critrevonc.2017.03.018 [Epub Mar 18, 2017]

[186] Dimopoulos MA, Moreau P, Palumbo A, Joshua D, Pour L, Hájek R, et al., ENDEAVOR Investigators. Carfilzomib and dexamethasone versus bortezomib and dexamethasone for patients with relapsed or refractory multiple myeloma (ENDEAVOR): A randomised, phase 3, open-label, multicentre study. The Lancet Oncology. 2016;**17**(1):27-38. DOI: 10.1016/S1470-2045(15)00464-7. [Epub Dec 5, 2015]

[187] Yadav P, Cook M, Cockwell P. Current trends of renal impairment in multiple myeloma. Kidney Diseases (Basel). 2016;**1**(4):241-527. DOI: 10.1159/000442511 [Epub Feb 3, 2016]

[188] Gaballa MR, Laubach JP, Schlossman RL, Redman K, Noonan K, Mitsiades CS, et al. Management of myeloma-associated renal dysfunction in the era of novel therapies. Expert Review of Hematology. 2012;**5**:51-66 (quiz 67-8). DOI: 10.1586/ehm.11.72

[189] Gavriatopoulou M, Terpos E, Kastritis E, Dimopoulos MA. Current treatments for renal failure due to multiple myeloma. Expert Opinion on Pharmacotherapy. 2016;**17**(16):2165-2177. DOI: 10.1080/14656566.2016.1236915 [Epub Sep 27, 2016]

[190] Parikh GC, Amjad AI, Saliba RM, Kazmi SM, Khan ZU, Lahoti A, et al. Autologous hematopoietic stem cell transplantation may reverse renal failure in patients with multiple myeloma. Biology of Blood and Marrow Transplantation. 2009;**15**:812-816. DOI: 10.1016/j.bbmt.2009.03.021

[191] Dimopoulos MA, Roussou M, Gkotzamanidou M, Nikitas N, Psimenou E, Mparmparoussi D, et al. The role of novel agents on the reversibility of renal impairment in newly diagnosed symptomatic patients with multiple myeloma. Leukemia. 2013;**27**:423-429. DOI: 10.1038/leu.2012.182 [Epub Jul 5, 2012]

[192] Terpos E, Kleber M, Engelhardt M, Zweegman S, Gay F, Kastritis E, et al., European Myeloma Network. European Myeloma Network guidelines for the management of multiple myeloma-related complications. Haematologica. 2015;**100**(10):1254-1266. DOI: 10.3324/haematol.2014.117176

[193] Raghavan R, Jeroudi A, Achkar K, Gaber AO, Patel SJ, Abdellatif A. Bortezomib in kidney transplantation. Journal of Transplantation. 2010. DOI: 10.1155/2010/698594 [Epub Sep 27, 2010]

[194] Heher EC, Rennke HG, Laubach JP, Richardson PG. Kidney disease and multiple myeloma. Clinical Journal of the American Society of Nephrology. 2013;**8**(11):2007-2017. DOI: 10.2215/CJN.12231212 [Epub Jul 18, 2013]

[195] Penfield JG. Multiple myeloma in end-stage renal disease. Seminars in Dialysis. 2006;**19**:329-334. DOI: 10.1111/j.1525-139X.2006.00181.x

[196] Heher EC, Goes NB, Spitzer TR, Raje NS, Humphreys BD, Anderson KC, et al. Kidney disease associated with plasma cell dyscrasias. Blood. 2010;**116**:1397-1404. DOI: 10.1182/blood-2010-03-258608 [Epub May 12, 2010]

[197] Bansal T, Garg A, Snowden JA, McKane W. Defining the role of renal transplantation in the modern management of multiple myeloma and other plasma cell dyscrasias. Nephron. Clinical Practice. 2012;**120**:228-235. DOI: 10.1159/000341760 [Epub Oct 5, 2012]

[198] Al-Anazi KA, Bacal J, Mokhtar N, Kawari M, AlHashmi H, Kalogiannidis P, et al. A young patient with refractory multiple myeloma and dialysis-dependent renal failure has been cured by non-cryopreserved autologous stem cell transplantation followed by live-related kidney transplantation. Journal of Stem Cell Biology and Transplantation. 2017;**1**(2):13. DOI: 10.21767/2575-7725.100013

[199] Baraldi O, Grandinetti V, Donati G, Comai G, Battaglino G, Cuna V, et al. Hematopoietic cell and renal transplantation in plasma cell dyscrasia patients. Cell Transplantation. 2016;**25**:995-1005. DOI: 10.3727/096368915X688560 [Epub Jul 8, 2015]

[200] Doney KC, Mielcarek M, Stewart FM, Appelbaum FR. Hematopoietic cell transplantation after solid organ transplantation. Biology of Blood and Marrow Transplantation. 2015;**21**:2123-2128. DOI: 10.1016/j.bbmt. 2015.08.004 [Epub Aug 10, 2015]

[201] Kawai T, Sachs DH, Sprangers B, Spitzer TR, Saidman SL, Zorn E, et al. Long-term results in recipients of combined HLA-mismatched kidney and bone marrow transplantation

without maintenance immunosuppression. American Journal of Transplantation. 2014;**14**:1599-1611. DOI: 10.1111/ajt.12731 [Epub Jun 5, 2014]

[202] Chen YB, Kawai T, Spitzer TR. Combined bone marrow and kidney transplantation for the induction of specific tolerance. Advances in Hematology. 2016;**2016**:6471901. DOI: 10.1155/2016/6471901 [Epub Apr 30, 2016]

[203] Spitzer TR, Sykes M, Tolkoff-Rubin N, Kawai T, McAfee SL, Dey BR, et al. Long-term follow-up of recipients of combined human leukocyte antigen-matched bone marrow and kidney transplantation for multiple myeloma with end-stage renal disease. Transplantation. 2011;**91**:672-676. DOI: 10.1097/TP.0b013e31820a3068

[204] Kawai T, Chen Y-B, Sykes M, Benedict C, Tolkoff-Rubin N, Day B et al. HLA identical or haploidentical combined kidney and bone marrow transplantation for multiple myeloma with end-stage renal failure. American Transplant Congress. June 13, 2016; (abstract number: 187)

[205] Ruiz-Delgado GJ, León-Peña AA, Medina-Ceballos E, Vargas-Espinosa J, León-González M, Ruiz-Argüelles GJ, et al. Double transplant in a patient with multiple myeloma: Bone marrow and kidney. Revista de Hematología (Mex.). 2015;**16**:333-337

[206] Khoriaty R, Otrock ZK, Medawar WA, Khauli RB, Bazarbachi A. A case of successful double sequential bone marrow and kidney transplantations in a patient with multiple myeloma. Nephrology, Dialysis, Transplantation. 2006;**21**:3585-3358. DOI: 10.1093/ndt/gfl403 [Epub Sep 12, 2006]

Chapter 7

The Role of Radiology and Radiotherapy for Multiple Myeloma

Milda Rudzianskiene, Viktoras Rudzianskas,
Ruta Dambrauskiene and Rolandas Gerbutavicius

Additional information is available at the end of the chapter

http://dx.doi.org/10.5772/intechopen.75397

Abstract

Skeletal-related events occur in 80% of patients with multiple myeloma (MM). Osteoporosis, osteoclastic destructions, pathological fractures of the bone, spinal cord and compression can impair patients' quality of life and reduce survival. Many imaging techniques can be used for the detection of MM bone lesions. Many clinical studies suggest modern imaging techniques for their greater sensitivity. Radiotherapy is a treatment of choice for solitary plasmacytoma of the bone and extramedullary plasmacytomas. However, radiation treatment of MM can be used as a palliative approach for uncontrolled pain, impending pathological fractures and in the cases of spinal cord compression. Radiotherapy induces analgesic effect in 75–100% of patients and promotes a recalcification in 40–60%. In patients with spinal cord compression, radiation therapy is given along with dexamethasone, and up to half of patients may experience improvement. It is well known that pain perception, response to analgesics and pain relief effect of radiotherapy are quite different for multiple myeloma patients. Clinical, laboratory and genetic factors may influence the pain perception and analgesic effect of radiotherapy. Side effects of radiation are generally mild, are limited to the radiotherapy site and can be predicted.

Keywords: multiple myeloma, bone disease, analgesic effect, palliative radiotherapy, radiation dose

1. Introduction

Skeletal-related events are one of the signs of multiple myeloma (MM) [1, 2]. Osteoclastic destructions increase the risk of pathologic fractures and spinal cord compression syndrome, which reduces patients' quality of life, increases treatment costs and worsens patient survival [3]. Radiotherapy is a treatment approach used in patients with solitary plasmacytomas. However, the role of radiation treatment of MM is palliative: to induce an analgesic effect in osteolytic lesions, to promote recalcification in the sites of impending pathological fractures and symptom control in spinal cord compression [4].

Despite the enormous development in MM treatment approaches and response to systemic therapy, patients are often in need of pain control due to slow repair of bone lesions. Chemotherapy treatment alone is insufficient for patients suffering from pain caused by osteolytic bone destruction or in case of an impending fracture at the destruction site. Seventy percent of patients receive radiation at least once during their MM therapy [5]. Where radiotherapy is applied, pain can be reduced by 75–100% from the starting level [5–12]. Recalcification of bone destructions caused by MM is observed in 40–60% of the cases after radiation treatment [5, 7, 12, 13]. Good results in the treatment of bone damages due to MM can be achieved when applying other supportive therapy measures, such as bisphosphonates, vertebroplasty and surgery methods, alongside radiation therapy.

It has been known for a long time that pain perception is not the same for all patients. The response to analgesics, pain relief and the effect of radiotherapy are very individual. The above can be determined by a different secretion of anti-inflammatory cytokines (IL-6, IL-10, TNFα, IL-1), which participate in the pathogenesis of the pain caused by a chronic disease and their concentration in blood serum. Circulating cytokines and inflammatory proteins are related to pain, cognitive functions, depression, fatigue and sleep disturbances [14–16]. The secretion of anti-inflammatory cytokines is regulated genetically. Cytokine genes are very polymorphous. Polymorphisms in regulatory regions, including promoters and non-transmittable areas, in a majority of the cases can change the gene expression in vitro [15]. Thus, the above has an impact on the secretion of cytokines and their concentration in blood serum, which determines the pain perception threshold and a different response of patients to analgesics and radiotherapy.

2. The role of imaging

Around 70–80% of patients have osteolytic lesions at diagnosis of MM, and up to 90% develop lytic lesions during the course of the disease [17]. The International Myeloma Working Group updated criteria for the diagnosis of symptomatic MM and revealed the value of modern imaging such as computed tomography (CT), whole-body low-dose computed tomography (LDCT), positron emission tomography/computed tomography (PET/CT) and magnetic resonance imaging (MRI) [18]. Modern imaging techniques had a greater sensitivity than conventional radiographic skeletal survey for the detection of MM bone lesions with as many as 80% or more lesions detected by the newer imaging techniques [18]. A summary of different imaging techniques is detailed in **Table 1**.

2.1. Conventional radiographic skeletal survey

Whole-body X-rays imagine (including plain radiographs of the whole skeleton) have been widely used for the detection of bone lesions at diagnosis and during the course of the disease. Osteolytic bone lesions are more common in the scull, vertebrae, ribs and pelvis. Although the

Imaging technique	Advantages	Limitations
Whole-body skeletal survey	Low cost	Low sensitivity
	Available in many centres	Only advance bone disease could be detected
	Validated technique	Reduced for the differential diagnosis between malignant and benign fractures
		Difficulty to assess certain areas
		Lack of detection of lytic lesions response to the treatment
		Dependent on the observer
		Imaging process is long and not well tolerable for patients
Whole-body low-dose computed tomography	A higher diagnostic sensitivity for the detection of osteolytic bone lesions	More expensive then whole-body skeletal survey
	Higher-quality images for planning biopsies and therapeutic interventions	Approach is available in some centres
	A low radiation dose compared with standard CT	Reduced for the differential diagnosis between malignant and benign fractures
	Superiority in estimating fracture risk and bone instability	Unclear prognostic significance
	Shorter duration of the examination	
Magnetic resonance imaging	A high sensitivity for the early detection of marrow infiltration by myeloma cells	High cost
	More sensitive in detecting multiple bone lesions and exclude asymptomatic myeloma	Imaging process is long and not well tolerable for patients
	The ability to detect spinal cord or nerve compression and the presence of soft-tissue masses	Unsuitable for patients with metal objects, contrast contraindicated
	Higher-quality images for planning biopsies and therapeutic interventions	
	Valuable for differential diagnosis between malignant and benign fractures	
	Prognostic significance	
	No radiation exposure	
Positron emission tomography/ computed tomography	A higher accuracy approach for the early detection of lesions and exclude asymptomatic myeloma	High cost
	Useful to evaluate disease activity before and after treatment	Lack of availability in many centres
	Detects osseous and extramedullary disease	Limited by false-positive results of inflammation
	A better definition of complete response and minimal residual disease	Lack of standardisation
	Prognostic significance	

Table 1. A summary of different imaging techniques for multiple myeloma patients.

whole-body X-ray was the standard of care for many years, it has several limitations: for a lytic lesion to become apparent, more than 30% loss of trabecular bone must occur; it is difficult to assess certain areas, such as the pelvis and the spine; there are limitations: the detection of lytic lesion response to anti-myeloma therapy because of a delayed evidence of healing; specificity is reduced for the differential diagnosis of myeloma-related fracture and benign fracture (very important, particularly in cases of new vertebral compression fractures in the absence of other criteria of relapse); it is dependent on the observer, and studies are long and often not tolerable for patients in severe pain [19].

2.2. Whole-body low-dose computed tomography

Whole-body LDCT allows the detection of osteolytic bone lesions in the whole skeleton with a greater sensitivity and a low radiation dose compared with standard CT. Advantages of whole-body LDCT over conventional skeletal survey include a higher diagnostic sensitivity for the detection of osteolytic lesions, especially in areas where the whole-body X-ray detection rate is low (i.e. pelvis and spine); superiority in estimating fracture risk and bone instability; shorter duration of the examination, which is an important issue for patients in pain; the production of higher-quality images for planning biopsies and therapeutic interventions; and the demonstration of unsuspected manifestations of myeloma or other diseases [19]. Major deficiencies of whole-body LDCT are the lack of specificity for the differential diagnosis between malignant and osteoporotic fractures and also the fact that this diagnostic approach is available in some centres only. In several studies, whole-body LDCT was found to be superior to whole-body X-ray for the detection of osteolytic lesions [19]. In one retrospective study, the total number of bone lesions detected by whole-body LDCT was 968 and the number of bone lesions detected by whole-body X-ray was only 248 ($p < .001$), which means that 61% of patients with normal whole-body skeleton X-ray images had more than one osteolytic bone lesion on the whole-body LDCT scan, and such patients should receive antimyeloma therapy [20]. This was confirmed by another prospective study, where whole-body LDCT revealed osteolytic bone lesions in 23% of patients with negative conventional radiographic skeletal X-ray scans, especially in the axial skeleton ($p < .001$) [21]. The same study proved that whole-body LDCT is superior in detecting lesions in patients with osteopaenia and osteoporosis [21].

2.3. Magnetic resonance imaging

MRI has been established as a valuable technique for imaging multiple myeloma because of its superior soft-tissue contrast resolution. MRI has a high sensitivity for the early detection of marrow infiltration by myeloma cells. Five MRI patterns of marrow involvement have been recognised in multiple myeloma: a focal pattern that consists of localised areas of myeloma cell infiltration of 5 mm or greater in diameter, a diffuse pattern characterised by an almost complete replacement of normal marrow by myeloma cells, a combined diffuse and focal pattern, a normal bone marrow pattern and a variegated or "salt and pepper" pattern with innumerable small bone marrow focal lesions [19].

Several studies showed that MRI is generally more sensitive in detecting multiple lesions compared to conventional radiographic skeletal survey. The systematic review of studies compared modern and conventional imaging techniques in the detection of bone lesions and confirmed the superiority of MRI over conventional skeletal X-ray, mainly in the axial skeleton [22].

Because of its high sensitivity in revealing bone marrow involvement, MRI is now used for the discrimination between smouldering and symptomatic multiple myeloma. Several studies have shown that approximately 40–50% of patients with normal whole-body X-ray scan had abnormal findings on MRI examinations [19].

MRI has the ability to detect spinal cord or nerve compression and the presence of soft-tissue masses and is recommended in patients with extraosseous lesions. MRI is the approach to define the degree of involvement and to evaluate for cord compression for surgical intervention or radiation therapy. Unfortunately, almost any skeletal tumour has the same signal-intensity profile as multiple myeloma. MRI is not disease-specific, and additional tests should be used to establish the diagnosis of multiple myeloma. MRI is also recommended for patients with a solitary bone plasmacytoma. MRI may demonstrate unsuspected bone lesions, and for such patients, systemic treatment must be given instead of radiation therapy, which is the treatment of choice for solitary bone plasmacytoma.

MRI also can provide important information for prognosis. Patients with diffuse MRI pattern experienced a poorer overall survival (OS) compared with patients with focal or normal patterns [19]. One study of 611 multiple myeloma patients showed that the presence of more than seven focal lesions was an independent predictor of poorer prognosis and that resolution of all focal lesions was an indicator of superior survival [23].

The major advantage of MRI over the whole-body LDCT or conventional CT is the discrimination between myelomatous and normal marrow. This is extremely helpful to differentiate myeloma from osteoporotic fractures in more than 90% of cases [19].

2.4. Positron emission tomography/computed tomography

PET/CT is a new imaging technique, which can be applied in the diagnosis, stage and prognosis of tumour and to evaluate the efficacy of the treatment. PET/CT provides information about the sites and number of lesions, hypermetabolic activity of the involved area (depending on F-18 fluorodeoxyglucose (FDG) uptake). Furthermore, PET/CT detects osseous and extramedullary disease in patients at diagnosis and relapse. PET/CT is a higher accuracy approach than traditional imaging techniques in the diagnosis of multiple myeloma. However, there is no uniform conclusion about the diagnostic accuracy of PET/CT for multiple myeloma because of the controversy on the variety of results.

The large meta-analysis has shown that PET/CT is more sensitive compared with conventional skeletal X-ray for the detection of bone lesions in multiple myeloma [22]. The higher detection rate of PET/CT over conventional skeletal X-ray scan for the presence of osteolytic lesions is especially important for patients with smouldering multiple myeloma. In the studies related to smouldering multiple myeloma, 16–39% of patients with normal whole-body X-ray had positive PET/CT results [19]. The probability of progression to symptomatic multiple myeloma within 2 years was 58–75% for patients with a positive PET/CT [19].

PET/CT may be used for the diagnosis of solitary bone plasmacytoma and extramedullary disease. It is not clear whether PET/CT or MRI is more preferable. PET/CT also has a value for patients with nonsecretory or oligosecretory MM for the detection of active lesions.

PET/CT has been tested for a better definition of complete response (CR) to MM therapy and as an independent factor for survival prognosis at diagnosis and after treatment. Approximately 30% of patients at CR had a positive PET/CT. In addition, PET/CT negativity was an independent predicted factor for prolonged PFS and OS in patients with a CR, patients with a positive PET/CT in CR and median PFS was 50 months compared to 90 months for patients with a negative PET/CT [24].

However, PET/CT remains a high-cost method, and there is lack of availability in many centres and may be limited by false-positive results caused by inflammation from other underlying diseases.

3. Radiotherapy for solitary plasmacytomas

The solitary plasmacytoma is a localised accumulation of monoclonal plasma cells without systemic plasma cell disease manifestation. Regarding location, it can be classified into solitary plasmacytoma of bone (SBP) and extramedullary plasmacytoma (EMP) [25]. SBP generally occurs in the vertebra and skull; however, EMP is most frequently observed in head and neck [25]. Plasmacytomas are radiosensitive neoplasms, and radiotherapy has a potentially curative effect for both SBP and EMP [4].

3.1. Radiotherapy for solitary plasmacytoma of bone

Radiotherapy with a curative intent is the treatment of choice, resulting in local control in more than 80% of patients with SBP [25, 26]. In some cases, as bone instability, rapid progression of neurological symptoms and surgical intervention are required, the results of surgery alone are not optimal and carry high rates of local relapse [27]. Currently, the standard of treatment for SBP is radiotherapy. Optimal-dosing guidelines have not been established due to the absence of prospective randomised studies. The United Kingdom Myeloma Forum recommend radiotherapy at least 40 Gy in 20 fractions [28]. For bulky disease (>5 cm), a higher-dose 50 Gy in 25 fractions was recommended [28]. Approximately 30% of patients who received higher doses than 50 Gy remained without evidence of any local disease failures [25]. In clinical practice, a radiation dose of 45–50 Gy in 20–25 fractions is recommended for the treatment of SBP.

The optimal target volume for radiotherapy planning in SBP is to encompass the tumour volume plus a margin of at least 1.5–2 cm on the tumour detectable by MRI [25, 26]. In case of vertebral involvement, fields typically include one to two uninvolved vertebrae above and below the affected level [25]. Prophylactic regional lymph node irradiation is not necessary in SBP.

3.2. Radiotherapy for extramedullary plasmacytoma

Like SBP, EMPs are highly radiosensitive; almost all patients (80–100%) achieve local control, and approximately 50–65% of patients remain free of disease longer than 10 years [26]. Due to a lesser number of patients and the absence of randomised prospective studies, the optimal dose of radiotherapy is not established. Current evidence-based recommendations by the United Kingdom Myeloma forum are similar to those for SBP [28]. The recommendations include radiotherapy dose of 40 Gy in 20 fractions for tumours of <5 cm and up to 50 Gy in 25 fractions for tumours of ≥5 cm with at least a 2-cm margin encompassing the primary tumour [28]. If cervical nodes are involved (or in Waldeyer's ring tumours), these should be included in the radiotherapy field [28].

Surgery may be an acceptable treatment method combined with radiotherapy. A combination of a higher dose of radiation and surgery predicted for better PFS [25]. Surgical procedures of the head and neck are not recommended, but surgery may be considered for other sites of the disease [26].

4. Indications for radiotherapy in multiple myeloma

Radiotherapy can produce a curative effect for both solitary plasmacytoma of bone and extramedullary plasmacytomas; however, its role in the treatment of MM patients is only palliative. The most common indications for radiotherapy in MM are pain relief in the sites of bone destructions, the prevention of pathological fractures or to decrease the pain in the fracture site, to evoke the recalcification, the management of spinal cord compression syndrome and the treatment of extramedullary disease.

4.1. Palliation for pain

Pain is the most common symptom experienced by MM patients. Up to 67% of patients report pain at diagnosis, and it may be present for several months before the diagnosis [29]. Local radiotherapy is effective for pain relief. It produces an analgesic effect by inhibiting chemical pain mediators and causing tumour shrinkage. There is a debate on the effect of radiation dose on pain relief.

Results of randomised clinical studies revealed the same effect of pain relief when applying two different radiotherapy regimens (8 Gy/1 fr and 3 Gy × 10 fr) for the treatment of patients with solid tumour metastases, though the application of a single fraction of 8 Gy treatment produces more recurrent treatment episodes [30–33]. The earlier data, however, cannot be directly applied in the treatment of patients with MM, since their future prospects are better (the average survival reaches 30–40 months), whereas the average survival among the patients with solid tumour metastases in bones is about 9 months [5]. In the meta-analyses by Sze et al. [34] and Wu et al. [35], no significant difference in the overall and complete response in pain reduction between single- (SF) and multiple-fraction (MF) palliative radiotherapy was observed. Chow et al. in the systematic review analysed 16 randomised trials comparing SF versus MF for bone metastases: no significant difference was found regarding response rates [30]. An increased risk for pathological fractures and spinal cord compressions was observed in the SF regimen, which was statistically insignificant, while retreatment in the SF regimen was 2.5-fold higher [30]. The role of different palliative radiotherapy regimens for MM is not well established due to lack of clinical trials. Medical literature provides only a small number of studies dealing with various radiotherapy regimens for the treatment of patients with multiple myeloma as well as impact of the radiotherapy regimen on pain relief at the sites of bone destructions [5–12]. However, final recommendations concerning the choice of the radiation therapy regime have not been presented yet.

Some clinical studies did not find a significant difference between the radiation dose and pain relief after radiotherapy [5, 8, 10, 12]; however, Adamietz et al. [6] and Minova et al. [11] reported that for adequate pain relief, higher doses would be obtained. Pain relief occurred in 80–92% [6, 11]. Adamietz et al. affirmed that local long-term palliation effect can only be achieved by a high radiation dose [6], whereas Leigh et al. analysed 101 patients and observed pain reduction in 97% of patients (complete in 26%) with a median dose 3–60 Gy. Only 6% of patients were retreated for the relapse which occurred after a median interval of 16 months [10]. This study showed the durable symptom relief after a mean total dose of 10 Gy [10].

Clinical, laboratory and genetic factors may influence pain perception and analgesic effects of radiotherapy. Retrospective studies published by Adamietz et al. [6] and Mose et al. [12] indicated that the incidence of pain relief was higher in patients treated with concurrent chemotherapy which had a significant impact on a positive response to radiotherapy, but other studies did not show this relationship [5, 10]. Mose et al. reported that not only concurrent chemotherapy but also the Karnofsky performance above 70% had a significant impact on a positive analgesic response to radiation treatment, whereas the total radiation dose, gender, age, irradiated site and bisphosphonates had no effect on pain relief [12]. In other study performed by Stolting et al., significant parameters for pain relief in the multivariate analysis were completeness of therapy, patients younger than 60 years and a single dose of 2 Gy; other parameters like Karnofsky index, concurrent chemotherapy and total dose were insignificant [5].

Medical literature provides several studies which have revealed that the polymorphism of inflammatory cytokine genes influences pain perception and analgesics dose. Furthermore, the altered levels of fatigue, depression and response to analgesics in pancreatic, lung or breast cancer have been described [15, 36–43]. These types of studies, however, have not been conducted for patients with multiple myeloma, though during the formation of bone destructions, anti-inflammatory cytokines are emitted by plasma cells and bone marrow stroma cells. No study has been performed worldwide, which would deal with the impact of polymorphism of genes encoding for cytokines in response to radiotherapy.

Hundred and one patients were involved in a randomised prospective clinical study performed at the Lithuanian University of Health Sciences [44]. Two different radiation treatment regimens of bone destructions due to multiple myeloma were compared. MF radiotherapy regime (3 Gy × 10 fr) was applied to 58 patients and SF (8 Gy × 1 fr) regime was applied to 43 patients. Pain relief was obtained in 84.5% of patients in MF regimen group (complete response 69.4%) and 74.4% of patients in SF regimen group (complete response 68.8%). No significant differences were observed in analgesic response between the groups. No significant differences were observed in the period of time before reaching the analgesic effect of radiotherapy: in both groups, analgesic effect was achieved in the first 4 weeks.

Univariate statistical analysis revealed that the age under 65 years ($p = 0.016$), stage II of the disease (according to Durie-Salmon classification) ($p = 0.03$) and recalcification in the irradiated site ($p = 0.011$) were significant parameters for analgesic response after radiotherapy, whereas other parameters (gender, Karnofsky index, paraprotein type, haemoglobin level, surgery, pain score at the admission, total radiation dose, bisphosphonates and concurrent chemotherapy) were not significant.

All parameters mentioned earlier were included in binary logistic regression model for the analysis of their influence to pain relief. Using a stepwise variable removal method (backward conditional), it was found that the following attributes have a significant impact on analgesic response after radiation treatment for pain relief: female gender, age under 65, IgG MM type and the presence of recalcification in the irradiated site. Other factors analysed, including the total radiation dose, were not significant for pain relief after radiation treatment. Results of analgesic response from clinical trials of palliative radiotherapy in the treatment of MM patients are shown in **Table 2**.

The study performed by Rudzianskiene et al. involved analysis of 12 gene polymorphisms of six cytokines (IL-6, IL-10, TNFα, IL-1α, IL-1β and IL-1RA) participating in the pathogenesis of the pain syndrome in bone destruction sites. The aim was to evaluate the influence of interleukins on the perception of pain and response to radiotherapy in MM patients [44].

Univariate statistical analysis was used to assess associations between severe pain status (8–10 points on VAS) before radiation treatment and genotype groups of each cytokine gene studied. None of the genotypes analysed was found to be significant for the perception of severe pain before treatment; yet, a marginal relation was observed that patients with GG genotype of IL1RN c.1812G > A polymorphism more often indicated severe pain before radiotherapy, compared to patients with GA and AA genotypes (relative risk (RR) 0.43; 95% confidence interval (CI) 0.18–1.06; $p = 0.068$) [44].

Multivariate logistic analysis included all the earlier clinical, demographic and symptom factors, as well as genotype groups of each cytokine gene analysed. Based on multivariate logistic regression, the following factors were determined to have a significant impact on severe pain before radiation treatment: Karnofsky index ≥60% and IL1RN c.1812G > A polymorphism GG genotype. Other factors analysed were not significant for the perception of severe pain before radiation treatment [44].

A comparison of a decrease in pain perception points before radiotherapy and during the monitored period, that is, after 4, 12 and 24 weeks, among patients with different genotypes was carried out. The analysis revealed that patients with IL-1α-encoding gene IL1A c.889C > T CC genotype had a significantly better response to radiation therapy and indicated milder pain after 12 and 24 weeks, compared to patients with TT and CT genotypes. Furthermore, patients with IL-1β-encoding gene IL1B c. 3953C > T CC genotype indicated significantly more often milder pain scores after radiotherapy in 12 and 24 weeks, compared to patients with TT and CT genotypes. Patients with IL-1RA-encoding gene IL1RN c.11100 T > C CC genotype had a faster response to radiation therapy, that is, a significant decrease in pain points was observed after 4 weeks, compared to patients with TT and CT genotypes [44].

Clinical study	Number of patients	Number of irradiated sites	Total dose (Gy)	Overall response (%)	Complete response (%)	Comments
Adamietz et al. [6]	70	70	2–30	39.6–80*	n/a	Local long-term palliation effect can only be achieved by high radiation dose and concurrent chemotherapy.
Leigh et al. [10]	101	306	3–60	91	n/a	There was no significance difference between analgesic response and higher radiation dose, and there was no influence of concurrent chemotherapy.
Mose et al. [12]	42	71	18–45	85	34.3	There was no significance difference between analgesic response and higher radiation dose, response is better with concurrent chemotherapy.
Yaneva et al. [9]	87	87	17–20	89.6	26.9	The total dose relationship with an analgesic response has not been evaluated. Radiotherapy has no influence on overall survival.
Stolting et al. [5]	138	272	2–60	85.3	22.2	There was no significance difference between analgesic response and higher radiation dose, and there was no influence of concurrent chemotherapy.
Minowa et al. [11]	29	53	4–60	92	n/a	Longer analgesic response was after higher radiation dose treatment.
Balducci et al. [7]	52	52	16–50	91	51.2	The total dose and concurrent chemotherapy relationship with an analgesic response has not been evaluated.
Rudzianskiene et al. [44]	101	101	8 Gy vs. 30 Gy	74.4 vs. 84.5	68.8 vs. 69.4	There was no significant difference between analgesic response and higher radiation dose, and there was no influence of concurrent chemotherapy.

*Without concurrent chemotherapy.

Table 2. A summary of published data on palliative radiotherapy analgesic response in the treatment of patients with MM.

4.2. To evoke the recalcification

Multiple myeloma is a disease inducing osteolytic process which leads to an increased risk of pathologic fracture or spinal cord compression and severe pain with a negative impact on the quality of life. According to the study, recalcification is achieved after some months and occurs in 40–50% of the irradiated bone destructions in patients with multiple myeloma [5, 7, 12, 13]. Palliative radiotherapy can be applied to avoid the impending or actual pathological fracture. However, the high-risk lesions should be first stabilised by orthopaedic measures and combined with post-operative radiation treatment for the improvement of pain and local control. Several retrospective studies, a majority of which included small patients' cohorts, have demonstrated that there is no relation between the total radiation dose and recalcification in the sites of bone destructions.

Mose et al. found that the stabilisation of the irradiated bone could be achieved in 46.4% of cases, and concurrent chemotherapy reinforces this effect [12]. Also, Stolting et al. reported a recalcification rate of 44.7% and the importance of concurrent chemotherapy for recalcification [5]. The study performed by Rudzianskiene et al. showed an overall response of recalcification with single-fraction radiotherapy of 35.9%, and in multi-fraction radiotherapy group, the response rate was 32.1% [44]. Binary logistic regression did not show a significant impact of concurrent chemotherapy on recalcification [44].

Koswig and Budach [45] found that an MF regimen (3 Gy × 10) significantly increases the bone density in the area of metastases from solid tumours compared with single fraction (8 Gy) in contrast to pain relief effect; also, Stolting et al. reported that recalcification was detected at total doses of >40 Gy for MM patients [5]. Balducci et al. found recalcification in 50% cases with a median total dose of 38 Gy and reported the importance of the early using of radiotherapy to avoid pathological fractures [7]. However, the studies published by Mose et al. [12] and Rudzianskiene et al. [44] did not show any influence of the total radiation dose on recalcification.

Mose et al. reported that not only concurrent chemotherapy but also the Karnofsky index above 70% and bisphosphonates had a significant impact on a positive recalcification effect to radiation treatment [12]. Also, in a clinical study performed by Rudzianskiene et al., the Karnofsky index more than 60% has a positive impact on recalcification in the irradiated site [44]. This study also founded that a haemoglobin level of less than 80 g/l, clinical stage II according to Durie-Salmon and a decrease in pain in the irradiated site are significant parameters for the recalcification [44].

The clinical study performed by Mose et al. showed that higher recalcification rates depend on the usage of bisphosphonates [12], but other study did not demonstrate such a relation [5]. In the clinical study reported by Rudzianskiene et al., the use of bisphosphonates was also an insignificant parameter but this may be due to the small sample of patients (only 18%) taking bisphosphonates [44].

Results of recalcification response from clinical trials of palliative radiotherapy in the treatment of MM patients are shown in **Table 3**.

4.3. The treatment of spinal cord compression

Epidural spinal cord compression that can cause pain and neurological impairment occurs in 5–20% of all patients with multiple myeloma at various disease stages and leads to disability [46, 47]. Pain is the first and more common presenting symptom followed by motor

Clinical study	Number of patients	Number of irradiated sites	Total dose (Gy)	Overall response (%)	Comments
Stolting et al. [5]	138	272	2–60	44.7	There was no significance difference between recalcification response and higher radiation dose, usage of bisphosphonates, concurrent chemotherapy increase response of recalcification.
Balducci et al. [7]	52	52	16–50	50	The influence of total radiation dose, concurrent chemotherapy and bisphosphonates was not evaluated.
Mose et al. [12]	42	71	18–45	46.4	There was no significance difference between recalcification response and total radiation dose, concurrent chemotherapy and bisphosphonates increase response of recalcification.
Rudzianskiene et al. [44]	101	101	8 Gy vs. 30 Gy	35.9 vs. 32.1	There was no significant difference between recalcification response and higher radiation dose, usage of bisphosphonates and there was no influence of concurrent chemotherapy.

Table 3. A summary of published data on palliative radiotherapy recalcification response in the treatment of patients with MM.

deficiency, sensory symptoms and bowel and bladder dysfunction [48]. Immediate diagnosis and treatment are very important in the preservation of neurological function in patients with spinal cord compression. Pain control, relief of spinal cord compression and improvement of neurologic function are the main goals of treatment. High-dose steroids must soon be initiated upon spinal cord compression diagnosed to obtain an antineoplastic and an antioedema effect [49]. In patients with neurologic symptoms directly due to cord compression, radiation therapy is given along with dexamethasone, and up to half of patients may have improvement of motor function [50]. In the largest retrospective studies, radiotherapy alone improves motor function in 75% of patients with spinal cord compression due to MM. A 1-year local control was 100% and a 1-year survival was 94% [51].

Radiation treatment can be used as fractionated external beam radiotherapy (EBRT) or stereotactic body RT (SBRT). Both methods are effective for palliative treatment and local tumour control. SBRT is a non-invasive treatment option for spinal disease in the absence of a high-grade spinal cord compression. SBRT allows the treatment of small- or moderate-sized tumours, even in close proximity to the spinal cord, in either a single or a limited number of dose fractions [48]. SBRT with a single 24 Gy fraction gives excellent tumour control [48].

Since myeloma is a very radiosensitive tumour, EBRT is an appropriate approach for patients who are not considered surgical treatment and it is also indicated after decompression intervention. There was no randomised trial that compared radiotherapy alone to radiotherapy plus upfront neurosurgery. Thus, radiotherapy alone is considered the standard treatment of

SCC from myeloma [52]. Several fractionation regimens: single-fraction, short-course multi-fraction and longer-course multi-fraction regimens are used for the treatment of spinal cord compression. Radiotherapy either 30 Gy in 10 fractions or lower radiation doses must be provided as an optimal approach causing the long-lasting local control [50]. Several clinical studies have examined the impact of multi-fraction regimens versus single-fraction regimens on pain relief and functional outcomes, local tumour control and overall survival [12, 52–55]. Rades et al. compared short-course 8 Gy in one fraction or 20 Gy in five fraction regimens with long-course 30–40 Gy in 10–20 fraction regimens [53]. There were no significant differences in functional or overall survival between the groups. However, a better local control (77 vs. 61%) and a 12-month progression-free survival (72 vs. 55%) were significantly better in long-course radiotherapy regimen group [53]. A phase III randomised multicentre Italian trial demonstrated a similar effect in functional outcomes and overall survival between two fractions of 8 Gy (16 Gy total dose) or a single dose of 8 Gy radiotherapy in patients with spinal cord compression and a short life expectancy [54].

Multiple myeloma patients with spinal cord compression have a comparably good survival, living for years after treatment in the era of novel drugs [55]. Only very few clinical studies can be found in the study, investigating radiotherapy of spinal cord compression in MM patients [12, 52, 55], and the appropriate radiotherapy regimen for the treatment of spinal cord compression in MM patients has not been defined yet. Rades et al. reported that the improvement of motor function was more frequent after long-course radiotherapy than after short-course at 6 months (67 vs. 43%) and at 12 months (76 vs. 40%) [55]. However, Mose et al. demonstrated that 65% of patients with spinal cord compression after radiotherapy experienced neurological improvement, and Karnofsky index, gender, age, site of myelocompression and the total radiation dose did not influence this effect [12].

One retrospective study was performed to find a predictive tool that allows the estimation of overall survival (OS) of elderly myeloma patients (aged ≥65 years) presenting with myeloma-induced spinal cord compression [52]. Rades et al. found that myeloma type (HR 3.31; 95% CI 1.75–6.49; $p < 0.001$), ECOG-PS (HR 5.33; 95% CI 2.67–11.11; $p < 0.001$), ambulatory status (HR 2.71; 95% CI 1.65–4.57; $p < 0.001$) and age (HR 1.95; 95% CI 1.03–3.78; $p = 0.040$) were significantly associated with survival, but fractionation regimen was not a predictive tool for OS [52].

The choice of radiotherapy regimen in the treatment of spinal cord compression should be based on the expectancy of patient's life. Longer-course programs, which result in a better local control than single-fraction and short-course programs, are the preferred treatment for patients with a more favourable survival prognosis. By contrast, patients with a poor prognosis are better candidates for multi-fraction short-course or single-fraction radiotherapy [52].

5. Surgery and radiation treatment

Surgical management of MM-related bone lesions sometimes is carried out due to disease sensitivity of radiation treatment and chemotherapy. The most common indications for surgical procedures are unstable fractures and spinal cord compression when bone fragments protrude from a vertebral fracture [49]. Vertebroplasty and kyphoplasty are carried out by fibroscopic percutaneous injection of polymethylmethacrylate into the fractured vertebrae in order to relieve pain. These procedures should be considered for symptomatic vertebral compression fractures, and this is a procedure of choice to improve the quality of life [3]. Vertebroplasty combined with post-operative radiotherapy is an effective approach in the pain palliation, maintaining the stability of vertebral column and improving the quality of life of patients. Some randomised clinical studies demonstrated that surgery and post-operative radiotherapy are more effective in the treatment of vertebral fractures than radiotherapy alone [56, 57]. Treating these patients with radiotherapy before surgery procedure allows for tumour shrinkage and can enable these patients to become candidates for vertebroplasty [58]. The study performed by Hirsch et al. reported that the timing of radiotherapy, before or after vertebroplasty, did not significantly impact outcomes of these procedures [58].

6. Side effects

Radiotherapy is generally well tolerated. The external beam localised fields' radiotherapy offers advantage of few acute and late toxicities. The potential side effects of radiotherapy are related to the fraction dose, total radiation dose, volume of the target, toxicities from other treatment approaches and the radiosensitivity of healthy surrounding tissues. The radiotherapy planning process uses established tolerance doses to avoid irreversible damage of critical organs, such as the lung, kidney, liver and spinal cord. Organ tolerances are based on the conventional radiotherapy (1.8–2 Gy per fraction daily, five times a week). When unconventional

Acute side effects	
	Clinical manifestation
Systemic side effects	Fatigue, anorexia, nausea/vomiting
Skin	Erythema, itching, dry desquamation, blister formation, hair loss in the treatment area
Mouth, oesophagus	Sore throat, dry mouth, trouble swallowing, taste loss
Small/large intestine	Loose stools/diarrhoea, cramps, bleeding, incontinence, rectal irritation
Haematologic	Neutropaenia, anaemia, thrombocytopaenia
Bladder	Bladder spasms, cystitis, urinary frequency, incontinence, haematuria
Late side effects	
Skin	Telangiectasia, atrophy, ulceration, pigmentation changes
Mouth, oesophagus	Xerostomia, sialitis, difficulty in swallowing, ulceration, trismus, osteoradionecrosis, fistula
Small/large intestine	Diarrhoea, cramping/colic, bowel movement, obstruction, bleeding, fistula, necrosis
Bladder	Haematuria, epithelial atrophy, reduction in bladder capacity

Table 4. A summary of most common side effects of radiation treatment.

fractionation regimens are introduced, the total radiation dose must be adjusted to avoid high risk of side effects, as lower total doses limit acute toxicity. In general, palliative radiotherapy doses are delivered with a larger dose per fraction. These hypofractionated regimens may provide the benefit of earlier response but with a greater risk of late side effects [59]. Late side effects occur from months to years after radiation treatment, and patients with a short life expectancy may not live long enough to experience such risks.

Side effects of radiation are generally mild, limited to the radiotherapy site and can be predicted. Most acute side effects arising within 90 days are self-limited, lasting days to weeks and resolve within few weeks with supportive care. Acute toxicities as fatigue, nausea/vomiting, mucositis, oesophagitis and bowel irritation are often easily managed and reversible. The more critical side effects are late side effects, emergent from cellular and vascular atrophy, and lead to the reduction of normal tissue function and organ dysfunction, which may develop months to years later, but they are very rare.

In 1982, the Radiation Therapy Oncology Group (RTOG) developed the Radiation Morbidity Scoring Criteria to classify radiotherapy effects. RTOG score has been widely employed and is accepted and acknowledged by medical communities [60].

Skin reactions are usually nominal during radiation treatment for bone metastases and are treated similar to burns. Patients treated with large volumes including pelvis, epigastrium or thoracolumbar spine region may experience nausea and/or vomiting. Prophylactic antiemetics can be administered 30–60 min prior to radiotherapy and continued on as needed. Hematologic side effects are mild and transient, but bone marrow suppression may occur if the patients are receiving treatment to large targets, when the total radiation dose is moderate or high, and a significant proportion of marrow is included, especially in heavily pretreated patients. Mucositis and oesophagitis causing difficult and painful swallowing occur after treatment to the head and neck or thorax. It should be treated with dietary modifications, oral rinses, antifungals, analgesics and cytoprotective agents. Radiation enteritis manifested by cramping; frequent, loose stools and occasionally bleeding may occur if large amounts of small intestine are included. Treating the pelvis may also result in short-lived diarrhoea [61]. A summary of clinical manifestations of the most common side effects of radiation treatment is shown in **Table 4**.

No significant differences were observed between SF and MF radiotherapy for bone metastases of solid tumours in the systematic review performed by Chow et al. [30]. Only two studies reported more acute toxicities (characterised as grades 2–4) in the group of MF regimens than in SF [30].

Based on the analysis of medical literature, the side effects of radiotherapy in multiple myeloma patients were generally mild. Balducci et al. [7] identified 44% of patients (n = 23) with side effects (grades 1–2): haematological toxicity in 48%, gastroenteric toxicity in 26%, pharyngeal toxicity in 9% and cutaneous toxicity in 17% patients. Mose et al. [12] reported about 54% side effects mostly of grades 1–2; grade 3 in 4% (haematological side effects, mucositis, creatinine level). These data correspond with Matuschek et al. [62] as this study reported 37% side effects with 50% grade 1 and 47.2% grade 2 and one patient grade 3 dysphagia.

7. Conclusions

Radiotherapy continues to be an effective palliative treatment approach in the management of bone disease in MM patients inducing an analgesic effect in osteolytic lesions, promoting recalcification in the sites of impending pathological fractures and controlling the symptoms in spinal cord compression without significant toxicity. No difference in the efficacy for pain relief and recalcification has been observed using different radiotherapy regimens. However, the choice of radiotherapy regimen in the treatment of spinal cord compression should be based on the expectancy of patient's survival. Multi-fraction regimens, which result in a better local control, are the preferred treatment for patients with a more favourable survival prognosis.

Conflict of interest

M. Rudzianskiene, V. Rudzianskas, R. Dambrauskiene and R. Gerbutavicius declare that they have no competing interests.

Author details

Milda Rudzianskiene*, Viktoras Rudzianskas, Ruta Dambrauskiene and Rolandas Gerbutavicius

*Address all correspondence to: milda.rudzianskiene@gmail.com

Oncology Institute of Lithuanian University of Health Sciences, Kaunas, Lithuania

References

[1] Raab MS, Podar K, Breitkreutz I, Richardson PG, Anderson KC. Multiple myeloma. Lancet. 2009;**374**:324-339

[2] Raje N, Roodman GD. Advances in the biology and treatment of bone disease in mutiple myeloma. Clinical Cancer Research. 2011;**17**:1278-1286

[3] Terpos E, Morgan G, Dimopoulos MA, Drake MT, Lentzsch S, et al. International myeloma working group recommendations for the treatment of multiple myeloma – Related bone disease. Journal of Clinical Oncology. 2013;**31**:2347-2357

[4] Talamo G, Dimaio C, Abbi KK, Pandey MK, Malysz J, et al. Current role of radiation therapy for multiple myeloma. Frontiers in Oncology. 2015;**5**:40

[5] Stolting T, Knauerhase H, Klautke G, Kundt G, Fietkau R. Total and single doses influence the effectiveness of radiotherapy in palliative treatment of plasmocytoma. Strahlentherapie Oncology. 2008;**184**:465-472

[6] Adamietz IA, Schober C, Schulte RW, Peest D, Renner K. Palliative radiotherapy in plasma cell myeloma. Radiotherapy and Oncology. 1991;**20**:111-116

[7] Balducci M, Chiesa S, Manfrida S, Rossi E, Za T, et al. Impact of radiotherapy on pain relief and recalcification in plasma cell neoplasms: Long-term experience. Strahlentherapie und Onkologie. 2011;**187**:114-119

[8] Bosch A, Frias Z. Radiotherapy in the treatment of the multiple myeloma. International Journal of Radiation Oncology, Biology, Physics. 1988;**15**:1363-1369

[9] Yaneva MP, Goranova-Marinova V, St G. Palliative radiotherapy in patients with multiple myeloma. Journal of BUON. 2006;**11**:43-48

[10] Leigh BR, Kurtts TA, Mack CF, Matzner MB, Shimm DS. Radiation therapy for the palliation of multiple myeloma. International Journal of Radiation Oncology, Biology, Physics. 1993;**801-4**(25):25

[11] Minowa Y, Sasai K, Ishigaki T, Nagata Y, Hiraoka M. Palliative radiation therapy for multiple myeloma. Nihon Igaku Hōshasen Gakkai Zasshi. 1996;**56**:1056-1060

[12] Mose S, Pfitzner D, Rahn A, Nierhoff C, Schiemann M, et al. Role of radiotherapy in the treatment of multiple myeloma. Strahlenther. Oncologia. 2000;**176**:506-512

[13] Manfrida S, Chiesa S, Rossi E et al. Impact of radiotherapy on pain relief and recalcification in patients affected by plasma cell neoplasms: a long term experience. Journal of Clinical Oncology. 2010;**28**(suppl): abstr e18558

[14] Lee BN, Dantzer R, Langley KE, Bennett GJ, Dougherty PM, et al. A cytokine-based neuroimmunologic mechanism of cancer-related symptoms. Neuroimmunomodulation. 2004; **11**:279-292

[15] Reyes-Gibby CC, Wang J, Spitz M, Wu X, Yennurajalingam S, et al. Genetic variations in interleukin-8 and interleukin-10 are associated with pain, depressed mood, and fatigue in lung cancer patients. Journal of Pain and Symptom Management. 2013;**46**:161-172

[16] Reyes-Gibby CC, Wu X, Spitz M, Kurzrock R, Fisch M, et al. Molecular epidemiology, cancer-related symptoms, and cytokines pathway. The Lancet Oncology. 2008;**9**:777-785

[17] Terpos E, Berenson J, Raje N, Roodman GD. Management of bone disease in multiple myeloma. Expert Review of Hematology. 2014;**7**(1):113-125

[18] Rajkumar SV, Dimopoulos MA, Palumbo A, Blade J, Merlini G, et al. International myeloma working group updated criteria for the diagnosis of multiple myeloma. The Lancet Oncology. 2014;**15**(12):e538-e548

[19] Terpos E, Dimopoulos MA, Moulopoulos LA. The role of imaging in the treatment of patients with multiple myeloma in 2016. American Society of Clinical Oncology Educational Book. 2016;**35**:e407-e417

[20] Princewill K, Kyere S, Awan O, Mulligan M. Multiple myeloma lesion detection with whole body CT versus radiographic skeletal survey. Cancer Investigation. 2013;**31**(3): 206-211

[21] Wolf MB, Murray F, Kilk K, Hillengass J, Delorme S, et al. Sensitivity of whole-body CT and MRI versus projection radiography in the detection of osteolyses in patients with monoclonal plasma cell disease. European Journal of Radiology. 2014;**83**(7):1222-1230

[22] Regelink JC, Minnema MC, Terpos E, Kamphuis MH, Raijmakers PG, et al. Comparison of modern and conventional imaging techniques in establishing multiple myeloma-related bone disease: A systematic review. British Journal of Haematology. 2013;**162**(1):50-61

[23] Walker R, Barlogie B, Haessler J, Tricot G, Anaissie E, et al. Magnetic resonance imaging in multiple myeloma: diagnostic and clinical implications. Journal of Clinical Oncology. 2007;**25**(9):1121-1128

[24] Zamagni E, Nanni C, Mancuso K, Tacchetti P, Pezzi A, et al. PET/CT improves the definition of complete response and allows to detect otherwise unidentifiable skeletal progression in multiple myeloma. Clinical Cancer Research. 2015;**21**(19):4384-4390

[25] Kilciksiz S, Karakoyun-Celik O, Agaoglu FY, Haydaroglu A. A review for solitary plasmacytoma of bone and extramedullary plasmacytoma. ScientificWorldJournal. 2012;**2012**: 895765

[26] Weber DM. Solitary bone and extramedullary plasmacytoma. Hematology. American Society of Hematology. Education Program. 2005:373-376

[27] Ozsahin M, Tsang RW, Poortmans P, Belkacémi Y, Bolla M, et al. Outcomes and patterns of failure in solitary plasmacytoma: A multicenter rare cancer network study of 258 patients. International Journal of Radiation Oncology, Biology, Physics. 2006;**64**(1): 210-217

[28] Soutar R, Lucraft H, Jackson G, Reece A, Bird J et al. Guidelines on the diagnosis and management of solitary plasmacytoma of bone and solitary extramedullary plasmacytoma. British Journal of Haematology. 2004;**124**(6):717-726

[29] Snowden JA, Ahmedzai SH, Ashcroft J, D'Sa S, Littlewood T, et al. Guidelines for supportive care in multiple myeloma 2011. British Journal of Haematology. 2011;**154**(1):76-103

[30] Chow E, Harris K, Fan G, Tsao M, Sze WM. Palliative radiotherapy trials for bone metastases: A systematic review. Journal of Clinical Oncology. 2007;**25**:1423-1436

[31] Foro Arnalot P, Fontanals AV, Galcerán JC, Lynd F, Latiesas XS, et al. Randomized clinical trial with two palliative radiotherapy regimens in painful bone metastases: 30 Gy in 10 fractions compared with 8 Gy in single fraction. Radiotherapy and Oncology. 2008;**89**:150-155

[32] Sande TA, Ruenes R, Lund JA, Bruland OS, Hornslien K, et al. Long-term follow-up of cancer patients receiving radiotherapy for bone metastases: Results from a randomised multicentre trial. Radiotherapy and Oncology. 2009;**91**:261-266

[33] Vairaktaris E, Yapijakis C, Serefoglou Z, Derka S, Vassiliou S, et al. The interleukin-10 (−1082A/G) polyorphism is strongly associated with increase risk for oral squamous cell carcinoma. Anticancer Research. 2008;**28**:309-314

[34] Sze WM, Shelley MD, Held I, Wilt TJ, Mason MD. Palliation of metastatic bone pain: Single fraction versus multifraction radiotherapy--a systematic review of randomized trials. Clinical Oncology. 2003;**15**:345-352

[35] Wu JS, Wong R, Johnston M, Bezjak A, Whelan T, et al. Meta-analysis of dose-fractionation radiotherapy trials for the palliation of painful bone metastases. International Journal of Radiation Oncology, Biology, Physics. 2003;**55**:594-605

[36] Illi J, Miaskowski C, Cooper B, Levine JD, Dunn L, et al. Association between pro- and anti- inflammatory cytokine genes and a symptom cluster of pain, fatigue, sleep disturbance, and depression. Cytokine. 2012;**58**:437-447

[37] McCann B, Miaskowski C, Koetters T, Baggott C, West C, et al. Associations between pro- and anti- inflammatory cytokine genes and breast pain in women prior to breast cancer surgery. The Journal of Pain. 2012;**13**:425-437

[38] Rausch SM, Clark MM, Ch P, Liu H, Felten S, et al. Relationship between cytokine gene single nucleotide polymorphism and symptom burden and quality of lifeinlungcancer-survivors. Cancer. 2010;**116**:4103-4113

[39] Reyes-Gibby CC, ElOsta B, Spitz MR, Parsons H, Kurzrock R, et al. The influence of tumor necrosis factor-alpha −308 G/a and IL-6 -174 G/C on pain and analgesia response in lung cancer patients receiving supportive care. Cancer Epidemiology, Biomarkers & Prevention. 2008;**17**:3262-3267

[40] Reyes-Gibby CC, Shete S, Yennurajalingam S, Frazier M, Bruera E, et al. Genetic and non genetic covariates of pain severity in patients with adenocarcinoma of the pancreas: Assess ing the influence of cytokine genes. Journal of Pain and Symptom Management. 2009;**38**:894-902

[41] Reyes-Gibby CC, Spitz M, Wu X, Merriman K, Etzel C, et al. Cytokine genes and pain severity in lung cancer: Exploring the influence of TNF–alpha-308 G/a IL6-174G/C and IL8-251T/a. Cancer Epidemiology, Biomarkers & Prevention. 2007;**16**:2745-2751

[42] Reyes-Gibby CC, Spitz MR, Yennurajalingam S, Swartz M, Gu J, et al. Role of inflammation gene polymorphisms on pain severity in lung cancer patients. Cancer Epidemiology, Biomarkers & Prevention. 2009;**18**:2636-2642

[43] Světlík S, Hronová K, Bakhouche H, Matoušková O, Slanař O. Pharmaco genetics of chronic pain and its treatment. Mediators of Inflammation. 2013;**2013**:864319

[44] Rudzianskiene M, Inciura A, Gerbutavicius R, Rudzianskas V, Macas A, et al. Single vs. multiple fraction regimens for palliative radiotherapy treatment of multiple myeloma: A prospective randomised study. Strahlentherapie und Onkologie. 2017;**193**(9):742-749

[45] Koswig S, Budach V. Remineralization and pain relief in bone metastases after after different radiotherapy fractions (10 times 3 Gy vs. 1 time 8 Gy). A prospective study. Strahlentherapie und Onkologie. 1999;**175**:500-508

[46] Kyle RA, Gertz MA, Witzig TE, Lust JA, Lacy MQ, et al. Review of 1,027 patients with newly diagnosed multiple myeloma. Mayo Clinic Proceedings. 2003;**78**:21-33

[47] Prasad D, Schiff D. Malignant spinal cord compression. The Lancet Oncology. 2005;**6**(1): 15-24

[48] Sen E, Yavas G. The Management of spinal cord compression in multiple myeloma. Annals of Hematology and Oncology. 2016;**3**(5):1090

[49] Tosi P. Diagnosis and treatment of bone disease in multiple myeloma: Spotlight on spinal involvement. Scientifica (Cairo). 2013;**2013**:104546

[50] Flouzat-Lachaniette CH, Allain J, Roudot-Thoraval F, Poignard A. Treatment of spinal epidural compression due to hematological malignancies: A single institution's retrospective experience. European Spine Journal. 2013;**22**(3):548-555

[51] Rades D, Veninga T, Stalpers LJ, Basic H, Rudat V, et al. Outcome after radiother apy alone for metastatic spinal cord compression in patients with oligometastases. Journal of Clinical Oncology. 2007;**25**:50-56

[52] Rades D, Conde-Moreno AJ, Cacicedo J, Veninga T, Gebauer N, et al. A predictive tool particularly designed for elderly myeloma patients presenting with spinal cord compression. BMC Cancer. 2016;**16**:292

[53] Rades D, Lange M, Veninga T, Rudat V, Bajrovic A, et al. Preliminary results of spinal cord compression recurrence evaluation (score-1) study comparing short-course versus long-course radiotherapy for local control of malignant epidural spinal cord compression. International Journal of Radiation Oncology, Biology, Physics. 2009;**73**:228-234

[54] Maranzano E, Trippa F, Casale M, Costantini S, Lupattelli M, et al. 8Gy single-dose radiotherapy is effective in metastatic spinal cord compression: Results of a phase III randomized multicentre Italian trial. Radiotherapy and Oncology. 2009;**93**:174-179

[55] Rades D, Hoskin PJ, Stalpers LJA, Schulte R, Ph P, et al. short course radiotherapy is not optimal for spinal cord compression due to myeloma. International Journal of Radiation Oncology, Biology, Physics. 2006;**64**:1452-1457

[56] Gerszten PC, Monaco EA 3rd. Complete percutaneous treatment of vertebral body tumors causing spinal canal compromise using a transpedicular cavitation, cement augmentation, and radiosurgical technique. Neurosurgical Focus. 2009;**27**(6):E9

[57] Patchell RA, Tibbs PA, Regine WF, Payne R, Saris S, et al. Direct decompressive surgical resection in the treatment of spinal cord compression caused by metastatic cancer: A randomised trial. Lancet. 2005;**366**(9486):643-648

[58] Hirsch AE, Jha RM, Yoo AJ, Saxena A, Ozonoff A, et al. The use of vertebral augmentation and external beam radiation therapy in the multimodal management of malignant vertebral compression fractures. Pain Physician. 2011;**14**(5):447-458

[59] Lutz S, Chow E. Palliative radiotherapy: Past, present and future-where do we go from here? Annals of Palliative Medicine. 2014;**3**(4):286-290

[60] Cox JD, Stetz J, Pajak TF. Toxicity criteria of the radiation therapy oncology group (RTOG) and the European Organization for Research and Treatment of cancer (EORTC). International Journal of Radiation Oncology, Biology, Physics. 1995;**31**(5):1341-1346

[61] Fairchild A, Hird A, Chow E. Pain control with palliative radiotherapy in bone metastases. Bone cancer. Progression and Therapeutic Approaches. 2010, Pages 295, 297-311 Academic press

[62] Matuschek C, Ochtrop TA, Bölke E, Ganswindt U, Fenk R, et al. Effects of radiotherapy in the treatment of multiple myeloma: A retrospective analysis of a single institution. Radiation Oncology. 2015 Mar 28;**10**:71

Chapter 8

Infections in Patients with Multiple Myeloma in the Era of Novel Agents and Stem Cell Therapies

Asma M. Al-Jasser and Khalid Ahmed Al-Anazi

Additional information is available at the end of the chapter

http://dx.doi.org/10.5772/intechopen.81683

Abstract

Multiple myeloma is a common hematologic malignancy that is associated with reduced cellular as well as humoral immunity ultimately causing various infectious complications. The recent advances in the management of myeloma have led not only to prolonged survival but also to shifts in the incidence as well as the spectrum of infections encountered. This book chapter will be an updated review on the infectious complications in patients with multiple myeloma in the era of novel agents, stem cell therapies, and monoclonal antibodies. It will cover causes of immunosuppression, timing, and types as well as management of the various infections reported with various therapeutic modalities that are currently utilized in the management of myeloma patients.

Keywords: multiple myeloma, hematopoietic stem cell transplantation, novel therapies, monoclonal antibodies, infectious complications

1. Introduction to multiple myeloma

Multiple myeloma (MM), the second most common hematologic malignancy (HM), is a plasma cell neoplasm characterized by production of a monoclonal immunoglobulin that ultimately leads to several complications including anemia, renal dysfunction, bone disease, immunodeficiency, and various infections [1–5].

Over the past two decades, the outcomes of patients with MM have improved substantially due to the following: (1) the widespread utilization of high-dose (HD) chemotherapy followed by autologous stem cell transplantation (HSCT), (2) the introduction of several novel therapies and monoclonal antibodies, (3) the evolution of advanced technology that facilitated understanding of the biology of the disease and helped in the diagnosis, risk stratification and follow-up of patients, (4) the evolution of new therapeutic strategies such as consolidation and maintenance treatments as well as total and continuous therapy, and (5) improvements in supportive care and antimicrobial therapies [1, 3–12]. Currently, the following novel therapies are available for patients with MM: (1) immunomodulatory agents such as thalidomide, lenalidomide, and pomalidomide; (2) proteasome inhibitors such as bortezomib, carfilzomib, and ixazomib; (3) monoclonal antibodies such as daratumumab and elotuzumab; and (4) histone deacetylase inhibitors such as panobinostat and vorinostat [1, 3, 4, 6, 9, 11]. Unfortunately, despite the remarkable progress achieved in the diagnostics and therapeutics and the plethora of therapeutic modalities, MM remains incurable [1, 4, 5, 7, 11]. The numerous treatment modalities that are available for patients with MM have shown their effectiveness, but they have their own adverse effects including bone marrow (BM) suppression and infectious complications that may be life-threatening [13–15].

The standard induction therapy in patients with newly diagnosed MM is the triplet regimen of bortezomib, lenalidomide, and dexamethasone [4, 16]. Autologous HSCT is the standard of care for transplant-eligible patients either upfront or at relapse [4, 10, 16]. Studies have shown that post-HSCT consolidation and maintenance treatments can further improve the outcome of patients with MM [10, 16, 17]. Monitoring disease response at various stages of treatment is essential and studies have shown that monitoring of minimal residual disease is associated with longer progression-free survival (PFS) and overall survival (OS) [18, 19].

2. Early mortality in MM

In patients with MM, several studies have shown that risk factors for early mortality include male gender, age >75 years, poor performance status, presence of comorbid medical conditions such as renal failure and hypertension, low platelet count, low serum albumin level, elevated serum levels of calcium and lactic dehydrogenase, low body mass index, presentation with primary plasma cell leukemia, advanced stage of disease at presentation, and infectious complications [20–25]. Two major studies that included 451 and 299 patients with MM showed that 65 and 45% of early deaths were attributable to infections [20, 21].

Despite the use of prophylactic antimicrobials, infections remain a leading cause of mortality and morbidity in patients with MM [26]. In patients with MM, approximately 45% of deaths occurring within 60 days of diagnosis are caused by various infections, predominantly pneumonia and sepsis [20, 26].

3. Reduced immunity in patients with MM

In patients with MM, causes of immunosuppression include: (1) the immunosuppressive effects of the disease or the direct immunosuppression caused by tumor cells, particularly in advanced stage or refractory disease, (2) therapeutic interventions to control MM, such as corticosteroids, cytotoxic chemotherapy, and the novel therapies such as thalidomide, lenalidomide and bortezomib reduce the immunity further by different mechanisms including neutropenia and mucositis, (3) old age and its immunosuppressive effects, (4) impairment of the capacity of the immune system to mount effective responses or challenges to infection or vaccination, (5) further suppression of the immune system by the administration of HD chemotherapy (melphalan) followed by autologous HSCT, and (6) presence of comorbid medical conditions [14, 27–31].

In patients with MM, the risks of infectious complications and disease progression are enhanced by following forms of dysfunction of the immune system: reduced antigen presentation, high cytokine levels and increased suppressive cells such as CD8 Tregs [32, 33]. Both cellular and humoral components of the immune system are suppressed in patients with MM [28, 34, 35]. Hypogammaglobulinemia or immunoparesis is associated with unfavorable prognosis in newly diagnosed patients with MM [34]. In a Danish study that included 2558 patients with MM, immunoparesis at diagnosis was not confirmed to be an independent prognostic factor for OS, but quantitative immunoparesis was found to be associated with a shorter PFS [34].

Patients with MM have increased susceptibility to infections due to the profound B-cell dysfunction or the depression in humoral immunity [36]. These patients are 10 times more prone to infections than patients with Waldenstrom's macroglobulinemia and 5 times more prone to infections than individuals with monoclonal gammopathy of undetermined significance [36]. MM patients have increased susceptibility to severe pneumococcal infections, and they respond poorly to pneumococcal vaccination [35, 36].

The highest risk of infection occurs within the first month after the diagnosis of MM, particularly in patients with renal failure [14, 36]. The infections that are encountered in patients with MM include urinary tract infection, pneumonia, septicemia, fungal infections, and viral infections such as *influenza virus* and *varicella zoster virus* (VZV) infections [14, 36]. However, bacterial infections predominate particularly those caused by: *Staphylococcus aureus*, *Streptococcus pneumonia*, *Haemophilus influenzae*, and *Escherichia coli* [14, 36]. The advent of autologous HSCT and the introduction of novel therapies in patients with MM have led to a shift in the spectrum of infections with increased incidence of viral and fungal infections [13, 36]. In a recent study, mitogen stimulation of cytokine release profiling for interleukin (IL)-5, IL-13, Th1, and Th2 was used to predict the risk of infections in patients with MM during maintenance therapy, but only IL-5 response was found to be predictive of infection on multivariate analysis [37].

4. Infectious complications in MM

The risk factors for infectious complications in patients with MM can be divided into patient-related factors, disease-related factors, and treatment-related factors as shown in **Table 1** [13, 14, 38–45]. However, the infections encountered in patients with MM include: (1) bacterial infections, predominantly involving respiratory and urinary tract, caused by *Streptococcus pneumonia*, *Staphylococcus aureus*, *Haemophilus influenzae*, *Klebsiella pneumonia*, *Escherichia coli*,

1 Patient-related factors:
- Female gender
- Old age
- Poor performance status and poor general condition
- Presence of comorbid medical conditions
- Hyperglycemia and uncontrolled diabetes mellitus
- Renal dysfunction/failure
- Increased serum ferritin level

2 Disease-related factors:
- Active disease
- Advanced disease; stage III according to international staging system
- Relapsed and refractory disease
- Immune dysfunction:
    - Suppression of cellular and humoral immunity including hypogammaglobulinemia
    - Low CD4+ cell count
    - Dysfunction of natural killer cells

3 Treatment-related factors:
- High-dose chemotherapy: melphalan, cyclophosphamide
- Novel therapies:
    - Immunomodulatory agents: thalidomide, lenalidomide, pomalidomide
    - Proteasome inhibitors: bortezomib, carfilzomib
    - Monoclonal antibodies: daratumumab, elotuzumab
- Neutropenia and lymphopenia
- Mucositis
- Presence of central venous catheters
- Corticosteroids: high dose or prolonged duration of therapy
- Autologous hematopoietic stem cell transplantation
- Allogeneic hematopoietic stem cell transplantation

Table 1. Risk factors for infectious complications in multiple myeloma.

Pseudomonas aeruginosa, and *Enterobacteriaceae*; (2) viral infections caused by *herpes simplex virus* (HSV), VZV, and *cytomegalovirus* (CMV); (3) fungal infections caused by *Candida* species and *Aspergillus* species; and (4) *Pneumocystis jiroveci pneumonia* (PJP) [14, 43, 44, 46–48].

The sites of infections in patients with MM include: (1) upper and lower respiratory tract with otitis, sinusitis, and pneumonia; (2) urinary tract; (3) brain with meningitis; (4) skin with VZV infection; (5) heart with endocarditis; (6) bone and joint infections; and (7) bacteremia [14, 43, 47–51]. Bacterial infections are the most frequent etiological agents. However, invasive fungal infections (IFIs) caused by molds such as *Aspergillus* species and *Fusarium* species have been increasingly reported [50]. The incidence of infections in MM patients has bimodal peaks: bacterial infections dominate 4–6 and 70–72 months after the diagnosis, while viral infections dominate 7–9 and 52–54 months after the diagnosis of MM [13].

In patients with MM having active disease, the following types of infections are common: bacteremia, pneumonia, sinusitis, otitis, meningitis, and IFIs [14, 50]. In active disease, Gram-negative bacterial (GNB) particularly encapsulated bacteria and fungi are common causes of infectious complications [14].

Patients with MM are at high risk of developing infections as infections in these patients have been reported to be 10 times more than that in healthy individuals. Also, the new novel therapies make patients with MM at higher risk of infectious complications than myeloma patients treated with cytotoxic chemotherapy [52, 53]. Even, prior to the diagnosis of MM, there is an underlying immune disturbance, which may predispose to various infections such as VZV, sinusitis, cystitis, and bronchitis that may be encountered during the disease evolution [54].

4.1. Neutropenia and febrile neutropenia

Neutropenia is a hematologic adverse event of medications characterized by an absolute neutrophil count (ANC) lower than 1500 cells/mL [55]. Neutropenia is a well-recognized complication of cytotoxic chemotherapy. Also, it develops in patients with MM receiving novel therapies or undergoing HSCT [55–57]. Prolonged and severe neutropenia increases the risk of febrile neutropenia (FN) and serious infections that may be life-threatening [57]. Persistent neutropenia causes not only delay in administration of chemotherapy or novel therapies, but also dose reductions in the next cycle of chemotherapy. Nevertheless, once the ANC reaches ≥1000 cells/mL, scheduled treatment may be resumed [55].

FN is a serious effect of chemotherapy, and it has the following adverse consequences: delay in administration of scheduled therapies, costs of hospitalization, and increased risk of morbidity and mortality in immunocompromised individuals [58]. Several studies have shown that the following risk factors for neutropenia and FN in patients with MM: (1) heavily pretreated disease and relapsed and refractory (R/R)-MM, (2) elderly patients with comorbid medical conditions, and (3) use of the following drugs particularly in combination with other agents such as lenalidomide, bendamustine, and the combination of bendamustine, bortezomib and dexamethasone [55, 58–60].

Management of patients with prolonged neutropenia and FN includes: (1) thorough physical evaluation for the site or source of infection, (2) taking enough cultures and septic screens, (3) administration of prophylactic and empirical antimicrobials, and (4) pre-emptive or prophylactic administration of granulocyte-colony stimulating factor (G-CSF) in patients who are expected to have prolonged or severe neutropenia [58, 59]. However, the choice of empirical antibiotic therapy in patients with HMs having FN depends on the risk stratification of the individual patient [61, 62]. In low-risk (LR) patients with FN, duration of neutropenia is <1 week and there are no comorbid medical conditions; while in high-risk (HR) patients with FN, the duration of neutropenia is >1 week and there are comorbid medical conditions [61, 62]. In case the patient is stratified as LR, oral antibiotics such as ciprofloxacin or levofloxacin are sufficient, while if the patient belongs to the HR group, intravenous (IV) antibiotics may need to be administered. IV ceftazidime, piperacillin-tazobactam, or a carbapenem can be given as single agents or in combination with either vancomycin or an aminoglycoside [62–65]. However, the fact that there is a recent increase in the incidence of Gram-positive bacteria (GPB) cultured from neutropenic patients with MM has to be taken into consideration [56]. Empirical antifungal therapy can be used in patients with persistent fever despite the use of broad-spectrum antibiotics [61, 62, 66]. In addition, recombinant G-CSF is commonly used to reduce the incidence, duration, and severity of FN [57]. Studies have shown that the use of G-CSF as primary prophylaxis improves quality of life, is cost-effective as it reduces the: days of hospitalization, infectious complications, and incidence of chemotherapy interruptions [58, 59].

4.2. Bacterial and bloodstream infections in MM

Bloodstream infections (BSIs) are important causes of morbidity and mortality in patients with HMs, and they contribute to delayed administration of planned chemotherapy, increased length of hospitalization, and increased health care costs [29]. The risk factors for bacteremia or bacterial BSIs in patients with HMs include the primary disease, neutropenia induced by intensive chemotherapy, and mucositis due to the cytotoxic effects of chemotherapy on the cells of gastrointestinal tract [67, 68]. In recent years, there has been a shift in prevalence of the causative organisms for bacterial BSIs in patients with HMs from GPB to GNB. Also, there has been increasing frequency of antimicrobial resistance in GNB [69]. Therefore, in patients with HMs having FN, BSIs caused by GNB should initially be treated with non-carbapenem-based anti-pseudomonal therapy taking into consideration the antimicrobial stewardship [67].

In patients with MM undergoing autologous HSCT, mucositis and chemotherapy-induced neutropenia are risk factors for the development of bacteremia [67, 68]. In two retrospective studies on BSIs that included 421 patients with MM, the following results were obtained: (1) the independent risk factors for BSIs were: advanced stage of disease, poor performance status, and receipt of autologous HSCT; (2) GPB, mainly *Streptococcus pneumonia*, were responsible for the majority of BSIs during the induction phase of treatment while GNB, mainly *Escherichia coli*, were responsible for the majority of BSIs in progressive disease; (3) the highest incidence of BSIs was encountered during the first 3 months from the diagnosis and during disease progression; (4) admissions to the intensive care unit were required in 23% of patients with BSIs; and (5) mortality rates due to BSIs were 11.5% in patients with progressive disease and 50% in patients with newly diagnosed MM [29, 70].

Bacteremia may antedate the diagnosis of MM and may be related to the use of venous catheters used during stem cell collection or autologous HSCT [71, 72]. Polymicrobial or multiple microbiologically confirmed infections are frequent and may cause serious consequences in recipients of HSCT [73]. Several studies have shown that the use of ciprofloxacin or levofloxacin prophylaxis in patients with MM undergoing autologous HSCT is associated with significant reduction in the incidence of FN, bacteremia, and pneumonia [68, 74, 75]. On the contrary, a randomized phase III study that included 212 MM patients undergoing induction therapy showed that the prophylactic use of antibiotics did not decrease the incidence of serious bacterial infections, thus obviating the need for the routine use of antibacterial prophylaxis in patients with MM receiving induction therapy [76]. However, other studies have shown that the addition of doxycycline to ciprofloxacin and the sequential use of levofloxacin followed by ertapenem in patients with MM subjected to autologous HSCT reduce the frequency of FN episodes, bacteremia, and documented bacterial infections without increasing the rate of serious complications [77, 78].

4.3. Viral infections in MM

Reactivation of CMV after autologous HSCT performed for patients with MM is relatively common and is mainly encountered in patients receiving tandem rather than single HSCT; HD-melphalan conditioning therapy; and induction with combination therapy particularly bortezomib, thalidomide, and dexamethasone [79]. Also, reactivation of *human herpes virus*-6 is relatively common following autologous HSCT and is usually associated with postengraftment fever [80]. Several studies performed in patients with MM have shown that the risk factors for reactivation of VZV, HSV, and *hepatitis-B virus* (HBV) include (1) progressive disease, (2) treatment with proteasome inhibitors such as bortezomib, (3) treatment with immunomodulatory agents particularly lenalidomide, and (4) HSCT [81–87].

Viremia caused by CMV is common and is often associated with fever, while CMV disease with biopsy proven tissue infiltration is rare in patients with MM receiving autologous HSCT [79]. CMV surveillance should be considered in patients with MM subjected to autologous HSCT, particularly those receiving tandem transplants, HD-melphalan and combination therapies for induction [79]. Acyclovir of valacyclovir prophylaxis should be offered to HR patients including recipients of HSCT, patients with progressive disease, and patients treated with bortezomib or lenalidomide [81–87].

4.4. Fungal infections in MM

Candidemia and IFIs are major complications in patients with HMs who develop prolonged and severe neutropenia. Additionally, IFIs are difficult to diagnose in these severely immunocompromised patients [88–91]. In patients with MM prior to the introduction of novel therapies, IFIs were encountered in patients treated with traditional intensive cytotoxic chemotherapeutic regimens and mortality rates due to IFIs were reaching 60% [91]. In the era of novel therapies, IFIs are associated with mortality rate of approximately 44% and are mainly encountered in MM patients having: (1) progressive disease, (2) $\geq$ 3 lines of therapy administered, (3) received HSCT, particularly in the early post-transplant period, and (4) history of IFI treated [91–93].

Over the past two decades, the spectrum of *Candida* species infections has shifted to *non-albicans* species, which frequently exhibit decreased susceptibility to fluconazole [89]. Empirical antifungal agents are recommended in patients with HMs having neutropenia and persistent or recurrent fever despite appropriate antibiotic therapy [88]. In patients with candidemia or invasive infection caused by *Candida* species, echinocandins such as caspofungin, liposomal amphotericin-B, and voriconazole are the treatments of choice, while voriconazole is the treatment of choice for IFIs caused by *Aspergillus* species [67, 89, 90, 92]. However, fluconazole is still the most common antifungal agent used for prophylaxis in HR patients and in recipients of HSCT [91, 92].

4.5. Tuberculosis in patients with MM

Tuberculosis (TB) is the most common cause of death from a single infectious agent worldwide [94]. In patients with HMs and in recipients of HSCT living in geographic locations that are endemic for TB, these infections are uncommon, but they cause significant morbidity and mortality [95, 96]. Early diagnosis, prompt administration of anti-TB chemotherapy, and adherence to treatment schedules are associated with successful outcome, while delayed management, drug resistance, and presence of disseminated infection are associated with poor prognosis and high mortality rates [95, 96].

The incidence of TB infection is higher in patients with MM than in the general population. Also, patients with MM have higher risk of mortality compared to MM patients without TB [97]. The risk factors for TB infection in patients with MM include: (1) the disease itself with its associated immunological abnormalities that include hypogammaglobulinemia as well as abnormal T cell-mediated and humoral immunities, (2) treatment of MM that includes corticosteroids, cytotoxic chemotherapy, and novel therapies such as bortezomib, (3) old age, (4) alcohol use disorder, (5) poor socioeconomic conditions, (6) HSCT, and (7) presence of comorbid medical conditions such as diabetes mellitus and malnutrition [94–104].

TB infections in patients with MM can be primary infections or reactivation of old or latent TB infections [94, 100, 101]. Reactivation of TB may by induced by (1) HD corticosteroids, (2) cytotoxic chemotherapy, (3) administration of novel therapies, and (4) autologous as well as allogeneic HSCT [95, 104]. In patients with MM receiving bortezomib-containing regimens, TB infections are uncommon [94]. In a retrospective analysis of 115 patients with MM treated with bortezomib-based therapy: TB infection was diagnosed in 7% of cases, bortezomib therapy was interrupted in 50% of the patients treated for TB and this affected outcome of patients significantly, but none of the patients died because of uncontrolled TB infection. In these patients, early diagnosis and prompt anti-TB treatment were essential to avoid further worsening of the outcome [94].

TB infections may be diagnosed at the time of diagnosis of MM or may evolve during or after treatment of MM [98–100, 105]. In patients with MM, TB infections have been reported to involve: (1) lungs with pulmonary infiltration, lung nodules, and bronchiectasis; (2) spine causing paraspinal masses and spinal cord compression; and (3) meninges with TB meningitis [98–100, 105]. However, spinal TB is the most serious form of TB infections [100]. TB infections in MM patients may coexist with infections caused by other microorganisms such as *Staphylococcus aureus* [99].

TB infections are 10–40 times more common in recipients of HSCT than in the general population. Also, approximately 80% of *Mycobacterium tuberculosis* infections encountered in recipients of HSCT have been reported in allograft recipients [96, 103, 104]. Patients with MM having latent TB or history of treated TB infection planned for novel therapies or subjected to cytotoxic chemotherapy or HSCT should receive isoniazid prophylaxis to prevent reactivation of their TB infections [95, 96, 101].

4.6. Bone and joint infections in MM

Bone and joint infections are uncommon in patients with MM. These infections manifest as: osteomyelitis, septic arthritis, and prosthetic joint infections [51, 106]. The pathogens encountered are similar to those cultured in patients without myeloma, although GPB predominate and polymicrobial infections occur less frequently [51]. In patients with MM treated with radiotherapy or IV bisphosphonates, there is a risk of developing osteonecrosis of the jaw [106, 107]. Patients with osteonecrosis of the jaw are at risk for developing infections and often require long-term antimicrobial therapy [108]. Having history of jaw osteonecrosis is not a contraindication for HSCT as the outcome of these patients is not worsened by HSCT itself [108].

5. Infections associated with use of novel agents

Infections represent a significant cause of morbidity and a leading cause of death in patients with MM [13, 53]. The novel therapies that have been introduced over the past decade have improved the survival of patients with MM [53, 109]. Consequently, management of disease complications such as infections has become an important issue as patients with MM survive longer [53]. The pattern of infection and the risk factors for infection in MM patients have shifted due to the evolution of new therapies and the widespread use of HSCT [13, 43].

Several studies have shown that the use of immunomodulatory agents such as thalidomide and lenalidomide and proteasome inhibitors such as bortezomib, particularly if they are used in drug combinations that include corticosteroids in the treatment of MM at any stage, induction, relapse, or maintenance, are associated with increased risk of infectious complications, thus making the use of antimicrobial prophylaxis with fluoroquinolones, acyclovir, cotrimoxazole, and fluconazole essential [13, 52, 110, 111]. Also, in a meta-analysis that included 13 clinical trials, with 2402 patients participating, the use of daratumumab and elotuzumab in the treatment of R/R-MM was associated with myelosuppression in the form of neutropenia and lymphopenia and subsequent risk of infectious complications such as pneumonia [109].

5.1. Infections associated with use of thalidomide

Thalidomide is not significantly myelotoxic, so the risk of infection in patients with MM receiving thalidomide alone is very low [14]. However, severe infections have been encountered once thalidomide is used in combination with other drugs in the treatment of MM. Therefore, antibiotic prophylaxis is needed once thalidomide is used in combination with other drugs such as dexamethasone [112].

5.2. Infections associated with use of lenalidomide

Lenalidomide has more potent costimulatory effects on CD4+ and CD8+ cells than thalidomide, and it causes neutropenia as part of myelosuppression, which is highest during the initial cycles of therapy and then it decreases thereafter [14, 31, 113].

Serious infections and even deaths have been encountered with the use of lenalidomide [31]. Several studies have shown the following results once lenalidomide is combined with dexamethasone: (1) various infections are prone to occur, and (2) these infectious complications may be severe to the extent that the patients need hospitalization to receive G-CSF and IV antimicrobial therapy, (3) respiratory tract infections are common, and (4) viral infections such as VZV may be encountered requiring treatment as well as prophylaxis with acyclovir [14, 82, 113–116].

5.3. Infections associated with use of pomalidomide

Pomalidomide causes neutropenia [44, 116, 117]. When combined with dexamethasone in the treatment of patients with MM, severe infections may develop and pneumonia is a commonly encountered infection [44, 116, 117].

Infection is the second most common cause of death, after disease progression, in MM patients treated with pomalidomide [44]. Patient receiving pomalidomide therapy may have interruption of their scheduled treatment in case of severe infection and may need: G-CSF administration, antimicrobial prophylaxis with quinolones and cotrimoxazole, and even revaccination [44, 116, 117].

5.4. Infections associated with use of bortezomib

Bortezomib causes decreased lymphocytic count and imbalance in T-lymphocyte subsets due to its potent immunosuppressive effect on T cells [14, 118–120]. Several studies have shown that the use of bortezomib in the treatment of patients with MM is associated with development of the following infectious complications: (1) viral infections such as HSV and VZV infections mainly in patients with IgG type of myeloma, (2) fungal infections, (3) bacterial infections, mainly in IgG type of MM, and (4) TB reactivation, which is more pronounced in patients receiving other drugs, such as thalidomide and cyclophosphamide, in combination with bortezomib [14, 118, 119, 121]. However, one study found that *Epstein–Barr virus* (EBV)-positive B-cells were more susceptible to killing by bortezomib. Hence, the drug could represent a novel strategy for the treatment of certain EBV-associated lymphomas [122].

5.5. Infections associated with use of carfilzomib

Carfilzomib causes BM suppression that includes lymphopenia [123, 124]. The use of carfilzomib in the treatment of MM has been associated with the following infections: bacterial pneumonia, viral respiratory tract infections, and bacterial sepsis [123, 124].

5.6. Infections associated with use of daratumumab

Daratumumab has the following effects: neutropenia, lymphopenia, hyperglycemia, and decrease in natural killer cells, which play a major role in the immune clearance of virally infected cells [125, 126]. The use of daratumumab in the treatment of MM patients is associated with the following infections: nasopharyngitis, pneumonia, and viral infections such as VZV [125–128].

http://dx.doi.org/10.5772/intechopen.81683

5.7. Infections associated with use of elotuzumab

Elotuzumab can cause neutropenia, lymphopenia, and hyperglycemia [129–132]. Several studies have shown that its use in the treatment of patients with MM is associated with the following infections: pneumonia, sepsis, and even leishmaniasis [129–131, 133].

5.8. Infections related to corticosteroids and bisphosphonates

Corticosteroids predispose to infectious complications by causing immune suppression and hyperglycemia [13, 14, 39]. The following infections have been reported in patients with MM receiving corticosteroid therapy: (1) *Candida albicans* and *non-albicans Candida*; (2) *Mycobacteriaceae*; (3) viruses such as HSV, VZV, CMV, and respiratory viruses; (4) encapsulated bacteria such as *Staphylococcus aureus*, *Streptococcus pneumonia*, *Pseudomonas aeruginosa*, and *Enterobacter aerogenes*; and (5) PJP [13, 14, 39]. The use of bisphosphonates in patients with MM is associated with osteomyelitis and osteonecrosis of the jaw [14].

6. Infections related to HSCT in MM

Prior to the era of novel therapies for MM, studies in patients with HMs receiving autologous HSCT showed that there was no significant difference in incidence, type of infection, and clinical course of infection between patients with MM and patients with other HMs [134, 135]. However, a recent study showed that in-hospital mortality in patients with MM receiving autologous HSCT was approximately 1.5% and that there was no significant difference in mortality between elderly individuals and young patients [136]. Nevertheless, elderly patients were more likely to develop complications such as pneumonia, septic shock, acute respiratory failure needing endotracheal intubation, acute renal failure, and cardiac arrhythmias [136].

In patients with MM having dialysis-dependent renal failure are at higher risk of FN and infectious complications such as septic shock compared to patients without renal failure [137]. Patients with MM subjected to autologous HSCT are at higher risk of developing bacterial meningitis, which is associated with high rates of mortality and morbidity [138]. MM patients having MBL2 (mannan-binding lectin, which is part of the innate immune system that protects against severe infections during autologous HSCT) polymorphism are at risk of severe infections particularly after receiving HD-melphalan and autologous HSCT [139]. In addition to the administration of prophylactic antimicrobials in patients with HR-MM and in recipients of HSCT, strategies to reduce the incidence of infectious complications include administration of IV immunoglobulins and vaccination despite the likelihood of vaccination failure [140, 141].

During stem cell mobilization, infections related to central venous catheters are likely to occur with predominance of GPB [142]. Conditioning therapy with HD-melphalan causes mucositis and myelosuppression with neutropenia [14]. The use of melphalan is associated with colitis, pneumonia, and bacteremia, and these infections are usually caused by the following encapsulated bacteria, *Candida* species and *Aspergillus* species [14].

During the post-transplant period, organisms such as *Clostridium difficile*, CMV, HSV, VZV, PJP, and other opportunistic organisms dominate [13, 14, 141]. The sites of infection during this period are gastrointestinal, respiratory, and urinary tracts [13, 14]. In the pre-engraftment period of time: bacteremia, pneumonia, cellulitis, and gastrointestinal infections with *Clostridium difficile* occur, while VZV, CMV, *Clostridium difficile*, and PJP with gastrointestinal tract, lung and skin infections dominate in the post-engraftment period of time [14]. Bacteremia in recipients of autologous HSCT is associated with previous bortezomib therapy and elevated beta-2 microglobulin level [141]. Recently, a significant increase in the incidence of infections caused by multidrug resistant organisms (MDROs) has been encountered [143]. Also, colonization with MDROs in recipients of autologous HSCT has negative impact on OS due to the profound immunosuppression caused by the HMs and their treatments [143].

Reactivation of HBV is a well-recognized complication in patients with chronic HBV infection undergoing cytotoxic chemotherapy or immunosuppressive treatment [144]. In patients undergoing autologous HSCT, reverse seroconversion of HBV is not a rare complication and this poses concerns about possible complications in such severely immunocompromised individuals [144]. There is an extremely low incidence of PJP in recipients of autologous HSCT; thus, routine PJP prophylaxis should not be offered routinely to this population group. However, patients who require systemic corticosteroid therapy in the post-transplant period are candidates for PJP prophylaxis [145].

7. Conclusions and future directions

The introduction of the novel agents in the treatment of patients with MM has led to unprecedented improvements in survival rates. However, these novel therapies have their own toxicities that include BM suppression and various infectious complications. These infections include bacterial, viral, fungal, mycobacterial, and parasitic infections. Also, they can be local or disseminated and can affect the bloodstream and may invade internal organs, thus causing life-threatening illnesses.

As these infectious complications vary according to the stage of the disease and the specific agents used, prospective and multicentric studies are needed to explore the real extent of these infections in order to establish guidelines for the use of antimicrobial agents in the prophylaxis as well as the treatment of the various infections that can be encountered.

Author details

Asma M. Al-Jasser[1] and Khalid Ahmed Al-Anazi[2]*

*Address all correspondence to: kaa_alanazi@yahoo.com

1 Riyadh Regional Laboratory, Ministry of Health, Riyadh, Saudi Arabia

2 Department of Adult Hematology and Hematopoietic, Stem Cell Transplantation, Oncology Center, King Fahad Specialist Hospital, Dammam, Saudi Arabia

References

[1] Naymagon L, Abdul-Hay M. Novel agents in the treatment of multiple myeloma: A review about the future. Journal of Hematology & Oncology. 2016;**9**(1):52. DOI: 10.1186/s13045-016-0282-1

[2] Holstein SA, McCarthy PL. Immunomodulatory drugs in multiple myeloma: Mechanisms of action and clinical experience. Drugs. 2017;**77**(5):505-520. DOI: 10.1007/s40265-017-0689-1

[3] Larocca A, Mina R, Gay F, Bringhen S, Boccadoro M. Emerging drugs and combinations to treat multiple myeloma. Oncotarget. 2017;**8**(36):60656-60672. DOI: 10.18632/oncotarget.19269 (eCollection Sep 1, 2017)

[4] Raza S, Safyan RA, Rosenbaum E, Bowman AS, Lentzsch S. Optimizing current and emerging therapies in multiple myeloma: A guide for the hematologist. Therapeutic Advances in Hematology. 2017;**8**(2):55-70. DOI: 10.1177/2040620716680548

[5] Mimura N, Hideshima T, Anderson KC. Novel therapeutic strategies for multiple myeloma. Experimental Hematology. 2015;**43**(8):732-741. DOI: 10.1016/j.exphem.2015.04.010

[6] Orlowski RZ, Lonial S. Integration of novel agents into the care of patients with multiple myeloma. Clinical Cancer Research. 2016;**22**(22):5443-5452. DOI: 10.1158/1078-0432.CCR-16-0861

[7] Dingli D, Ailawadhi S, Bergsagel PL, Buadi FK, Dispenzieri A, Fonseca R, et al. Therapy for relapsed multiple myeloma: Guidelines from the Mayo stratification for myeloma and risk-adapted therapy. Mayo Clinic Proceedings. 2017;**92**(4):578-598. DOI: 10.1016/j.mayocp.2017.01.003

[8] Kharfan-Dabaja MA, Hamadani M, Reljic T, Nishihori T, Bensinger W, Djulbegovic B, et al. Comparative efficacy of tandem autologous versus autologous followed by allogeneic hematopoietic cell transplantation in patients with newly diagnosed multiple myeloma: A systematic review and meta-analysis of randomized controlled trials. Journal of Hematology & Oncology. 2013;**6**:2. DOI: 10.1186/1756-8722-6-2

[9] Anderson KC. Progress and paradigms in multiple myeloma. Clinical Cancer Research. 2016;**22**(22):5419-5427. DOI: 10.1158/1078-0432.CCR-16-0625

[10] Gay F, Engelhardt M, Terpos E, Wäsch R, Giaccone L, Auner HW, et al. From transplant to novel cellular therapies in multiple myeloma: European Myeloma Network guidelines and future perspectives. Haematologica. 2018;**103**(2):197-211. DOI: 10.3324/haematol.2017.174573

[11] Sonneveld P, De Wit E, Moreau P. How have evolutions in strategies for the treatment of relapsed/refractory multiple myeloma translated into improved outcomes for patients? Critical Reviews in Oncology/Hematology. 2017;**112**:153-170. DOI: 10.1016/j.critrevonc.2017.02.007

[12] Danylesko I, Beider K, Shimoni A, Nagler A. Novel strategies for immunotherapy in multiple myeloma: Previous experience and future directions. Clinical & Developmental Immunology. 2012;**2012**:753407. DOI: 10.1155/2012/753407

[13] Teh BW, Harrison SJ, Worth LJ, Spelman T, Thursky KA, Slavin MA. Risks, severity and timing of infections in patients with multiple myeloma: A longitudinal cohort study in the era of immunomodulatory drug therapy. British Journal of Haematology. 2015;**171**(1):100-108. DOI: 10.1111/bjh.13532

[14] Nucci M, Anaissie E. Infections in patients with multiple myeloma in the era of high-dose therapy and novel agents. Clinical Infectious Diseases. 2009;**49**(8):1211-1225. DOI: 10.1086/605664

[15] Mai EK, Haas EM, Lücke S, Löpprich M, Kunz C, Pritsch M, et al. A systematic classification of death causes in multiple myeloma. Blood Cancer Journal. 2018;**8**(3):30. DOI: 10.1038/s41408-018-0068-5

[16] Rajkumar SV. Multiple myeloma: 2016 update on diagnosis, risk-stratification, and management. American Journal of Hematology. 2016;**91**(7):719-734. DOI: 10.1002/ajh.24402

[17] Facon T. Maintenance therapy for multiple myeloma in the era of novel agents. Hematology. American Society of Hematology. Education Program. 2015;**2015**:279-285. DOI: 10.1182/asheducation-2015.1.279

[18] Landgren O, Rajkumar SV. New developments in diagnosis, prognosis, and assessment of response in multiple myeloma. Clinical Cancer Research. 2016;**22**(22):5428-5433. DOI: 10.1158/1078-0432.CCR-16-0866

[19] Fulciniti M, Munshi NC, Martinez-Lopez J. Deep response in multiple myeloma: A critical review. BioMed Research International. 2015;**2015**:832049. DOI: 10.1155/2015/832049

[20] Augustson BM, Begum G, Dunn JA, Barth NJ, Davies F, Morgan G, et al. Early mortality after diagnosis of multiple myeloma: Analysis of patients entered onto the United Kingdom Medical Research Council trials between 1980 and 2002—Medical Research Council Adult Leukaemia Working Party. Journal of Clinical Oncology. 2005;**23**(36):9219-9226. DOI: 10.1200/JCO.2005. 03.2086

[21] Hsu P, Lin TW, Gau JP, Yu YB, Hsiao LT, Tzeng CH, et al. Risk of early mortality in patients with newly diagnosed multiple myeloma. Medicine (Baltimore). 2015;**94**(50):e2305. DOI: 10.1097/MD.0000000000002305

[22] Costa LJ, Gonsalves WI, Kumar S. Early mortality in multiple myeloma: Risk factors and impact on population outcomes. Blood. 2014;**124**(21):1320

[23] Ríos-Tamayo R, Sáinz J, Martínez-López J, Puerta JM, Chang DY, Rodríguez T, et al. Early mortality in multiple myeloma: The time-dependent impact of comorbidity: A population-based study in 621 real-life patients. American Journal of Hematology. 2016;**91**(7):700-704. DOI: 10.1002/ajh.24389

[24] Jung SH, Cho MS, Kim HK, Kim SJ, Kim K, Cheong JW, et al. Korean Multiple Myeloma Working Party (KMMWP). Risk factors associated with early mortality in patients with

multiple myeloma who were treated upfront with a novel agents containing regimen. BMC Cancer. 2016;**16**:613. DOI: 10.1186/s12885-016-2645-y

[25] Terebelo H, Srinivasan S, Narang M, Abonour R, Gasparetto C, Toomey K, et al. Recognition of early mortality in multiple myeloma by a prediction matrix. American Journal of Hematology. 2017;**92**(9):915-923. DOI: 10.1002/ajh.24796

[26] Karlsson J, Andréasson B, Kondori N, Erman E, Riesbeck K, Hogevik H, et al. Comparative study of immune status to infectious agents in elderly patients with multiple myeloma, Waldenstrom's macroglobulinemia, and monoclonal gammopathy of undetermined significance. Clinical and Vaccine Immunology. 2011;**18**(6):969-977. DOI: 10.1128/CVI.00021-11

[27] Tete SM, Bijl M, Sahota SS, Bos NA. Immune defects in the risk of infection and response to vaccination in monoclonal gammopathy of undetermined significance and multiple myeloma. Frontiers in Immunology. 2014;**5**:257. DOI: 10.3389/fimmu. 2014.00257 (eCollection 2014)

[28] Schütt P, Brandhorst D, Stellberg W, Poser M, Ebeling P, Müller S, et al. Immune parameters in multiple myeloma patients: Influence of treatment and correlation with opportunistic infections. Leukemia & Lymphoma. 2006;**47**(8):1570-1582. DOI: 10.1080/10428190500472503

[29] Huang CT, Liu CJ, Ko PS, Liu HT, Yu YB, Hsiao LT, et al. Risk factors and characteristics of blood stream infections in patients with newly diagnosed multiple myeloma. BMC Infectious Diseases. 2017;**17**(1):33. DOI: 10.1186/s12879-016-2155-1

[30] Safdar A, Armstrong D. Infections in patients with hematologic neoplasms and hematopoietic stem cell transplantation: Neutropenia, humoral, and splenic defects. Clinical Infectious Diseases. 2011;**53**(8):798-806. DOI: 10.1093/cid/cir492

[31] Ying L, YinHui T, Yunliang Z, Sun H. Lenalidomide and the risk of serious infection in patients with multiple myeloma: A systematic review and meta-analysis. Oncotarget. 2017;**8**(28):46593-46600. DOI: 10.18632/oncotarget.16235

[32] Giannopoulos K, Kaminska W, Hus I, Dmoszynska A. The frequency of T regulatory cells modulates the survival of multiple myeloma patients: Detailed characterisation of immune status in multiple myeloma. British Journal of Cancer. 2012;**106**(3):546-552. DOI: 10.1038/bjc.2011.575

[33] Muthu Raja KR, Kubiczkova L, Rihova L, Piskacek M, Vsianska P, Hezova R, et al. Functionally suppressive CD8 T regulatory cells are increased in patients with multiple myeloma: A cause for immune impairment. PLoS One. 2012;**7**(11):e49446. DOI: 10.1371/journal.pone.0049446

[34] Sørrig R, Klausen TW, Salomo M, Vangsted AJ, Frølund UC, Andersen KT, et al. Immunoparesis in newly diagnosed multiple myeloma patients: Effects on overall survival and progression free survival in the Danish population. PLoS One. 2017; **12**(12):e0188988. DOI: 10.1371/journal.pone.0188988 (eCollection 2017)

[35] Karlsson J, Hogevik H, Andersson K, Roshani L, Andréasson B, Wennerås C. Pneumococcal vaccine responses in elderly patients with multiple myeloma, Waldenstrom's

macroglobulinemia, and monoclonal gammopathy of undetermined significance. Trials in Vaccinology. 2013;**2**:31-38. DOI: 10.1016/j.trivac. 2013.09.001

[36] Karlsson J, Roalfe L, Hogevik H, Zancolli M, Andréasson B, Goldblatt D, et al. Poor correlation between pneumococcal IgG and IgM titers and opsonophagocytic activity in vaccinated patients with multiple myeloma and Waldenstrom's macroglobulinemia. Clinical and Vaccine Immunology. 2016;**23**(4):379-385. DOI: 10.1128/CVI. 00654-15

[37] Teh BW, Harrison SJ, Allison CC, Slavin MA, Spelman T, Worth LJ, et al. Predicting risk of infection in patients with newly diagnosed multiple myeloma: Utility of immune profiling. Frontiers in Immunology. 2017;**8**:1247. DOI: 10.3389/fimmu.2017.01247 (eCollection 2017)

[38] Nucci M. Infection in multiple myeloma. Revista Brasileira de Hematologia e Hemoterapia. 2009;**31**(2):32-34. DOI: 10.1590/S1516-84842009000800010

[39] Jung SH, Jang HC, Lee SS, Ahn JS, Yang DH, Kim YK, et al. The impact of hyperglycemia on risk of severe infections during early period of induction therapy in patients with newly diagnosed multiple myeloma. BioMed Research International. 2014;**2014**:413149. DOI: 10.1155/2014/413149

[40] Hyun SY, Han SH, Kim SJ, Jang JE, Kim Y, Cho H, et al. Pretreatment lymphopenia, poor performance status, and early courses of therapy are risk factors for severe bacterial infection in patients with multiple myeloma during treatment with bortezomib-based regimens. Journal of Korean Medical Science. 2016;**31**(4):510-518. DOI: 10.3346/jkms.2016.31.4.510

[41] Hyun SY, Jang JE, Kim Y, Hwang DY, Kim SJ, Kim YR, et al. Risk factors for the development of severe bacterial infection in patients with multiple myeloma during chemotherapy with bortezomib containing regimens. Blood. 2013;**122**(21):5370

[42] Goranov S. Clinical problems of infectious complications in patients with multiple myeloma. Folia Medica (Plovdiv). 1994;**36**(1):41-46

[43] Valković T, Gačić V, Ivandić J, Petrov B, Dobrila-Dintinjana R, Dadić-Hero E, et al. Infections in hospitalised patients with multiple myeloma: Main characteristics and risk factors. Turkish Journal of Haematology. 2015;**32**(3):234-242. DOI: 10.4274/tjh.2013.0173

[44] Dimopoulos MA, Leleu X, Palumbo A, Moreau P, Delforge M, Cavo M, et al. Expert panel consensus statement on the optimal use of pomalidomide in relapsed and refractory multiple myeloma. Leukemia. 2014;**28**(8):1573-1585. DOI: 10.1038/leu.2014.60

[45] de la Rubia J, Cejalvo MR, Ribas P. Infectious complications in patients with newly diagnosed multiple myeloma: A complication from the past? Leukemia & Lymphoma. 2015;**57**(2):258-268. DOI: 10.3109/10428194.2015.1088647

[46] Norden CW. Infections in patients with multiple myeloma. Archives of Internal Medicine. 1980;**140**(9):1150-1151. DOI: 10.1001/archinte.1980.00330200026012

[47] Kalambokis GN, Christou L, Tsianos EV. Multiple myeloma presenting with an acute bacterial infection. International Journal of Laboratory Hematology. 2009;**31**(4):375-383. DOI: 10.1111/j.1751-553X. 2009.01154.x

[48] Doughney KB, Williams DM, Penn RL. Multiple myeloma: Infectious complications. Southern Medical Journal. 1988;**81**(7):855-858

[49] Todaro J, Bollmann PW, Nussbacher A, Camargo LF, Santos BF, Alvarenga D, et al. Multiple myeloma complicated with pseudomonas endocarditis. Einstein (Sao Paulo). 2012; **10**(4):498-501

[50] Nucci M, Anaissie E. Infections in patients with multiple myeloma. Seminars in Hematology. 2009;**46**(3):277-288. DOI: 10.1053/j.seminhematol. 2009.03.006

[51] Phuoc V, Abad C, Tande A, Tosh PK, Kapoor P, Sia I, et al. Bone and joint infections in multiple myeloma: A retrospective review of patients at Mayo clinic. Blood. 2016; **128**(22):5636

[52] Offidani M, Corvatta L, Bringhen S, Gentili S, Gay F, Maracci L, et al. Infection complications in 476 patients with newly diagnosed multiple myeloma treated with lenalidomide or bortezomib combinations. Blood. 2015;**126**(23):5365

[53] Blimark C, Holmberg E, Mellqvist UH, Landgren O, Björkholm M, Hultcrantz M, et al. Multiple myeloma and infections: A population-based study on 9253 multiple myeloma patients. Haematologica. 2015;**100**(1):107-113. DOI: 10.3324/haematol.2014.107714

[54] McShane CM, Murray LJ, Engels EA, Landgren O, Anderson LA. Common community-acquired infections and subsequent risk of multiple myeloma: A population-based study. International Journal of Cancer. 2014;**134**(7):1734-1740. DOI: 10.1002/ijc.28479

[55] Palumbo A, Bladé J, Boccadoro M, Palladino C, Davies F, Dimopoulos M, et al. How to manage neutropenia in multiple myeloma. Clinical Lymphoma, Myeloma & Leukemia. 2012;**12**(1):5-11. DOI: 10.1016/j.clml.2011.11.001

[56] Fernández-Mosteirín N, Salvador-Osuna C, Gimeno Lozano JJ, Marco Lamata ML, Blasco Alberdi M, Rubio Félix D, et al. Incidence of febrile episodes in patients with multiple myeloma undergoing autologous peripheral blood stem cell transplantation. Anales de Medicina Interna 2005;**22**(5):213-216

[57] Leleu X, Gay F, Flament A, Allcott K, Delforge M. Incidence of neutropenia and use of granulocyte colony-stimulating factors in multiple myeloma: Is current clinical practice adequate? Annals of Hematology. 2018;**97**(3):387-400. DOI: 10.1007/s00277-017-3191-7

[58] Cerchione C, Catalano L, Peluso I, Nappi D, Di Perna M, Salvatore D, et al. Managing neutropenia by pegfilgrastim in patients affected by relapsed/refractory multiple myeloma treated with bendamustine-bortezomib-dexamethasone. Supportive Care in Cancer. 2016;**24**(12): 4835-4837

[59] Sun HL, Atenafu EG, Yeboah E, Reece DE, Trudel S, Kukreti V, et al. Intermittent granulocyte colony-stimulating factor for neutropenia management in patients with relapsed or refractory multiple myeloma treated with lenalidomide plus dexamethasone. Leukemia & Lymphoma. 2015;**56**(2):407-414. DOI: 10.3109/10428194.2014.915544

[60] Mitani Y, Usami E, Kimura M, Nakao T, Okada K, Matsuoka T, et al. Risk factors for neutropenia with lenalidomide plus dexamethasone therapy for multiple myeloma. Die Pharmazie. 2016;**71**(6):349-351

[61] Villafuerte-Gutierrez P, Villalon L, Losa JE, Henriquez-Camacho C. Treatment of febrile neutropenia and prophylaxis in hematologic malignancies: A critical review and update. Advances in Hematology. 2014;**2014**:986938. DOI: 10.1155/2014/986938

[62] Wingard JR. Treatment of neutropenic fever syndromes in adults with hematologic malignancies and hematopoietic cell transplant recipients (high-risk patients). In: Bow E, Thorner AR, editors. Up To Date 2018

[63] Cooper MR, Durand CR, Beaulac MT, Steinberg M. Single-agent, broad-spectrum fluoroquinolones for the outpatient treatment of low-risk febrile neutropenia. The Annals of Pharmacotherapy. 2011;**45**(9):1094-1102. DOI: 10.1345/aph.1Q147

[64] He L, Zhou C, Zhao S, Weng H, Yang G. Once-daily, oral levofloxacin monotherapy for low-risk neutropenic fever in cancer patients: A pilot study in China. Anti-Cancer Drugs. 2015;**26**(3):359-362. DOI: 10.1097/CAD.0000000000000187

[65] Aguilar-Guisado M, Espigado I, Martín-Peña A, Gudiol C, Royo-Cebrecos C, Falantes J, et al. Optimisation of empirical antimicrobial therapy in patients with haematological malignancies and febrile neutropenia (How Long study): An open-label, randomised, controlled phase 4 trial. Lancet Haematology. 2017;**4**(12):e573-e583. DOI: 10.1016/S2352-3026(17)30211-9

[66] Gea-Banacloche J. Evidence-based approach to treatment of febrile neutropenia in hematologic malignancies. Hematology. American Society of Hematology. Education Program. 2013;**2013**:414-422. DOI: 10.1182/asheducation-2013.1.414

[67] Gedik H, Şimşek F, Kantürk A, Yildirmak T, Arica D, Aydin D, et al. Bloodstream infections in patients with hematological malignancies: Which is more fatal-cancer or resistant pathogens? Therapeutics and Clinical Risk Management. 2014;**10**:743-752. DOI: 10.2147/TCRM. S68450

[68] Satlin MJ, Vardhana S, Soave R, Shore TB, Mark TM, Jacobs SE, et al. Impact of prophylactic levofloxacin on rates of bloodstream infection and fever in neutropenic patients with multiple myeloma undergoing autologous hematopoietic stem cell transplantation. Biology of Blood and Marrow Transplantation. 2015;**21**(10):1808-1814. DOI: 10.1016/j.bbmt.2015.06.017

[69] Trecarichi EM, Pagano L, Candoni A, Pastore D, Cattaneo C, Fanci R. Current epidemiology and antimicrobial resistance data for bacterial bloodstream infections in patients with hematologic malignancies: An Italian multicentre prospective survey. Clinical Microbiology and Infection. 2015;**21**(4):337-343. DOI: 10.1016/j.cmi.2014. 11.022

[70] Teh BW, Harrison SJ, Slavin MA, Worth LJ. Epidemiology of bloodstream infections in patients with myeloma receiving current era therapy. European Journal of Haematology. 2017;**98**(2):149-153. DOI: 10.1111/ ejh.12813

[71] Shahani S, Shahani L. Streptococcus pneumoniae bacteraemia leading to the diagnosis of multiple myeloma. BMJ Case Reports. 2014;**2014**:bcr2014204472. Published 2014 Sep 19. DOI: 10.1136/bcr-2014-204472

[72] Lee MN, Huh HJ, Kim B, Kang CI, Kim K, Ki CS, et al. A case of catheter-related Kocuria marina bloodstream infection in a patient with multiple myeloma. Lab Med Online. 2014;**4**(1):51-54. DOI: 10.3343/lmo.2014.4.1.51

[73] Trifilio S, Villa M, Mehta J. Polymicrobial and multiple microbiologically proven infections in HSCT recipients. Biology of Blood and Marrow Transplantation. 2013; **19**(2):S257-S258. DOI: 10.1016/ j.bbmt.2012.11.377

[74] Vaxman I, Rozovsky U, Shargian L, Moshe M, Sela-Navon M, Raanani P, et al. Antibacterial prophylaxis reduces the risk of bacteremia and febrile neutropenia in patients with multiple myeloma and lymphoma undergoing high-dose chemotherapy and autologous hematopoietic cell transplantation. Biology of Blood and Marrow Transplantation. 2017;**23**(3):S201. DOI: 10.1016/j.bbmt.2016.12.387

[75] Watts N, Chodavarapu A, Rahman M, Saad A, Costa LJ, Salzman D. The role of antibacterial prophylaxis in preventing central line-associated blood stream infections (CLABSIs) in multiple myeloma patients undergoing an autologous stem cell transplant. Biology of Blood and Marrow Transplantation. 2017;**23**(3):S199-S200. DOI: 10.1016/j.bbmt.2016.12.385

[76] Vesole DH, Oken MM, Heckler C, Greipp PR, Katz MS, Jacobus S, et al. University of Rochester Cancer Center and the Eastern Cooperative Oncology GroupOral antibiotic prophylaxis of early infection in multiple myeloma: A URCC/ECOG randomized phase III study. Leukemia. 2012;**26**(12):2517-2520. DOI: 10.1038/leu.2012.124

[77] Kim JH, Goulston C, Zangari M, Tricot G, Boyer MW, Hanson KE. Impact of a change in antibacterial prophylaxis on bacteremia and hospitalization rates following outpatient autologous peripheral blood stem cell transplantation for multiple myeloma. Transplant Infectious Disease. 2014;**16**(3):421-429. DOI: 10.1111/tid.12225

[78] Sivik JM, Davidson J, Hale CM, Drabick JJ, Talamo G. Addition of doxycycline to ciprofloxacin for infection prophylaxis during autologous stem cell transplants for multiple myeloma. Supportive Care in Cancer 2018. DOI: 10.1007/s00520-018-4165-6 (Epub ahead of print)

[79] Kim JH, Goulston C, Sanders S, Lampas M, Zangari M, Tricot G, et al. Cytomegalovirus reactivation following autologous peripheral blood stem cell transplantation for multiple myeloma in the era of novel chemotherapeutics and tandem transplantation. Biology of Blood and Marrow Transplantation. 2012;**18**(11):1753-1758. DOI: 10.1016/j.bbmt.2012.06.008

[80] Horowitz N, Oren I, Lavi N, Zuckerman T, Benyamini N, Kra-Oz Z, et al. New rising infection: Human herpesvirus 6 is frequent in myeloma patients undergoing autologous stem cell transplantation after induction therapy with bortezomib. Bone Marrow Research. 2012;**2012**:409765. DOI: 10.1155/2012/409765

[81] Teh BW, Slavin MA, Harrison SJ, Worth LJ. Prevention of viral infections in patients with multiple myeloma: The role of antiviral prophylaxis and immunization. Expert Review of Anti-Infective Therapy. 2015;**13**(11):1325-1336. DOI: 10.1586/14787210.2015.1083858

[82] König C, Kleber M, Reinhardt H, Knop S, Wäsch R, Engelhardt M. Incidence, risk factors, and implemented prophylaxis of varicella zoster virus infection, including complicated varicella zoster virus and herpes simplex virus infections, in lenalidomide-treated multiple myeloma patients. Annals of Hematology. 2014;**93**(3):479-484. DOI: 10.1007/s00277-013-1951-6

[83] Fukushima T, Sato T, Nakamura T, Iwao H, Nakajima A, Miki M, et al. Daily 500 mg valacyclovir is effective for prevention of Varicella zoster virus reactivation in patients with multiple myeloma treated with bortezomib. Anticancer Research. 2012;**32**(12):5437-5440

[84] Pour L, Adam Z, Buresova L, Krejci M, Krivanova A, Sandecka V, et al. Varicella-zoster virus prophylaxis with low-dose acyclovir in patients with multiple myeloma treated with bortezomib. Clinical Lymphoma & Myeloma. 2009;**9**(2):151-153. DOI: 10.3816/CLM.2009.n.036

[85] Kim JW, Min CK, Mun YC, Park Y, Kim BS, Nam SH, et al. Varicella-zoster virus-specific cell-mediated immunity and herpes zoster development in multiple myeloma patients receiving bortezomib- or thalidomide-based chemotherapy. Journal of Clinical Virology. 2015;**73**:64-69. DOI: 10.1016/j.jcv.2015.10.018

[86] Swaika A, Paulus A, Miller KC, Sher T, Almyroudis NG, Ball D, et al. Acyclovir prophylaxis against varicella zoster virus reactivation in multiple myeloma patients treated with bortezomib-based therapies: A retrospective analysis of 100 patients. The Journal of Supportive Oncology. 2012;**10**(4):155-159. DOI: 10.1016/ j.suponc.2011.10.006

[87] Vickrey E, Allen S, Mehta J, Singhal S. Acyclovir to prevent reactivation of varicella zoster virus (herpes zoster) in multiple myeloma patients receiving bortezomib therapy. Cancer. 2009;**115**(1):229-232. DOI: 10.1002/cncr.24006

[88] Nucci M. Use of antifungal drugs in hematology. Revista Brasileira de Hematologia e Hemoterapia. 2012;**34**(5):383-391. DOI: 10.5581/1516-8484.20120095

[89] Farmakiotis D, Tarrand JJ, Kontoyiannis DP. Efficacy and tolerability of micafungin monotherapy for candidemia and deep-seated candidiasis in adults with cancer. Antimicrobial Agents and Chemotherapy. 2014;**58**(6):3526-3529. DOI: 10.1128/AAC.00051-14

[90] Dewan E, Biswas D, Kakati B, Verma SK, Kotwal A, Oberoi A. Epidemiological and mycological characteristics of candidemia in patients with hematological malignancies attending a tertiary-care center in India. Hematology/Oncology and Stem Cell Therapy. 2015;**8**(3):99-105. DOI: 10.1016/j.hemonc.2015.06. 006

[91] Teh BW, Teng JC, Urbancic K, Grigg A, Harrison SJ, Worth LJ, et al. Invasive fungal infections in patients with multiple myeloma: A multi-center study in the era of novel myeloma therapies. Haematologica. 2015;**100**(1):e28-e31. DOI: 10.3324/haematol.2014.114025

[92] Liu J, Huang H, Li Y, Liu L, Li J, Liu Z, et al. Epidemiology and treatment of invasive fungal diseases in patients with multiple myeloma: Findings from a multicenter prospective study from China. Tumour Biology. 2016;**37**(6):7893-7900. DOI: 10.1007/s13277-015-4441-8

[93] Nadiminti K, Pilla SV, Singh Abbi KK, Mott SL, Ince D, Tricot GJ, et al. Incidence of fungal infections associated with the use of novel agents as part of conditioning regimen during autologous stem cell transplant in multiple myeloma; a single center experience at the university of Iowa. Biology of Blood and Marrow Transplantation. 2017;**23**(3): S193. DOI: 10.1016/j.bbmt.2016.12.374

[94] Ahn JS, Rew SY, Yang DH, Jung SH, Kang SJ, Kim MY, et al. Poor prognostic significance of Mycobacterium tuberculosis infection during bortezomib-containing chemotherapy in patients with multiple myeloma. Blood Research. 2013;**48**(1):35-39. DOI: 10.5045/br.2013.48.1.35

[95] Al-Anazi KA, Al-Jasser AM, Evans DA. Infections caused by mycobacterium tuberculosis in patients with hematological disorders and in recipients of hematopoietic stem cell transplant, a twelve year retrospective study. Annals of Clinical Microbiology and Antimicrobials. 2007;**6**:16. DOI: 10.1186/1476-0711-6-16

[96] Al-Anazi KA, Al-Jasser AM, Alsaleh K. Infections caused by Mycobacterium tuberculosis in recipients of hematopoietic stem cell transplantation. Frontiers in Oncology. 2014;**4**:231. DOI: 10.3389/fonc. 2014.00231 (eCollection 2014)

[97] Tsai CK, Huon LK, Ou SM, Kuan AS, Yeh CM, Lee YT, et al. Risk and impact of tuberculosis in patients with multiple myeloma. Leukemia & Lymphoma. 2017;**58**(11):2598-2606. DOI: 10.1080/10428194.2017.1312369

[98] Tsai YC, Wang HC, Hsiao HH, Liu TC. Tuberculosis meningitis in patient with multiple myeloma during bortezomib-containing therapy. The Kaohsiung Journal of Medical Sciences. 2016;**32**(10):531-532. DOI: 10.1016/j.kjms.2016.05.010

[99] Burton CH, Fairham SA, Millet B, DasGupta R, Sivakumaran M. Unusual aetiology of persistent back pain in a patient with multiple myeloma: Infectious discitis. Journal of Clinical Pathology. 1998;**51**(8):633-634

[100] Omoti CE, Ehimwenma O, Ogbeide OU. Osteosclerotic myeloma associated with spinal tuberculosis with neurological manifestation: A case report. American Journal of Case Reports. 2008;**9**:321-324

[101] Akı ŞZ, Sucak GT, Tunçcan ÖG, Köktürk N, Şenol E. The incidence of tuberculosis infection in hematopoietic stem cell transplantation recipients: A retrospective cohort study from a center in Turkey. Transplant Infectious Disease. 2018;**20**(4):e12912. DOI: 10.1111/tid.12912. Epub 2018 May 9

[102] Budak-Alpdogan T, Tangün Y, Kalayoglu-Besisik S, Ratip S, Akan H, Baslar Z, et al. The frequency of tuberculosis in adult allogeneic stem cell transplant recipients in Turkey. Biology of Blood and Marrow Transplantation. 2000;**6**(4):370-374

[103] Lee HJ, Lee DG, Choi SM, Park SH, Cho SY, Choi JK, et al. The demanding attention of tuberculosis in allogeneic hematopoietic stem cell transplantation recipients: High incidence compared with general population. PLoS One. 2017;**12**(3):e0173250. DOI: 10.1371/journal.pone.0173250 (eCollection 2017)

[104] García-Elorriaga G, Rey-Pineda GD. Tuberculosis and hematopoietic stem cell transplant: Review of a difficult and often underestimated problem. World Journal of Clinical Infectious Diseases. 2013;**3**(4):70-78. DOI: 10.5495/wjcid.v3.i4.70

[105] Yeshurun M, Laporte JP, Lesage S, Najman A. Spinal cord compression of dual etiology, multiple myeloma and spinal tuberculosis. Leukemia & Lymphoma. 2002;**43**(2):427-428. DOI: 10.1080/10428190290006279

[106] Hameed A, Brady JJ, Dowling P, Clynes M, O'Gorman P. Bone disease in multiple myeloma: Pathophysiology and management. Cancer Growth Metastasis. 2014;**7**:33-42. DOI: 10.4137/CGM.S16817

[107] Shah A, Latoo S, Ahmad I. Multiple myeloma and dentistry. In: Gupta A, editor. Multiple Myeloma—An Overview. Intech Open; 2012. DOI: 10.5772/31490

[108] Mawardi H, Glotzbecker B, Richardson P, Woo SB. Hematopoietic cell transplantation in patients with medication-related osteonecrosis of the jaws. Biology of Blood and Marrow Transplantation. 2016;**22**(2):344-348. DOI: 10.1016/j.bbmt.2015.08.021

[109] Zhang T, Wang S, Lin T, Xie J, Zhao L, Liang Z, et al. Systematic review and meta-analysis of the efficacy and safety of novel monoclonal antibodies for treatment of relapsed/refractory multiple myeloma. Oncotarget. 2017;**8**(20):34001-34017. DOI: 10.18632/oncotarget.16987

[110] Teh BW, Harrison SJ, Worth LJ, Thursky KA, Slavin MA. Infection risk with immunomodulatory and proteasome inhibitor-based therapies across treatment phases for multiple myeloma: A systematic review and meta-analysis. European Journal of Cancer. 2016;**67**:21-37. DOI: 10.1016/j.ejca.2016.07.025

[111] Miceli T, Colson K, Gavino M, Lilleby K, IMF Nurse Leadership Board. Myelosuppression associated with novel therapies in patients with multiple myeloma: consensus statement of the IMF Nurse Leadership Board. Clinical Journal of Oncology Nursing. 2008;**12**(3 Suppl):13-20. DOI: 10.1188/08.CJON.S1.13-19

[112] Offidani M, Corvatta L, Polloni C, Gentili S, Brioni A, Visani G, et al. Infectious complications in patients with multiple myeloma treated with new drug combinations containing thalidomide. Leukemia & Lymphoma. 2011;**52**(5):776-785. DOI: 10.3109/10428194.2011.555027

[113] Mariz JM, Esteves GV. Review of therapy for relapsed/refractory multiple myeloma: Focus on lenalidomide. Current Opinion in Oncology. 2012;**24**(Suppl 2):S3-S12. DOI: 10.1097/01.cco.0000410243.84074.dc

[114] Kukreti V, Masih-Khan E, Dean S, Kumar D, Mikhael JR, Trudel S, et al. Infectious complications in advanced relapsed/refractory multiple myeloma patients treated with lenalidomide (revlimid +/− corticosteroids). Blood. 2009;**114**:2876

[115] Reece D, Kouroukis CT, Leblanc R, Sebag M, Song K, Ashkenas J. Practical approaches to the use of lenalidomide in multiple myeloma: A Canadian consensus. Advances in Hematology. 2012;**2012**:621958. DOI: 10.1155/2012/621958

[116] Ríos-Tamayo R, Martín-García A, Alarcón-Payer C, Sánchez-Rodríguez D, de la Guardia AMDVD, García Collado CG, et al. Pomalidomide in the treatment of multiple myeloma: Design, development and place in therapy. Drug Design, Development and Therapy. 2017;**11**:2399-2408. DOI: 10.2147/DDDT.S115456 (eCollection 2017)

[117] Moreau P, Dimopoulos MA, Richardson PG, Siegel DS, Cavo M, Corradini P, et al. Adverse event management in patients with relapsed and refractory multiple myeloma taking pomalidomide plus low-dose dexamethasone: A pooled analysis. European Journal of Haematology. 2017;**99**(3):199-206. DOI: 10.1111/ ejh.12903

[118] Li J, Li Y, Huang B, Zheng D, Chen M, Zhou Z. Drug-induced modulation of T lymphocytes as a potential mechanism of susceptibility to infections in patients with multiple myeloma during bortezomib therapy. Cell Biochemistry and Biophysics. 2015;**71**:457-464. DOI: 10.1007/s12013-014-0224-x

[119] Basler M, Lauer C, Beck U, Groettrup M. The proteasome inhibitor bortezomib enhances the susceptibility to viral infection. Journal of Immunology. 2009;**183**(10):6145-6150. DOI: 10.4049/jimmunol. 0901596

[120] Jung S-H, Ahn J-S, Kang S-J, Yang D-H, Kim Y-K, Kim H-J, et al. Lymphocytopenia is associated with an increased risk of severe infections in patients with multiple myeloma treated with bortezomib-based regimens. Blood. 2012;**120**:5042

[121] Kim K, Kim SJ, Maeng CH. Relationship between bortezomib-containing regimens and the incidence of tuberculosis in patients with myeloma. Blood Research. 2013;**48**(3):233-234. DOI: 10.5045/br.2013.48.3.233

[122] Zou P, Kawada J, Pesnicak L, Cohen JI. Bortezomib induces apoptosis of Epstein-Barr Virus (EBV)-transformed B bells and prolongs survival of mice inoculated with EBV-transformed B cells. Journal of Virology. 2007;**81**(18):10029-10036. DOI: 10.1128/JVI.02241-06

[123] Harvey RD. Incidence and management of adverse events in patients with relapsed and/or refractory multiple myeloma receiving single-agent carfilzomib. Clinical Pharmacology. 2014;**6**:87-96. DOI: 10.2147/CPAA.S62512 (eCollection 2014)

[124] Badros AZ, Vij R, Martin T, Zonder JA, Kunkel L, Wang Z, et al. Carfilzomib in multiple myeloma patients with renal impairment: Pharmacokinetics and safety. Leukemia. 2013;**27**(8):1707-1714. DOI: 10.1038/leu.2013.29

[125] Casneuf T, Xu XS, Adams HC 3rd, Axel AE, Chiu C, Khan I, et al. Effects of daratumumab on natural killer cells and impact on clinical outcomes in relapsed or refractory multiple myeloma. Blood Advance. 2017;**1**(23):2105-2114. DOI: 10.1182/bloodadvances.2017006866. (eCollection Oct 24, 2017)

[126] Drgona L, Gudiol C, Lanini S, Salzberger B, Ippolito G, Mikulska M. ESCMID Study Group for Infections in Compromised Hosts (ESGICH) Consensus Document on the safety of targeted and biological therapies: An infectious diseases perspective (Agents targeting lymphoid or myeloid cells surface antigens [II]: CD22, CD30, CD33, CD38, CD40, SLAMF-7 and CCR4). Clinical Microbiology and Infection. 2018;**24**(Suppl 2):S83-S94. DOI: 10.1016/j.cmi.2018.03.022

[127] Lokhorst HM, Plesner T, Laubach JP, Nahi H, Gimsing P, Hansson M, et al. Targeting CD38 with daratumumab monotherapy in multiple myeloma. The New England Journal of Medicine. 2015;**373**(13):1207-1219. DOI: 10.1056/NEJMoa1506348

[128] Johnsrud JJ, Susanibar S, Jo-Kamimoto J, Johnsrud AJ, Kothari A, Burgess MJ, et al. Infection risk associated with daratumumab. Open Forum Infectious Diseases. 2017; **4**(suppl 1):S702-S703. DOI: 10.1093/ofid/ofx163.1884

[129] Laubach J, Nooka AK, Cole C, O'Donnell, Vij R, Usmani SZ, et al. An open-label, single arm, phase IIa study of bortezomib, lenalidomide, dexamethasone, and elotuzumab in newly diagnosed multiple myeloma. Journal of Clinical Oncology. 2017;**35**(suppl 15): 8002. DOI: 10.1200/JCO.2017.35.15_suppl.8002. Epub 2017 May 30

[130] Lonial S, Dimopoulos M, Palumbo A, White D, Grosicki S, Spicka I, et al. Elotuzumab therapy for relapsed or refractory multiple myeloma. The New England Journal of Medicine. 2015;**373**(7):621-631. DOI: 10.1056/NEJMoa1505654

[131] Suzuki K, Sunami K, Ohashi K, Iida S, Mori T, Handa H, et al. Randomized phase 3 study of elotuzumab for relapsed or refractory multiple myeloma: ELOQUENT-2 Japanese patient subanalysis. Blood Cancer Journal. 2017;**7**(3):e540. DOI: 10.1038/bcj.2017.18

[132] Taniwaki M, Yoshida M, Matsumoto Y, Shimura K, Kuroda J, Kaneko H. Elotuzumab for the treatment of relapsed or refractory multiple myeloma, with special reference to its modes of action and SLAMF7 signaling. Mediterranean Journal of Hematology and Infectious Diseases. 2018;**10**(1):e2018014. DOI: 10.4084/MJHID.2018.014 (eCollection 2018)

[133] Ziogas DC, Terpos E, Gavriatopoulou M, Migkou M, Fotiou D, Roussou M, et al. Coexistence of leishmaniasis and multiple myeloma in the era of monoclonal antibody (anti-CD38 or anti-SLAMF7) containing triplets: One shared story of two exceptional cases. Leukemia & Lymphoma. 2018;**59**(4):983-987. DOI: 10.1080/10428194.2017.1361031

[134] Reich G, Mapara MY, Reichardt P, Dörken B, Maschmeyer G. Infectious complications after high-dose chemotherapy and autologous stem cell transplantation: Comparison between patients with lymphoma or multiple myeloma and patients with solid tumors. Bone Marrow Transplantation. 2001;**27**(5):525-529. DOI: 10.1038/sj.bmt.1702822

[135] Auner HW, Sill H, Mulabecirovic A, Linkesch W, Krause R. Infectious complications after autologous hematopoietic stem cell transplantation: Comparison of patients with acute myeloid leukemia, malignant lymphoma, and multiple myeloma. Annals of Hematology. 2002;**81**(7):374-377. DOI: 10.1007/s00277-002-0484-1

[136] Sanchez L, Sylvester M, Parrondo R, Mariotti V, Eloy JA, Chang VT. In-hospital mortality and post-transplantation complications in elderly multiple myeloma patients undergoing autologous hematopoietic stem cell transplantation: A population-based study. Biology of Blood and Marrow Transplantation. 2017;**23**(7):1203-1207. DOI: 10.1016/j.bbmt.2017.03.012

[137] St Bernard R, Chodirker L, Masih-Khan E, Jiang H, Franke N, Kukreti V, et al. Efficacy, toxicity and mortality of autologous SCT in multiple myeloma patients with dialysis-dependent renal failure. Bone Marrow Transplant. 2015;**50**(1):95-99. DOI: 10.1038/bmt.2014.226

[138] van Veen KE, Brouwer MC, van de Ende A, van de Beek D. Bacterial meningitis in hematopoietic stem cell transplant recipients: A population-based prospective study. Bone Marrow Transplantation. 2016;**51**(11):1490-1495. DOI: 10.1038/bmt.2016.181

[139] Mølle I, Peterslund NA, Thiel S, Steffensen R. MBL2 polymorphism and risk of severe infections in multiple myeloma patients receiving high-dose melphalan and autologous stem cell transplantation. Bone Marrow Transplantation. 2006;**38**(8):555-560. DOI: 10.1038/sj.bmt.1705466

[140] Khalafallah A, Maiwald M, Cox A, Burns D, Bates G, Hannan T, et al. Effect of immunoglobulin therapy on the rate of infections in multiple myeloma patients undergoing autologous stem cell transplantation or treated with immunomodulatory agents. Mediterranean Journal of Hematology and Infectious Diseases. 2010;**2**(1):e2010005. DOI: 10.4084/MJHID.2010.005

[141] Park H, Youk J, Kim HR, Koh Y, Kwon JH, Yoon SS, et al. Infectious complications in multiple myeloma receiving autologous stem cell transplantation in the past 10 years. International Journal of Hematology. 2017;**106**(6):801-810. DOI: 10.1007/s12185-017-2313-2

[142] Jillella AP, Ustun C, Robach E, Sertkaya D, DiPiro C, Kallab AM, et al. Infectious complications in patients receiving mobilization chemotherapy for autologous peripheral blood stem cell collection. Journal of Hematotherapy & Stem Cell Research. 2003;**12**(2):155-160. DOI: 10.1089/152581603321628296

[143] Scheich S, Reinheimer C, Brandt C, Wichelhaus TA, Hogardt M, Kempf VAJ, et al. Clinical impact of colonization with multidrug-resistant organisms on outcome after autologous stem cell transplantation: A Retrospective Single-Center Study. Biology of Blood and Marrow Transplantation. 2017;**23**(9):1455-1462. DOI: 10.1016/j.bbmt.2017.05.016

[144] Uhm JE, Kim K, Lim TK, Park BB, Park S, Hong YS, et al. Changes in serologic markers of hepatitis B following autologous hematopoietic stem cell transplantation. Biology of Blood and Marrow Transplantation. 2007;**13**(4):463-468. DOI: 10.1016/j.bbmt.2006.11.019

[145] Raser K, McNulty ML, Yanik G, Goldstein SC, Magenau J, Pawarode A, et al. Routine prophylaxis of Pneumocystis jirovenci pneumonia in recipients of autologous hematopoietic stem cell transplantation. Biology of Blood and Marrow Transplantation. 2014; **20**:S104-S127

Chapter 9

Management of Multiple Myeloma in Developing Countries

Ogbonna Collins Nwabuko

Additional information is available at the end of the chapter

http://dx.doi.org/10.5772/intechopen.76500

Abstract

Multiple myeloma (MM) is one of the commonest hematological malignancies of public health importance especially in low-income countries (LICs) of Sub-Saharan Africa. The two major challenges in the management of MM in developing countries are in the diagnosis and treatment. It poses diagnostic dilemma to physicians, especially orthopedic surgeons, because of the skeletal related events (SREs). Lack of modern equipment for diagnosis is a key player in late diagnosis of MM, and the management follows a palliative approach in the region. There is a gross inadequacy in the palliative care of MM in developing countries. The definitive treatment still remains melphalan-prednisone (MP) combination regimen as against the standard bortezomib-lenalidomide-dexamethasone (RVD) triplet regimen used in developed countries. Stem cell transplantation is still a far cry in the treatment of MM in the region due to its high cost and unavailability in the region. About 7.6% of MM patients survive up to 5 years postdiagnosis in LICs. This is below estimated 5 years postdiagnosis overall survival of 44.9% recorded by SEER cancer statistics review of 1975–2007 in the USA. This chapter highlights management and some of the diagnostic and therapeutic challenges encountered by people living with MM in developing countries.

Keywords: multiple myeloma, management, developing countries

1. Introduction

Multiple myeloma (MM), otherwise known as plasma cell myeloma, is a malignant plasma cell disorder characterized by clonal proliferation of terminally differentiated B-lymphocytic cells in the bone marrow. This leads to overproduction of aberrant immunoglobulins in the blood, a condition known as paraproteinemia. It is one of the commonest hematological malignancies of public health importance in low-income countries of Sub-Saharan Africa. It accounts for 10–15% of all lymphohematopoietic cancers, 1% of all cancer diagnosis, and 0.9–2% of all cancer-related deaths globally [1]. According to 2009 cancer statistics, the cumulative incidence of MM in the United States is 20,580 cases with an estimated number of deaths of 10,580 and a case fatality rate greater than 51% [2]. The prevalence of MM is in the increase in African continent especially in the oil-rich Niger-Delta Nigeria where it accounts for about 8.2% of all hematological malignancies [3, 4]. The management of MM starts with a good history, which brings into limelight the epidemiology, pathogenesis, and the clinical features of the disease. This is followed by a series of investigations to make the diagnosis and to clinically stage the disease before therapeutic interventions. The major challenges in the management of MM in developing countries are in the diagnosis and treatment. The duo are majorly responsible for the complications, poor prognosis, and survival outcome of people living with MM in the region. This chapter highlights the management of multiple myeloma and some of the challenges encountered in the diagnosis and treatment of this disease in developing countries using Nigerian experience as a prototype.

2. Etiopathogenesis of multiple myeloma and its significance in its management

The etiology of multiple myeloma is unknown. However, previous studies have identified factors implicated as "potentially etiologic multiple myeloma risk factors" [5, 6]. These factors include increasing age (>65 years), male gender, black race, and positive family history (first-degree family relatives) of multiple myeloma. Other causes include environmental agents such as cumulative exposure to ionizing radiation and certain chemicals such as dioxin, herbicides, and pesticides. There is a hypothesis that these specific pesticides are causatively linked to myelomatogenesis through the hypothesized precursors of multiple myeloma such as essential monoclonal gammopathy (MGUS) and solitary multiple myeloma (SMM) [7, 8].

Physiologically, a plasma cell is an immunologically activated B-cell that produces antibody. A B-cell goes through series of rearrangement with the immunoglobulin gene to generate functional antibody. It can enter into the circulation to interact directly with antigen to differentiate into a short-lived plasma cell that lives for about 3 days. On the other hand, a myeloma cell is a postgerminal center plasma cell that has undergone immunoglobulin gene recombination, class switching, and somatic hypermutation, and homes to the bone marrow to become long-lived plasma cell (i.e., can live for ≥30 days) [9]. Cytogenetically, MM is divided into two groups based on karyotype gain or loss into hyperdiploid and non-hyperdiploid MM. The hyperdiploid MM, which constitutes about 55–60% of MM primary tumor, is characterized by hyperdiploid karyotype with chromosome range of 48–78 and trisomies of odd number chromosomes, including 15, 9, 5, 19, 3, 11, 7, and 21 (ordered by decreasing frequency). The hyperdiploid variants are typically the IgG kappa-types with bone involvements. The non-hyperdiploid karyotype accounts for the remaining 40–45% of MM primary tumor, and it includes the hypodiploid or near-tetraploid chromosome numbers (i.e., fewer than 48 or more than 74 chromosomes). Chromosomal translocations affect more commonly the non-hyperdiploid karyotypes. In terms of prognosis, hyperdiploid MM is better than non-hyperdiploid karyotype provided the former is not associated with deletion of chromosome 13 (RB1 gene and miRNA-15a/16-1 cluster dysregulation) and 17 (involving the TP53 locus) or amplification of chromosome 1q21 [9, 10]. The critical role of pathogenesis of MM is to give insight into the biology of the disease. Also, the pathways of the pathogenesis of the disease serve as potential sites for therapeutic interventions, especially the target therapies, which can utilize them for their actions.

3. Requirements for standard diagnosis and staging of multiple myeloma

The diagnosis of multiple myeloma is based on a constellation of hematologic, immunologic, histologic, and radiographic features. There are two methods of diagnosis of MM: the old and new methods. In the old method, a minimum of two major criteria, or one major criterion plus one minor criterion, or three minor criteria is used in making diagnosis of MM [11]. The major criteria are plasmacytoma on tissue biopsy, bone marrow infiltration with greater than 30% BMPCs, monoclonal globulin spike on serum electrophoresis, while the minor criteria include bone marrow infiltration with 10–30% BMPCs, paraprotein less than the defined quantity for major criteria, and lytic bone lesion. **Table 1** shows the criteria for diagnosis of MM using the old method. The newer method of diagnosis takes into cognizance of the popularly known criteria which uses the end-organ damage as defined using both the classic as "CRAB" criteria for hypercalcemia, renal failure, anemia, and bone lesions and additional criteria including recurrent bacterial infections (> 2 in 12 months), amyloidosis, or symptomatic hyperviscocity. In the newer method, initiation of therapy is an evidence of organ or tissue damage (end-organ damage) [9]. Diagnosis is made by clonal BMPCs of not less than 10% of biopsy-proven bony or extramedullary plasmacytoma or any evidence of myeloma-defining events. The myeloma-defining events in this context include any evidence of end-organ damage or presence of any one or more biomarkers of malignancy such as clonal BMPCs greater than 60%, serum-free

Major criteria:
I Plasmacytoma on tissue biopsy
II Bone marrow infiltration with >30% BMPCs
III Monoclonal globulin spike (paraprotein) on serum electrophoresis (IgG >35 g/L and IgA >20 g/L) or on concentrated urine electrophoresis (>1 g/24 h or kappa or lambda light chain)
Minor criteria:
A = Bone marrow infiltration with 10–30% plasma cells
B = Paraprotein less than the level defined earlier
C = Lytic bone lesions
D = Normal IgM <0.5 g/L, IgA <1 g/L or IgG <6 g/L
Abbreviations: MM, multiple myeloma; BMPC, bone marrow plasma cell; IgG, immunoglobulin G; IgA, immunoglobulin A; IgM, immunoglobulin M.

Table 1. Criteria for the diagnosis of MM (old method).

1. Clonal BMPCs ≥10% of biopsy-proven bony or extramedullary plasmacytoma
Any one of the following myeloma-defining events:

- Evidence of end-organ damage that can be attributed to the underlying plasma cell proliferative disorder, specifically:
  - **a.** Hypercalcemia: serum calcium >0.025 mmol/L (>1 mg/dL) higher than the upper limit of normal or >2.75 mmol/L (>11 mg/dL)
  - **b.** Renal insufficiency: creatinine clearance <40 mL per min or serum creatinine >177 μmol/L (>2 mg/mg/dL)
  - **c.** Anemia: hemoglobin value of 20 g/L below the lower limit of normal, or a hemoglobin value <100 g/L
  - **d.** Bone lesions: one or more osteolytic lesions on skeletal radiography, CT, or PET-CT
- Any one or more of the following biomarkers of malignancy:
  - **a.** Clonal bone marrow plasma cell percentage* ≥ 60%
  - **b.** Involved: uninvolved serum free light chain ratio ≥ 100
  - **c.** >1 focal lesions on MRI studies

*Clonal should be established by showing kappa/lambda-light-chain restriction on flow cytometry, immunohistochemistry, or immunofluorescence. BMPC percentage should preferably be estimated from a core biopsy specimen; in case of a disparity between the aspirate and core biopsy, the highest value should be used.
Source: In Table 107-2 [9].

Table 2. Criteria for diagnosis of MM (newer method).

1. All of the following

Hemoglobin >10.5 g/dL

Serum calcium normal

X-ray showing normal bone structure or solitary bone plasmacytoma only

Low paraprotein levels

IgG < 50 g/L

IgA < 30 g/L

Urinary light chain <4 g/24 h

2. Fitting neither stage I or stage III

3. One or more of the following:

Hemoglobin <8.5 g/dL

Serum calcium >3 mmol/L

Advanced lytic bone lesions (more than three lytic lesions)

High paraprotein levels

IgG >70 g/L

IgA >50 g/L

Urinary light chain >12 g/24 h

Subclassification

A. Serum creatinine <170 μmol/L

B. Serum creatinine ≥170 μmol/L

D-S, Durie-Salmon; IgG, immunoglobulin G; IgA, immunoglobulin A.

Table 3. D-S staging system.

light chain ratio greater than 100, and or greater than one focal lesions on magnetic resonance imagery studies. **Table 2** shows the current criteria of diagnosis of MM.

The staging of MM is another important step after diagnosis. The essence of staging is for decision-making on therapeutic interventions and for prognostication of the disease. There are two clinical staging systems for MM. They include the Durie-Salmon staging system and the international staging system (ISS). The Durie-Salmon (D-S) clinical staging system has been in use for more than 30 years, but it has been remodified to a newer staging system useful for the assessment of myeloma tumor mass [9, 12] The old D-S staging system has three stages (I, II, and III) and two subclassifications (A and B). Here, the staging of MM is based on five parameters viz.: the hemoglobin concentration, the serum calcium level, osteolytic bone lesions, serum, and urinary immunoglobulin quantification. The subclassification A in the staging connotes "normal renal status" (evidenced by normal serum creatinine level), while B connotes "abnormal renal state" (evidenced by deranged serum creatinine level). This is shown in **Table 3**. The modified Salmon-Durie assesses myeloma tumor mass using the old system to stage MM into high tumor mass (stage III), low tumor mass (I), and intermediate tumor mass myelomas (II), which is shown in **Table 4**. The ISS is based on two widely available parameters, serum beta-2 microglobulin and albumin. This staging system recognizes three stages and can be useful for prognostication of survival intervals of MM patients (**Table 5**) [13].

The standard assessment of MM requires a panel of investigations, which are carried out periodically postdiagnosis for prognostication and monitoring of the disease response to treatment. These investigations include complete blood count, blood chemistry, serum and

(I)	High tumor mass (stage III) (>1.2 × 10^{12} myeloma cells/m^2)*		
	One of the following abnormalities must be present		
	A.	Hemoglobin <8.5 g/dL, hematocrit <25%	
	B.	Serum calcium >12 mg/dL	
	C.	Very high serum or urine myeloma protein production rates:	
		1.	IgG peak >7 g/dL
		2.	IgA peak >5 g/dL
		3.	Urine light chains >12 g/24 h
	D.	More than three lytic bone lesions on bone survey (bone scan not acceptable)	
(II)	Low tumor mass (stage I) (<0.6 × 10^{12} myeloma cells/m^2)*		
	All of the following must be present:		
	A.	Hemoglobin >10.5 g/dl, or hematocrit >32%	
	B.	Serum calcium normal	
	C.	Low serum myeloma protein production rates:	
		1.	IgG peak <5 g/dl
		2.	IgA peak <3 g/dl
		3.	Urine light chains <4 g/24 h
	D.	No bone lesions or osteoporosis	
(III)	Intermediate tumor mass (stage II) (0.6 to 1.2 × 10^{12} myeloma cells/m^2)*		
	All patients who do not qualify for high or low tumor mass categories are considered to have intermediate tumor mass		
	A.	No renal failure (creatinine ≤2 mg/dl)	
	B.	Renal failure (creatinine >2 mg/dl)	

*Estimated number of neoplastic plasma cells.
Data adapted from Durie and Salmon [12]. A remodified D-S staging system.

Table 4. Assessment of myeloma tumor mass (Salmon-Durie).

Stage I	β_2M < 3.5 ALB ≥ 3.5
Stage II	β_2M < 3.5 ALB < 3.5 or β_2M 3.5–5.5
Stage III	β_2M > 5.5

ALB, serum albumin in g/dL; β_2M,serum β_2-microglobulin in mg/L.
Data from Greipp et al. [13].

Table 5. International staging system (ISS).

Complete Blood Count and differential count; examination of blood film
Chemistry screen, including calcium, creatinine, lactate dehydrogenase, BNP, proBNP
β_2-microglobulin; C-reactive protein
Serum protein electrophoresis, immunofixation, quantification of immunoglobulin, serum-free light chains
24-hour urine collection for protein electrophoresis, immunofixation, quantification of immunoglobulins, including light chains
Marrow aspirate and trephine biopsy with metaphase cytogenetics, FISH, immunophenotyping; gene array, and plasma labeling index (if available)
Bone survey and MRI; PET-CT
Echocardiogram with assessment of diastolic function and measurement of interventricular septal thickness; EKG (if amyloidosis suspected)

BNP, brain natriuretic peptide, CT, computed tomography; EKG, electrocardiogram; FISH, fluorescence in situ hybridization, MRI, Magnetic resonance imaging; PET, positron emission tomography; proBNP, prohormone B-type natriuretic peptide.
Source: In Table 107-4 [9].

Table 6. Assessment of myeloma.

urine monoclonal protein assay, C-reactive protein, beta-2 microglobulin test, marrow study, skeletal survey, echocardiogram, immunophenotyping, cytogenetic tests, etc. (**Table 6**).

4. Challenges in diagnosis of multiple myeloma

The prevalence of MM is on the increase in developing countries such as those found in Sub-Saharan Africa [3, 14]. The oil-rich regions are worse hit probably due to a wide range of environmental pollution, flaring of gases, water pollution, oil spillage, and lack of effective environmental policies [6]. This is understandable based on the hypothesis that occupation studies of chemical, petroleum, and radiation industry workers have provided inconsistent evidence of causal association with MM [5]. Another potential etiologic factor that could be a key player in the increasing prevalence is the median age of diagnosis. Studies in Nigeria, Africa's most populous black nation, have shown that the median age of diagnosis of multiple myeloma is 59.9 years (45–78 years) [14–17]. This age is less than the 65 years median age of diagnosis recorded by SEER cancer statistics review of 1975–2007 in the USA [18]. The implication of this early age of diagnosis is that more people may likely be diagnosed with MM by the time they attend the age of 65, hence increasing the burden of the disease. The male to female ratio of about 2:1 recorded by most of the studies shows a gender disparity of the disease. However, the later may not have much role to play on the increased prevalence of MM in developing countries.

There is a dearth of data on the diagnosis or prevalence of premalignant plasma cell disease in low- and some middle-income countries. The two known hypothesized precursors of MM are MGUS and smoldering MM. Based on retrospective data from Mayo clinic, MGUS is associated with 1% annual risk of progression to MM, while SMM has 10% annual risk of progression to MM. However, due to lack of resources for making diagnosis at this early stage, these premalignant diagnoses are missed. This ultimately leaves the attending physicians with MM patients who present at advanced stages of the disease.

The diagnosis of MM is made late, usually between Durie-Salmon stages II-A (intermediate myeloma mass) and III-B (high myeloma mass) in developing countries [14–17]. The mean duration from onset of symptoms to diagnosis in a study was 13.12 months (95% CI, 6.65–19.58) [6, 17]. In some geographic regions, the onset of symptoms to diagnosis can last as long as 10 years [17]. The lack of modern equipments for diagnosis and staging of the disease are the key players in the late diagnosis of MM in most developing countries including Nigeria [14]. Most health institutions in developing countries (especially the low-income) do not have the infrastructural and medical capacities to handle comprehensive assessment investigations for MM patients. In a recent study in Nigeria, it was found that only 72% of patients with a preliminary diagnosis of MM could afford basic assessment tests required for confirmation and staging of the disease. Out of this number, 43 and 55.7% could do immunoglobulin quantification and Bence Jones Protein tests, respectively.

The commonest assessment tests done by the patients are hematocrit, erythrocyte sedimentation rate, skeletal x-ray, bone marrow aspiration, and trephine biopsy in centers where there are hematologists [14–17]. About 56–60% of MM patients could afford serum electrolyte urea and creatinine assessment tests required for staging the disease [**Table 2**], while less than 50% of the patients could do serum protein, globulin, and albumin level estimation. The serum albumin is one of the analytes essential for international prognostic staging of MM. The β_2M, serum immunofixation test, marrow aspirate and trephine biopsy with metaphase cytogenetic, FISH, immunophenotyping, gene expression profiling (GEP), and plasma cell labeling index (PCLI) are myeloma assessment tests, which are not readily available in developing countries due to the cost and prevailing poverty in the countries. The implication of this is that most MM diagnosed in these regions are cytogenetically unknown and are not internationally staged. Hence, MM patients do not benefit from accurate risk stratification and prognostic assessments as offered to their counterparts in developed countries [19].

These challenges in diagnoses and disease staging contribute to the poor survival outcome of people living with MM in these regions. In a 10-year retrospective study of 26 MM patients in Niger-delta region of Nigeria, only one (3.8%) of the patients could do a marrow metaphase cytogenetic (FISH) test and this happened to be a high risk category (t(4,14) immunoglobulin A)multiple myeloma [3, 20]. In the study, only four subjects could afford immunofixation test, which showed IgA:IgG-type myeloma ratio of 1:3 and this was in keeping with previous study by Salawu and Durosimi [16].

5. Challenges due to skeletal related events (SREs) and other complications

MM poses a diagnostic dilemma for the orthopedic surgeons because of the frequent skeletal manifestations." It is usually misdiagnosed as an orthopedic disease when in the real sense it is a hematologic disease with orthopedic complications. At advanced stage, it causes multiple lytic bone lesions with severe osteoporosis and pathological fracture. A recent observational study in Nigeria [14] found that about 84.6% of newly diagnosed multiple myeloma patients in Nigeria presented with multiple bone lesions. Pathological fracture constitutes about 42.3% of SREs in the MM patients in the region. It is surprising to note that 84.6% of all newly diagnosed MM are referrals from orthopedic wards [3, 14]. The key players of the bone lesions in multiple myeloma are cytokines namely IL-6 (Interleukin-6), TNF-alpha (tumor necrosis factor), vascular endothelial growth factor (VEGF), platelet derived growth factor (PDGF), and insulin-like growth factor (IGF). These cytokines, especially VEGF and PDGF, have angiogenic effect on the bone marrow microenvironment and this effect favors the growth of myeloma cells in the bone. IL-6, an important osteoclast-activating cytokine, plays an important role in the pathogenesis of osteoporosis in MM [21]. Annibali et al. [22], in their pilot study, described the roles of these cytokines in bone tissue destruction and the effect of zoledronic acid (a bisphosphonate) on their chemical behaviors in MM patients. Other complications such as anemia, hemiplegia, nephropathy, and constipation accounted for 61.5%, 35%, 23%, and 19% of newly diagnosed MM patients in same study. Anemia in MM results from bone marrow invasion by abnormal plasma cells that secret erythropoiesis-suppressive cytokines, and this anemia is usually anemia of chronic disorder [23].

6. Challenges of multiple myeloma treatment

The last step in the management of multiple myeloma is the therapeutic intervention. The current standard treatment for MM is palliative care. This is a holistic treatment that offers supportive, definitive, and psychosocial care for people living with MM [24]. There is a gross inadequacy in the palliative care of MM in developing countries, hence the call to scale-up the care of people living with MM. This is because of the life-threatening nature and the suffering associated with the disease. A recent study has shown that inadequate palliative care accounts significantly for the low survival interval of MM patients [3]. The overall survival interval of MM patients in various studies in a developing country such as Nigeria showed a range of 3 months to 39.7 months [3, 15–17]. In one of the studies, it was found that only about 7.6% of MM patients survive up to 5 years postdiagnosis. This was far below the estimated 5-year period survival of 32 and 44.9% recorded by Ries et al. [25] and Altekruse et al. [26] in

Surveillance, Epidemiology, and End Results (SEER) cancer statistics review of 1975–2002 and 1975–2007, respectively, in the USA. The implication is that many LMICs are more than 40 years backward in terms of management of MM compared to high-income countries such as the USA. The two major challenges in the treatment of MM in developing countries are anchored on the supportive and definitive treatment of MM.

6.1. Challenges in supportive treatment of MM

The standard supportive care for MM patients at advanced stage of the disease, which include the use of analgesics, bisphosphonates (BPs), component blood therapy, antibiotics therapy, renal dialysis viz-a-viz renal transplant, radiotherapy, orthopedic care, is grossly inadequate. Chronic bone pain appears to be one of the commonest clinical features of MM, and analgesic drug is the first supportive therapy offered to patients with the disease. However, in the assessment and treatment of pain in MM patients in some low-income countries such as Nigeria, the WHO analgesic ladder for cancer pain control is not usually adhered to, as only few centers can access oral morphine and other opiate analgesics [27]. This leads to analgesic abuse (self-medication), most of which are nephrotoxic, hence, worsening the prognosis of the disease. A study showed that less than 40% of MM patients could afford BPs. BPs are useful in preventing, reducing, and delaying MM SREs such as bone pain, osteoporosis, and other lytic bone lesions. They can also help to control the growth of extramedullary tumors, hence the need to scale-up their usage in MM [22, 28].

There is a gross inadequate access to radiation therapy in LICs including Nigeria. Studies have shown that only about 3.8–20% (average 12%) of MM patients who need radiotherapy at one point or the other of the disease could access it [3, 17]. The major reason is that the megavoltage radiotherapy machine per population size is grossly inadequate (1-MV machine per 24 million population as against the International Atomic Energy Agency (IAEA) requirement of 1-MV machine per 250,000 population or per 350–400 new cancer patients in centers with excellent cancer registry) [29].

About 60% of MM patients seen in LICs such as Nigeria present with severe grade of anemia (hemoglobin <7 g/dL). The implication is that they will rely on blood transfusion therapy in order to improve the quality of their life. Unfortunately, many of the LICs do not practice safe blood transfusion. They depend majorly on commercial (paid) blood donation as against voluntary non-remunerated blood donation (VNRBD), thereby predisposing the patients to transfusion transmissible infectious diseases (TTIs) including HIV [30]. The facilities for component blood therapy (i.e., apheresis machines) are not available in most health centers. For instance, there was no documented beneficiary from component blood therapy in previous studies in Nigeria. All severely anemic patients that require blood transfusion benefited from either allogeneic whole blood transfusion (50%) or the use of erythroid growth factor such as human recombinant erythropoietin (38%) [3, 14].

Infection is one of the major killers in MM in LICs, especially when immune paresis has set in. About 11.1% of MM patients present with neutropenic sepsis in this region. Infection control is by the use of antibiotic therapy/prophylaxis and colony forming unit-granulocyte-monocyte agents (CFU-GM) such as filgrastim or neupogen. However, the later is usually expensive and only very few patients can afford it, hence worsening the survival outcome of the disease [3].

There is an increase in the incidence of nephropathy in MM in LICs. A range of 16–36% was recorded in previous studies in Nigeria [3, 17, 31] as against 20% in the USA [32]. A striking finding about the nephropathies in MM patients in LICs is their severity at presentation, which qualifies most of them for renal dialysis (or renal transplant). However, this is an expensive palliative intervention as only very few patients can comply with the courses of dialysis, which may not be available in some centers.

In African continent, the major complications that bring MM patients to the hospital for the first time are operable (surgical) complications. A recent study revealed that 56.7% of patients diagnosed with MM received different forms of surgery ranging from craniotomy (plasmacytoma of the skull), partial cystectomy (solitary plasmacytoma of bladder), to internal fixation of orthopedic pins due to SREs complications arising from myeloma cells. Surprisingly, these complications have set in long before diagnoses were made. The presence of extramedullary plasmacytoma indicates poor prognosis, and this is worsened further in the absence of involved field radiotherapy (IFR) [33].

6.2. Challenges in definitive treatment of MM

The standard definitive interventions for people living with MM are antimyeloma chemotherapy regimens and stem cell transplantation (autologous stem-cell transplantation (ASCT)). The antimyeloma chemotherapeutic regimens have undergone series of transformation and evolution over the years. The current antimyeloma therapeutic agents have changed the paradigm in the management of the disease. These agents have the best effect in improving the quality of life and overall survival intervals of MM patients. They have positively changed the course of the disease especially in high-income countries where they are relatively more available. This has been due in large part to a better understanding of the biology of the disease and the development of several highly effective therapies. They include proteasome inhibitors [PI] (bortezomib, carfilzomib, ixazomib, marizomib, and oprozomib), immunomodulatory [IMiD] agents (thalidomide, lenalidomide, and pomalidomide), monoclonal antibody therapies (elotuzumab, daratumumab, and siltuximab), Bcl inhibitor (navitoclax), FGFR3 inhibitor (dovitinib), and histone deacetylase (HDAC) inhibitors (panobinostat, romidepsin, vorinostat, and rocilinostat). These agents include those that target the myeloma itself, some that target the bone marrow microenvironment, and those that target both [34].Unfortunately, these agents are not readily available in low- and some middle-income countries (LMICs) including Nigeria. The huge disparity in income, health-care infrastructure, and access to novel drugs in LMICs hinders the delivery of optimum care to every patient with MM in the region [35] due to limitation in purchasing power.

There may be no "standard therapy" for MM treatment, based on the many novel therapies, which have emerged for the treatment of the disease. The treatment approaches that are often referred to as standard are usually those with strong evidence of clinical efficacy. Although a recent clinical trial has shown that a combination of PI and IMiD will make for a standard regimen when added with dexamethasone [36], the current opinion is in favor of individualized treatment options, which is based not only on cytogenetic risk classification, but also on host factors, disease stage, and a variety of other prognostic factors.

According to the National Comprehensive Cancer Network (NCCN) guidelines, the consensus standard of care in newly diagnosed MM who have no intention for ASCT is RVD (lenalidomide, bortezomib, and dexamethasone) [36]. This is because RVD has improved median overall survival (OS) compared to conventional RD (75 months versus 64 months; HR 0.709; two-sided $p = 0.025$), improved overall response rate [ORR] (82 versus 72%), and improved progressive-free survival (PFS) (43 months versus 30 months, HR 0.712; one-sided $p = 0.0018$) [37, 38].

This consensus standard of treatment of MM is yet to be achieved in many developing countries. Unlike in developed countries where treatment is beginning to be customized based on mapping of patient's genome, most low-income countries are yet to offer their patients such opportunities. In Nigeria, the major antimyeloma chemotherapy drug is the old conventional alkylating agent known as melphalan (M), which is usually combined with a steroid (i.e., prednisolone, P) as a double or triple-only combination regimen. MP is still the most accessible commonly used regimen for treating MM patients because of the cost and availability, long after it has been phased out for treating MM patients in developed countries. About 84% of newly diagnosed MM patients in some LICs still depend on MP doublet combination regimen [3].This is contrary to the standard RVD triplet regimen accepted worldwide as the current treatment of choice for MM. About 28% of MM patients from the group of patients already on MP could afford a "partial-standard" triplet regimen made up of either one PI (i.e., bortezomib-melphalan-prednisolone VMP (7.7%)) or one IMiD agent (i.e., thalidomide-melphalan-prednisolone TMP (19.7%). "Partial" in this context connotes combination of a target (novel) therapy with old conventional regimen (i.e., MP in this case). However, a recent study in Nigeria has shown that up to 16.7% of MM patients use bortezomib-thalidomide-dexamethasone (BTD) as their first-line regimen [39]. Although RVD has a better median overall survival (OS), progressive free survival (PFS) and overall response rate (ORR) compared to BTD, this is a move toward the right direction as the latter regimen is close to the standard regimen (RVD) in terms of the benefits derived from a PI and IMiD combination regimens [36]. But, again, this is a bad news for many developing countries as less than 20% of MM patients in the region could access close-to-standard (partial) antimyeloma regimen [40]. The remaining 16% constitute the MM patients who are either on unclassified (i.e., neither known old conventional nor new novel therapy) antimyeloma regimens (such as vincristine adriamycin dexamethasone VAD, CVP, and CVAP) or not on any cytotoxic chemotherapy [3].

Stem cell transplantation (i.e., ASCT) is not a common option of treatment of MM in most developing countries. The only patient (3.8%) who benefited from this intervention from a previous study was outside Nigeria and the patient died two years posttransplantation. There is paucity of data regarding stem cell transplantation in most LICs especially those from Sub-Saharan African region. For instance, no center offers ASCT in Nigeria presently. Although few successful attempts on allogeneic stem-cell transplantation have been made in a center in Southern Nigeria (on sickle cell disease), but it has not been sustainable due to technological inequalities, brain drain of health workers, lack of funding, and political-will from the government. The public health system does not guarantee health insurance coverage for oncology treatment and stem-cell transplantation. Transplant-eligible patients who require stem-cell transplantation usually pay out from their pockets, and this could add to another burden to the patients [41–43]. However, in high-income countries, the reverse is the case and the survival outcome is usually better.

7. Other challenges

7.1. National Cancer (MM) Registry

There is no standard National cancer (MM) registry or Surveillance Epidemiology End-Result (SEER) cancer statistics review center in most developing countries including Nigeria. This has hindered getting accurate statistics of the disease in most developing countries.

7.2. National Guideline for management of MM

There are no standard guidelines for the treatment of MM in many developing countries including Nigeria. This is responsible for the disparities in some of the outcomes. A lot of confounding issues have arisen as a result of disharmony in the management of the disease in many developing countries. There is a need to control all confounding issues that may arise as a result of heterogeneous management of the MM in developing countries. Each country is expected to design its own consensus guidelines that will best serve the patients putting international best practices in mind.

7.3. Psychosocial input

One of the components of a good palliative care of people living with terminal diseases such as MM is the psychosocial care. In developed countries, the social workers and the spiritualists have their roles to play in order to improve the quality of life of the patients. For instance, some patients who have financial challenges in procuring their treatment may not access social workers either because they are not there or they might be there but they are not functioning. This may create more health burden or even cause death of the patients in some cases.

8. Conclusion and recommendations

Late diagnosis and inadequate palliative care are the hallmarks of poor prognosis and overall survival outcome of MM in developing countries [3]. There is a need to educate the physicians, especially orthopedic surgeons, renal physicians, and gastroenterologists to exercise higher index of suspicion, as they are usually the first to see such patients [44].

The government, stakeholders in health institutions, and donor agencies who are passionate for MM have a role to play in its management toward improving the quality of life of people living with the disease. This is achievable by improved funding of MM research and treatment in developing countries. The public health system should as a matter of urgency provide health insurance coverage for the management of MM patients especially in LICs such as Nigeria where the over 62% of population lives on extreme poverty of less than two dollars per day [41].

There is also a need to build special centers designated for the treatment of MM where all relevant modern health-care facilities/equipments for diagnosis, risk assessments, and treatment of MM should be available, while taking into cognizance international best practices for the management of the disease.

Adequate access to radiation therapy is a crucial component of modern multidisciplinary cancer care including MM. There must be a strict adherence to the IAEA recommendation of one megavoltage machine per 400 new cancer patients in areas with excellent cancer registry or one per 250,000 population size in areas without excellent cancer registry. The implication is that in countries like Nigeria where there are barely five functioning radiotherapy machine, the number has to be scaled up between 260 and 840 megavoltage units taking into cognizance a population size of 210 million people (based on 2006 population census and average annual growth rate of 3.1%) [29].

Supportive care of people living with MM must take into cognizance psychosocial health of the individuals and their families. This is the only way forward in ensuring a holistic care and improved quality of life of these patients. Every component of palliative workforce including the social workers must be involved in realizing this goal.

There is a need to scale-up definitive treatment of MM in developing countries using stem-cell transplantation. Autologous non-cryopreserved stem-cell transplantation avoids the cost of establishing and maintaining a cryopreservation facility, and this can be feasible in transplant centers in economic-constrained regions [45, 46]. Studies have shown that high-dose melphalan with autologous stem-cell support improves the survival rate for patients with myeloma. Also, when they are carefully selected for treatment with ASCT, they can be managed with a brief initial hospitalization and outpatient follow-up, with low morbidity and mortality [47–50].

Also, efforts should be intensified to set up excellent cancer (MM) registries in developing countries so as to improve on the statistics and epidemiology of MM and other cancer diseases. Each country is expected to formulate its own consensus guidelines that will best serve the patients using international best practices.

Author details

Ogbonna Collins Nwabuko[1,2]*

*Address all correspondence to: ogbollins2002@yahoo.com

1 Department of Hematology, Federal Medical Center, Umuahia, Abia State, Nigeria

2 Department of Hematology, College of Health Sciences, Abia State University, Aba, Abia State, Nigeria

References

[1] Parkin DM, Bray F, Ferley J, Pisani P. Global cancer statistics. CA: A Cancer Journal for Clinicians. 2002;**55**(2):74-108

[2] Jemal A, Siegel R, Ward E, Hao Y, Xu J, Thun MJ. Cancer statistics, 2009. CA: A Cancer Journal for Clinicians. 2009;**59**(4):225-249

[3] Landgren O, Kyle RA, Pfeiffer RM, et al. Monoclonal gammopathy of undetermined significance (MGUS) consistently precedes multiple myeloma. A prospective study. Blood. 2009;**113**(22):5412-5417

[4] Kyle RA, Rajkumar SV. Epidemiology of the plasma-cell disorders. Clinical Haematology. 2007;**20**(4):637-636

[5] Alexander DD, Mink PJ, Adami H, et al. Multiple myeloma: A review of the epidemiologic literature. International Journal of Cancer. 2007;**120**(suppl 12):40-61

[6] Nwabuko OC, Igbigbi EE, Chukwuonye II, Nnoli MA. Multiple myeloma in Niger Delta, Nigeria: Complications and the outcome of palliative interventions. Cancer Management and Research. 2017;**9**:189-196. Available from: http://www.dovepress.com/doi.org/10.2147/CMAR.S126136 [Accessed: May 30, 2017]

[7] Rajkumar SV, Larson D, Kyle RA. Diagnosis of smouldering multiple myeloma. The New England Journal of Medicine. 2011;**365**(5):474-475 [Epub: August 5, 2011]

[8] Landgren O, Kyle RA, Hoppin JA, et al. Pesticide exposure and risk of monoclonal gammopathy of undetermined significance (MGUS) in the agriculture health study. Blood. 2009;**113**(25):6386-6391

[9] Myeloma. In: Litchman MA, Kaushansky K, Prchal JT, Marcel ML, Burns JL, Armitage JO, editors. Williams Manual of Hematology. 9th ed. New York: McGraw-Hill Education; 2017.pp. 634-662

[10] Ghobrial IM, Lacy MQ. Plasma cell disorders. In: McCrae KR, Steenma DP, editors. American Society of Hematology Self-Assessment Program. 5th ed. Richmond: Cadmos Communication; 2017. pp. 634-662

[11] Rajkumar SV, Kyle RA. Multiple myeloma: Diagnosis and treatment. Mayo Clinic Proceedings. 2005;**80**(10):1371-1382

[12] Durie BGM, Salmon SE. A Clinical staging system for multiple myeloma: Correlation of measured myeloma cell mass with presenting clinical features, response to treatment and survival. Cancer. 1975;**36**(3):75, 842-854

[13] Greipp PR, San Miguel J, Durie BG, et al. International staging system for multiple myeloma. Journal of Clinical Oncology. 2005 May 20;**23**(15):3412-3420

[14] Nwabuko OC, Igbigbi EE, Okoh DA. Plasma cell myeloma: Challenges in diagnosis in sub-Saharan Africa. Jokull Journal. 2015;**65**(1):254-266

[15] Omoti C, Halim NKD. Plasma cell myeloma in a tertiary Center in Niger-Delta Region of Nigeria: Clinico-immunologic analysis. Pakistan Journal of Medical Sciences. 2007;**23**(1): 27-32

[16] Salawu L, Durosimi MO. Myelomatosis: Clinical and laboratory features in Nigeria. West African Journal of Medicine. 2005;**24**(1):54-57

[17] Fasola FA, Eteng K, Akinyemi JO. Multiple myeloma: Challenges of management in a developing country. Journal of Medical Sciences. 2008:397-403

[18] Altekruse SF, Kosary CL, Krapch M. SEER. Cancer Statistics Review. 1975-2007. Bethesda: National Cancer Institute; 2010. Available from: seer.cancer.gov/statfacts/html/mulmy.html [Accessed: April 14,2017]

[19] Fonseca R, Blood E, Rue M, et al. Clinical and biologic implications of recurrent genomic aberrations in myeloma. Blood. 2003;**101**:4569-4575

[20] Avet-Loiseau H, Attal M, Moreau P, et al. Genetic abnormalities and survival in multiple myeloma: The experience of the Intergroupe francophone du Myelome. Blood. 2007;**109**: 3489-3495

[21] Garret JR, Durie BGM, Nedwin GE, et al. Production of lymphotoxin, a bone resorbing cytokine by cultured human myeloma cells. The New England Journal of Medicine. 1989; **317**(9):526-532

[22] Annibali AO et al. Cytokines behavior in multiple myeloma patients during Zoledronic acid treatment. Journal of Blood and Lymph. 2017;**7**(4):184

[23] Beguin Y, Yerna M, Loo M, Weber M, Fillet G. Erythropoiesis in multiple myeloma: Defective red cell production due to inappropriate erythropoietin production. British Journal of Haematology. 1992;**82**(4):648-653

[24] Sepulveda C, Marlin A, Yoshida T, Ulrich A. Palliative care: World Health Organization's global perspective. The Journal of Pain and Symptom Management. 2002;**24**:91-96

[25] Ries LAG, Eisner MP, Kosary CL, et al. SEER Cancer Statistics Review, 1975–2002, Bethesda, MD: National Cancer Institute; 2005. Based on November 2004 SEER data submission, posted to the SEER web site 2005; Myeloma section. Available from: http://seer.cancer.gov/csr/1975_2002/ [Accessed April 14, 2017]

[26] Altekruse SF, Kosary CL, Krapcho M. SEER Cancer Statistics Review. 1975–2007. Bethesda: National Cancer Institute; 2010. Reviewed from: seer.cancer.gov/statfacts/html/mulmy.html

[27] World Health Organization. Traitement de la douleur cancereuse. Geneva: World Health Organization; 1987

[28] Evangelos T, Gareth M, Meletios AD, et al. International myeloma working group recommendations for the treatment of multiple-myeloma related bone disease. Journal of Clinical Oncology. 2013;**31**(18):2347-2357

[29] Nwankwo KC, Dawotola DA, Sharma V. Radiotherapy in Nigeria: Current status and future challenges. The West African Journal of Radiology. 2013;**20**:84-88

[30] Nwokeukwu IH, Nwabuko OC, Chuku A, Ajuogu E, Okoh DA. Prevalence of human immunodeficiency virus, hepatitis B virus, hepatitis C virus, and syphilis in blood donors in a tertiary health facility in south eastern Nigeria. Hematology and Leukemia. 2014;**2**:4

[31] Madu AJ, Ochenis S, Nwagha TA, Ibegbulam OG, Anike US. Multiple myeloma in Nigeria: An insight to the clinical, laboratory features, and outcomes. Nigeria Journal of Clinical Practice. 2014;**17**(2):212-217

[32] Badros A, Barlogie B, Siegel E, Robert J, et al. Results of autologous stem cell transplant in multiple myeloma patients with renal failure. British Journal of Haematology. 2001;**114**(4): 822-829. DOI: 10.1046/j.1365-2141.2001.03033.x

[33] Kar M, Roy R, Chakraborty J, Das S. Extramedullary plasmacytoma—A rare presentation. Journal Indian Academy of Clinical Medicine. 2008;**9**(4):229

[34] Hideshima T, Mitsiades C, Tonon G, et al. Understanding multiple myeloma pathogenesis in the bone marrow to identify new therapeutic targets. Nature Reviews. Cancer. 2007;**7**: 585-598

[35] Darly T, Wee Joo C, Takaaki C, et al. Management of multiple myeloma in Asia: Resource-stratified guidelines. The Lancet. 2013;**14**(12):e571-e581

[36] Durie BG, Hoering A, Abidi MH, et al. Bortezomib with lenalidomide and dexamethasone versus lenalidomide and dexamethasone alone in patients with newly diagnosed myeloma without intent for immediate autologous stem-cell transplant (SWOG SO777): A randomized, open-label, phase 3 trial. Lancet. 2017;**389**:519-527

[37] Richardson PG, Weller E, Lonial S, et al. Lenalidomide, bortezomib, and dexamethasone combination therapy in patients with newly diagnosed multiple myeloma. Blood. 2010; **116**:679-686

[38] Anderson KC, Alsina M, Bensinger W, et al. Multiple myeloma. Journal of the National Comprehensive Cancer Network. 2011;**9**:1146-1183

[39] Korubo KI, Madu AJ, Okoye H, Nwogoh B. Bortezomib prescription pattern for the treatment of multiple myeloma by hematologists in Nigeria. Journal of Global Oncology. 2017. DOI: 10.1200/JGO.17.00033. Published online before print November 1, 2017

[40] Nwabuko OC, Nnoli MA, Okoh DA, John EJ, Chukwuonye II. Survival outcome of multiple myeloma patients on chemotherapeutic regimens in the Niger-Delta Nigeria. International Journal of Recent Scientific Research. 2015;**6**(6):4889-4893

[41] Uzochukwu BS, Ughasoro MD, Etiaba E, et al. Health care financing in Nigeria: Implications for achieving universal health coverage. Nigerian Journal of Clinical Practice. 2015;**18**:437-444

[42] Oyekunle AA. Haematopoietic stem cell transplantation: Prospects and challenges in Nigeria. Annals of Ibadan Postgraduate Medicine. 2006;**4**(1):17-27

[43] Bazuaye GN. Challenges of setting up the first stem cell transplantation Center in a Developing Country (Nigeria). International Journal of Tropical Disease and Health. 2013;**3**(4):292-299

[44] Olaniyi JA, Fowodu FO. Multiple myeloma: The burden and clinico-laboratory characteristics in a Nigerian foremost tertiary hospital. Journal of Applied Hematology. 2015;**6**(2): 58-63

[45] Wannesson L, Panzarella T, Mikhael J, Keating A. Feasibility and safety of autotransplant with noncryopreserved marrow or peripheral blood stem-cells: A systemic review. Annals of Oncology. 2007 (April 1);**18**(4):623-632. DOI: 10.1093/annal/mdm069

[46] Al-Anazi KA. Autologous hematopoietic stem cell transplantation for multiple myeloma without cryopreservation. Bone Marrow Research. 2012;**2012**:917361. DOI: 10.1155/2012/917361. Epub: May 28, 2012

[47] Jagannath S, Vesole DH, Zhang M, Desikan KR, Copeland N, Jagannath M, Bracy D, Jones R, Crowley J, Tricot G, Barlogie B. Feasibility and cost-effectiveness of outpatient autotransplants in multiple myeloma. Bone Marrow Transplantation. 1997 Sep;**20**(6):445-450

[48] Paul TM, Liu SV, Chong EA, et al. Outpatient Autologous Stem Cell Transplantation for Patients with Myeloma. Clinical Lymphoma, Myeloma and Leukemia. 2015 Sept; **15**(9): 536-540. DOI: 10.1016/j.clml.2015.05.006. Epub: June 16, 2015

[49] Graff TM, Singavi AK, Schmidt W, et al. Safety of outpatient autologous hematopoietic cell transplantation for multiple myeloma and lymphoma. Bone Marrow Transplantation. 2015 Jul;**50**(7):947-953. DOI: 10.1038/bmt.2015.46

[50] Holbro A, Ahmed I, Cohen S, et al. Safety and cost-effectiveness of outpatient autologous stem cell transplantation in patients with multiple myeloma. Biology of Blood and Marrow Transplantation. 2013 April;**19**(4):547-551. DOI: 10.1016/j.bbmt.2012.12.006